The Art of Living in Australia

Philip E. Muskett

Contents

THE ART OF LIVING
IN AUSTRALIA

BY

Philip E. Muskett

DEDICATION

AUSTRALIA--ONE AND UNITED. AS AN AUSTRALIAN I DEDICATE THIS VOLUME TO
THE PEOPLE OF AUSTRALIA WITH ONE ABIDING HOPE FOR THE DEVELOPMENT OF
ALL THE: GREAT NATURAL FOOD INDUSTRIES OF OUR COUNTRY.

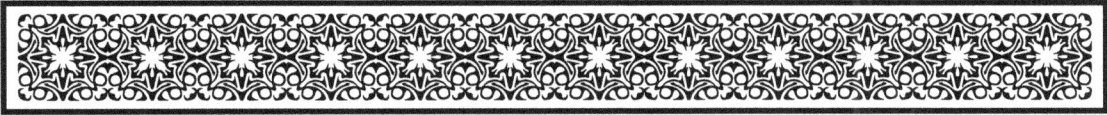

PREFACE.

Although this work fully deals with all the many matters connected with the art of living in Australia, its principal object is the attempt to bring about some improvement in the extraordinary food-habits at present in vogue. For years past the fact that our people live in direct opposition to their semi-tropical environment has been constantly before me. As it will be found in the opening portion of the chapter on School Cookery, the consumption of butcher's meat and of tea is enormously in excess of any common sense requirements, and is paralleled nowhere else in the world. On the other hand, there has been no real attempt to develop our deep-sea fisheries; market gardening is deplorably neglected, only a few of the more ordinary varieties being cultivated; salads, which are easily within the daily reach of every home, are conspicuous by their absence; and Australian wine, which should be the national beverage of every-day life, is at table--almost a curiosity.

Nearly three years have been occupied in the preparation of this volume, as several of the subjects it treats of have hitherto remained practically unexplored. This statement is not intended to excuse any shortcomings, but simply to explain the impediments which had to be overcome. There has been some little difficulty, therefore, in obtaining information in many instances. At the same time, it must be cheerfully recorded that assistance was freely forthcoming on the part of those from whom it was sought. Quite a number have been interviewed on the topics with which they were familiar; and on several occasions this has necessitated journeys out of Sydney on the writer's part. With the object of making inquiries into the fish supply of Melbourne, also, a special visit was paid to that city. And further, in order to gain an insight into vineyard work and cellar management, an instructive time was passed at Dr. T. Fiaschi's magnificent Tizzana vineyard on the Hawkesbury River.

It may seem to savour somewhat of boldness, yet I hazard the opinion that the real development of Australia will never actually begin till this wilful violation of her people's food-life ceases. For let us suppose that the semi-tropical character of our Australian life was duly appreciated by one and all. If such were the case--and I would it were so--there would be a wonderful change from the present state of affairs. But as it is, the manners and customs of the Australians are a perpetual challenge to the range of temperature in which they live. Indeed, the form of food they indulge in proves incontestably that they have never yet realized their semi-tropical environment. With a proper recognition of existing climatic surroundings there would be an overwhelming demand for more fish food; for something better than the present Liliputian supply; and for the creation of extensive deep-sea fisheries. Fish in Australia is nothing more than a high-priced luxury, although projects for the development of the deep-sea fisheries have been repeatedly suggested. Somehow or other we never get beyond this stage, and as a consequence the yield from our fisheries is simply pitiable. A widespread use of fish and an adequate fish supply would give employment to hundreds and to thousands. As I have pointed out in the chapter relating to this subject, the want of enterprise shown in starting our deep-sea fisheries is an inexplicable anomaly. If the Australian people had sprung from an inland race, this would not, perhaps, have been so difficult to understand. But coming, as we do, from a stock the most maritime the world has ever seen, such a defect is not to our credit as inheritors of the old traditions.

Nor can it be pretended that market gardening has ever been taken up seriously, if we apply the statement to Australia as a whole. It is true that Sydney and Melbourne, and possibly Adelaide and Brisbane, have made an attempt in this direction. But even with this admission there is not much reason for congratulation from an olitory point of view. Few--only very few--of the more commonly known varieties are grown. For if the potato and the cabbage were taken away, Australia would be almost bereft of vegetables. There are, however, many others, which are delicious and wholesome, which are easily grown, and which would make a pleasing addition to the present monotonously restricted choice. And there is something even more than all this. It is, that market gardening is a healthy and profitable calling; that it settles the people on the land; and that it creates a class of small landed proprietors--the very bone and sinew of any population.

In the chapter relating to Australian Food Habits it will be found that many of these desirable vegetables are enumerated. Their good qualities are highly appreciated on the Continent and elsewhere, and there is no earthly reason why they should not be grown here. The history of the introduction of the tomato into Australia is instructive in this connection. For years and years it struggled desperately, but unsuccessfully, for a place, and the attempt to bring it into use was on the point of being abandoned in consequence. But at last its undeniable merits were acknowledged, and to-day it is in universal request. Now, it is perfectly safe to assume that the same recognition would be awarded to many other vegetables vegetables at present practically unknown in Australia. For instance, sweet corn--which, however, must not be confused with Indian corn--is of exquisite flavour, almost melting in the mouth, while it possesses also eminently nourishing properties. It is a great favourite with Americans, and hundreds of acres are required annually for the New York markets alone.

But if there is one desirable form of food which we should expect to find in daily use by the whole Community, it is surely the salad. More than this, it deserves to meet with favour as a national dish. It takes pre-eminent rank in Southern Europe, and is certainly entitled to occupy a similar high position in the Australian food list. Unfortunately there is just the same story to tell, and the strange neglect of salads can only be expressed by the term incomprehensible. It is a waste-saving dish; it is wholesome, in that it is purifying to the blood; it is full of infinite variety; and its low price brings it within easy every-day reach even of the humblest dwelling. But, as things are, even the salad plants themselves are represented by a meagre list, and are confined to only few varieties. And as far as salad herbs are concerned, they are literally unknown.

Now, although I am strongly of opinion that a more widespread use of fish, vegetables, and salads in Australia would be attended by the happiest results (both by benefiting the national health and by developing Australia's food-industries), yet it must not be understood that I countenance vegetarianism. So far from being a vegetarian, I am one of those who firmly believe in the advantages derived from a mixed diet. But my assertion is that we in Australia habitually consume an injurious amount of meat to the exclusion of far more needed nourishment. The golden rule as far as the Australian dietary is concerned is a minimum of meat, and a relatively maximum amount of the other classes of food. The influence which food exercises upon health is a matter of far-reaching importance, in that it affects the daily life of the whole population. Amongst others, the following medical writers--Sir James Risdon Bennett, Dr. J. Milner Fothergill, Dr. T. King Chambers, and Dr. J.H. Bennett--have in the past contributed much to this subject. In the present day, Sir Henry Thompson, Sir William Roberts, Dr. T. Lauder Brunton, Dr. F.W. Pavy, Dr. Burney Yeo, and many more have given their advocacy to the same purpose. It is urged by all these authorities that there is a needless consumption of animal food even in the old country, and they all agree that an exaggerated value is attached to butcher's meat on the part of the public. If representative medical opinion thus protests against the use of an unnecessary amount of animal diet in the climatic conditions obtaining in the United Kingdom, how much more would the misuse of the same food in a semi-tropical climate like Australia be disapproved of! Indeed, I am perfectly certain, that were those who have given attention to food and dietetics in possession of the facts, they would unhesitatingly condemn the grotesque inversion of food-habits at present in vogue throughout Australia. There is one very important matter which unquestionably requires to have special attention drawn to it. I refer to the customary Australian mid-day meal. Strange to say, all through the hot season, as well as the rest of the year, this consists in most cases of a heavy repast always comprising meat. Why, even in the cooler months, a ponderous meal of this kind is not required! My own views are that meat in the middle of the day is quite unnecessary, and, indeed, during the hot months actually prejudicial. Most people in Australia, after a fair trial, will find that a lunch of some warm soup, with a course perhaps of some fish, and vegetables, or salad, or whatever it may be to follow, will not only be ample, but will give them a sensation of buoyancy in the afternoon they never before experienced. Among the recipes will be found many which may help to bring about a reform in this respect. The heavier meal should certainly be towards the evening after the sun-heat of the day is over, at which time it is more enjoyed and better digested.

Having thus far referred to our totally inadequate supply of fish food, of vegetables, and of salad plants and herbs, there is still the great Australian wine industry to consider. At present only in its swaddling clothes, it is destined before very long to enter upon its vigorous life. There was an eminent French naturalist, M.F. Peron, sent out to Australia by the Emperor Napoleon during the years 1801 to 1804 inclusive. A shrewd observer, he saw even at that early period of

Australian history that there were unequalled possibilities for her wine. In the course of his interesting narrations he remarks:--"By one of those chances which are inconceivable, Great Britain is the only one of the great maritime powers which does not cultivate the vine, either in its own territories or its colonies; notwithstanding, the consumption of wine on board its fleets and throughout its vast regions is immense."

In the whole of Australia the annual production of wine is only a little over three million gallons; but in France, as well as in Italy, it is nearly 800 million gallons. These two countries together, therefore, every year produce about 1,596 million gallons more wine than Australia. These stupendous figures reveal very plainly what an enormous expansion awaits our wine industry.

The colossal growth of the wool trade is in striking contrast to the puny dimensions of the wine industry. In 1805 the exportation of wool from Australia was "nil." In 1811 it reached to the modest amount of 167 lbs., while Spain exported 6,895,525 lbs. In 1861 the exportation of wool from Australia increased to 68,428,000 lbs., whilst from Spain it fell to 1,268,617 lbs. And lastly, in 1891 the amount of wool exported from Australia reached the majestic figures of 593,830,153 lbs., representing a value of 20,569,093 pounds. If New Zealand be included, the total export attains to 710,392,909 lbs., having a value of 24,698,779 pounds. It must be borne in mind that these figures represent only the wool actually exported, and do not include that kept back for Australian requirements. As I have pointed out in the beginning of the chapter on Australian wine, if the latter industry had increased in similar proportion, Australia's prosperity would be second to none in the world.

There are some other striking figures which are well worth referring to. The city of Paris alone requires nearly 300,000 gallons of wine daily. Now, the total yearly wine production of the whole of Australia is but a little over three million gallons. It will follow from the preceding, then, that the single city of Paris itself would consume in 12 days all the wine which the whole of Australia takes 12 MONTHS to make.

The future prosperity of Australia, at least to a very great extent, is wrapped up in her wine industry; for its development means much more than a large export trade to other countries. It means, in fact, the use of Australian wine as a national and every-day wholesome beverage; it means the covering of the land with smiling vineyards; it means employment and a healthy calling literally to thousands upon thousands; and, lastly, it means settlement upon the land, and a more diffused distribution of the population throughout Australia.

It must be remembered that the nervous system is far more susceptible to the effects of alcohol in a warm than in a cooler climate. It is said that in Southern Europe there are very few water drinkers, but that, on the other hand, there are very few who indulge in strong drink. The system does not feel to want the strong alcohol, so to speak. A weaker wine in a warm climate produces the same feeling of exhilaration that one of greater alcoholic strength does in colder countries. We shall not go far wrong in Australia if we stick to our own natural wines. As it will be found in the chapter on Australian wine, the every-day wine for Australian use is a wine of low alcoholic strength; a wine of which a tumblerful may be taken with benefit; a wine, indeed, which is beneficial, cheering, hygienic, restorative, and wholesome.

By reason of his semi-tropical climate the Australian is bathed in an atmosphere of sunshine. This has a distinct effect upon the blood, for the action of sunlight upon this fluid is to redden it--a fact which has for ages been dwelt upon by the poets. But for a scientific explanation of this effect of sunlight in reddening the blood we must turn to the spectrum analysis. The visible solar spectrum as shown through a prism by the ordinary sunbeam is made up of the seven different colours, namely, red, orange, yellow, green, blue, indigo, and violet. Instead of consisting simply of white light as a whole, it is now universally accepted that in this spectrum different properties belong to different parts. Light or luminous power to one portion; heat or calorific power to another; and chemical power or actinism to a third.

The visible solar or Newtonian luminous spectrum, resulting from the decomposition of white light by a prism, is only the middle portion of the whole solar spectrum. Beyond the red end there are rays possessing still greater-heating effect; and beyond the violet extremity there are rays endowed with far more powerful chemical action. The violet, and especially these latter ultra-violet rays, redden the life stream by increasing the haemoglobin--that crystallizable body which forms so large a portion of the coloured corpuscles of the blood. Sunlight, moreover, has not only this action upon the animal kingdom, but also upon the vegetable world as well Plants, like celery, which are subjected to blanching, become whitened under the process of etiolation. This is due to the absence of chlorophyll, the green colouring matter of plants, which can only be developed by the presence of light. The tops of celery, being unearthed, retain their green colour, while the stem embedded in the soil acquires its familiar whiteness.

Many philosophical writers, notably David Hume and Charles Comte, C. Montesquieu in his L'Esprit des Lois, and Henry Thomas Buckle in his HISTORY OF CIVILISATION IN ENGLAND, have dilated upon the influence
which climate exerts over race, and all their forceful opinions are to the effect that the character of a people is moulded by climatic

conditions. More than this, the same new was entertained by the classic writers; for we find the philosopher and orator Cicero recording his belief that "Athens has a light atmosphere, whence the Athenians are thought to be more keenly intelligent; Thebes a dense one, and the Thebans fat-witted accordingly." Again, Horace, the poet and satirist, has given us the famous passage:--" You would swear he (Alexander the Great) was born in the dense atmosphere of the Boeotians."

But the influence of climate is not confined to ordinary conditions alone, because without the shadow of a doubt it controls disease as well. As it is well known, certain diseases are peculiar to, and confined to, certain regions. And, moreover, a malady will vary in its type in different zones. Thus the disease known as rickets is in the old country marked in many cases by bending of the bones, giving rise to deformities of the limbs, &c. The Australian type of the disorder, however, is milder altogether, and is of a different character. The Australian child is straight-limbed almost without exception, yet the Australian type of rickety disease, as I pointed out in 1891, is quite a definite affection.

At the Congress of Naturalists and Physicians at Strasburg in 1885 the great German pathologist, Professor Virchow, called attention to a sphere of research in which, he alleged, neither the French nor the English had hitherto accomplished anything of importance, namely, the modifications of the organism, and particularly of the special alterations of each organ, connected with the phenomena of acclimatization. This reproach cannot be denied. We have not yet reached the stage in Australia of noting the effect which climate has upon the system in general, much less of inquiring into the changes which occur in such organs as the liver, spleen, &c. But apart from investigating the phenomena of acclimatization, it is very plain that the people of Australia have never given any heed to their semitropical climate, or else the food-faults now universally practised would have been rectified long before this.

It has always been a matter of interesting speculation as to what the characteristic type of the future Australian will be. But reflections of this kind can only be in the right direction by bearing in mind the ever-present climatic conditions. Climate is of all forces the most irresistible; for, on the one hand, the Great Desert of Sahara could not be crossed in an Arctic costume and on Esquimaux diet; nor, on the other, could the Polar regions be explored in a Hindoo garb and on Oriental fare. And though blood is thicker than water, yet the resistless influence of a semi-tropical range of temperature will be to imprint on the descendants of the present inhabitants of Australia some marked peculiarities of skin-colour, of facial expression, of lingual accent, and perhaps even of bodily conformation.

Quite recently an observing writer, in a keenly analytical if somewhat facetious article, gave it as his opinion that the coming Australians will be as follows:--"They will not be so entirely agricultural as the Americans were; they will be horsemen, not gig-drivers. Descended from adventurers, not from Puritans, and eager, as men of their climate must be, for pleasant lives, they will thirst for dependent possessions, for gardens where fortunes grow. The early Americans were men of austere temper, who led, on an ungrateful soil, lives of permanent hardship. They had to fight the sea, the snow, the forest, the Indians, and their own hearts. The Australians, with a warmer climate, without Puritan traditions, with wealth among them from the first, will be a softer, though not a weaker people; fonder of luxury, and better fitted to enjoy Art, with an appreciation of beauty which the Americans have never shown. They will be a people growing and drinking wine, caring much for easy society, addicted to conversation, and never happy without servants. The note of discontent which penetrates the whole American character will be absent."

From the climatic standpoint alone it is safe to predict that the future Australian will be more nearly akin to the inhabitants of Southern Europe than to his progenitors in the old country; though, naturally, there will be considerable diversity between the native born of the various regions, covering as they do such a vast extent of territory. The ample opportunities for outdoor life will do much towards ensuring physical development. And, finally, the imaginative faculties will be very active, and it is quite permissible to hope that in time there will be a long roll of artists, musicians, and poets.

As it will be seen, a considerable portion of this work is taken up with the practical side of living, as exemplified by the Australian Cookery Recipes. From the very first it was recognised that it was imperative to include them within its compass. It occurred to me, however, that this important department would better be undertaken by someone thoroughly conversant with the subject. With this object in view, therefore, I submitted to Mrs. H. Wicken what I required. I knew Mrs. Wicken to be well qualified for the task from the following facts, namely, that she had previously been successful in her culinary writings; that she was a Diplomee of the National Training School for Cookery, South Kensington; and that she occupied the responsible post of lecturer to the Technical College, Sydney. My propositions were that the recipes were to be written purely for Australian use, and that they were to be of the strictly economical order. Mrs. Wicken accepted the task, and it can only be hoped that her efforts will meet with the approbation they deserve.

In their original form the three chapters on Australian Food Habits, Australian Fish and Oysters, and on Salads, appeared in THE DAILY TELEGRAPH, Sydney. I take this opportunity, therefore, of expressing my sense of obligation to the Proprietors thereof for their courtesy in permitting me to make complete use of these three contributions. As they now appear in chapters they have been revised, considerably altered, and materially added to, for the purposes of reproduction in book form.

143, Elizabeth Street
Hyde Park, Sydney
September 1893

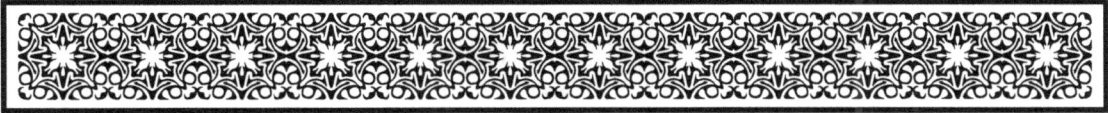

EPIGRAPH

A farmer being on the point of death, and wishing to show his sons the way to success in farming, called them to him and said--"My children I am now departing this life, but all that I have to leave you, you will find in the vineyard." The sons, supposing that he referred to some hidden treasure, as soon as the old man was dead, set to work with their spades and ploughs and every implement that was at hand, and turned up the soil over and over again. They found indeed no treasure; but the vines, strengthened and improved by this thorough tillage, yielded a finer vintage than they had ever yielded before, and more than repaid the young husbandmen for all their trouble. So truly is industry in itself a treasure.--THE FABLES OF AESOP.

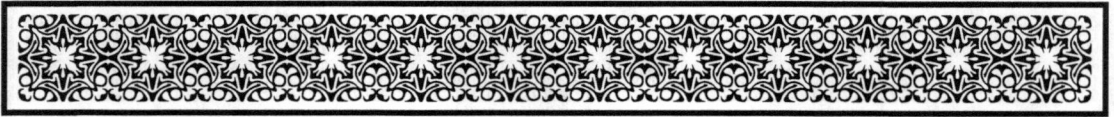

PART I.
THE ART OF LIVING IN AUSTRALIA

CHAPTER I. THE CLIMATE OF AUSTRALIA.

Australia, forming as it does a vast island continent in the Southern world, lies to some extent within the tropical range, for the Tropic of Capricorn traverses its northern part. At present, however, its most densely populated portion lies just outside the tropics, and it is this semi-tropical part of Australia with which we have mostly to do. And apart, too, from the mere fact of Australia being between certain parallels of latitude, which makes its climate tropical or semi-tropical, as the case may be, its position is peculiar in that it forms this enormous ocean-girt continent already described.

One of the most extraordinary circumstances in connection with the Australian people is, that they have never yet realized their semi-tropical environment. It would naturally be supposed that a dominating influence of this kind would have, from the very first, exercised an irresistible effect on their mode of living. But, on the contrary, the type of the Australian dwelling-house, the clothing of the Australian people, and, what is more significant than anything else, their food habits, prove incontestably that they have never recognised the semi-tropical character of their climate all over the rest of the world it will be found that the inhabitants of different regions adapt themselves to their surroundings. For instance, the Laplander and the Hindoo live in such a widely different manner, that one can scarcely believe they belong to the same human family.

It has, however, been reserved for Australia, strange even from the first, to prove an exception to this universal law. Yes, strange even from the first! For did not the earliest arrivals find that the seasons came at the wrong time of the year; that Christmas-tide came with sunshine, and that the middle of the year was its coolest part? Were there not found in it curious animals, partly quadruped, partly bird, and partly reptile? Were there not discovered, also, other animals who carried their young in a pouch? Moreover, did Dot these first settlers see that the trees shed their bark, and not their leaves; and that the stones were on the outside, not the inside, of the cherries?

But even admitting these peculiarities of season, of FAUNA and of flora it may be asked, How is it that the people of Australia have never adapted themselves to their climatic surroundings? The answer, or rather answers, to such an interrogation must largely consist of matters of opinion. This being the case, therefore, I call do no more than attempt to give my own explanation of this singular anomaly. It must be remembered that the one great impetus to colonisation in Australia was the discovery of gold in 1851. Up till that time settlement had been proceeding steadily, it is true. Indeed, one may go 80 far as to say that the development of the country was progressing, although slowly, on safe and natural lines. But the announcement of the finding of gold, which was continually being corroborated by successive reports, acted as an electric stimulus throughout the whole civilized world. As a consequence shipload after shipload of new comers flocked to Australia, all aflame with the same ardent desire--gold. Amongst them were certainly many of the picked men of the earth, whose spirit will leaven the whole of Australasia for all time to come. Yet even at the present day we still see the influence of this gold period at work, in the readiness with which men are caught by any plausible mining prospectus. They have only to be told that a company is being formed to extract gold out of road metal, and they are ready to believe it, and, what is more, prepared to put money into it.

But far better than all this eagerness to amass wealth by some fortunate COUP, would be the natural development of the country. Agriculture and market-gardening, vine-growing and wine-making, the deep-sea fisheries and all the other comparatively neglected opportunities, only await their expansion into vast sources of wealth. What wonder, then, that a continent with so much that is wanting in connection with its food life should be living in a manner distinctly opposed to its climatological necessities! In the case of America there is a far different history. Settlement began there in a small way at first, to gradually expand as time went on. There was no sudden event, with the exception of the short-lived Californian gold rush of 1849-50, to set men flocking to its shores in countless legions. No, in America the inland territory has been peopled, steadily and slowly at first, but in after years by leaps and bounds, so that its development has been on a perfectly natural basis.

But there must be something even more than this to explain the want of adaptation to climate shown in Australia, and it is, I think, to be found in the following. It must be remembered that Australia has been peopled chiefly by the Anglo-Saxon race. In such a stock the traditional tendencies are almost ineradicable, and hence it is that the descendants of the new comers believe as their fathers, did before them. It's in the blood. For there can be no doubt but that the Anglo-Saxon thinks there is only one way of living in every part of the world--no matter whether the climate be tropical, semi-tropical, or frigid. Those in the old country live in a certain manner, and all the rest of the globe have every right to follow their example.

These two facts that Australia was peopled in part by the influx which followed the discovery of gold, and that its inhabitants belong essentially to the Anglo-Saxon race, have unquestionably exercised a great influence over our Australian food-habits. But notwithstanding these powerful underlying factors, there still remains that most extraordinary circumstance, to which I at first referred, namely, that the Australian people have never realized their semi-tropical environment. In order to assign to this latter the prominence it deserves, it seems desirable to make special inquiry into the peculiarities of the climate in its different parts. With that object in view, therefore, I wrote for certain information to the observatories of the four principal Australian metropolitan centres, namely, Sydney, Melbourne, Adelaide, and Brisbane. As has always been the case, I received the fullest answers to my requests from Mr. H.C. Russell, Government Astronomer of New South Wales; from Mr. R.L.J. Ellery, Government Astronomer of Victoria; from Sir Charles Todd, Government Observer of South Australia; and from Mr. Clement L. Wragge, Government Meteorologist of Queensland. And it is with a feeling of considerable indebtedness to these gentlemen that I acknowledge their uniform kindness. And yet it is important to remember that the annual temperature, by itself, of any given locality may afford no indication whatever of its climatic peculiarities. Take for instance the climate of the North-Eastern portion of the United States. That region is characterized by intense heat during the summer, and extreme cold in the winter. In New York, for example, the mean summer temperature ranges as high as 70.9 degrees, while the mean winter temperature is as low as 30.1 degrees; yet the mean temperature of the whole year is 53.2 degrees, affording no indication of these extremes. The mean annual temperature alone, therefore, would be entirely misleading, as it would give no idea of these alternations of heat and cold. Such being the case, the actual character of any climate will be far better realized by placing in juxtaposition the mean annual temperature, the mean temperature of the hot, and the mean temperature of the cooler months. First of all, then, I purpose showing the mean annual temperature, and also the mean temperatures for the hot and cooler months, of the four largest Australian centres.

TABLE showing the Mean Annual Temperature, and also the Mean Temperatures
for the Hot and Cooler Months, of Sydney, Melbourne, Adelaide, and Brisbane.

Capital.	Mean Annual Temeperature	Mean Temperature for the Hot Months	Mean Temperature for the Cold Months
Sydney	62.9	70	58.7
Melbourne	57.5	64.9	53.8
Adelaide	63.1	72.4	58.4
Brisbane	67.74	75.2	64.3

Much will be gained by a comparison of these temperatures of the Australian capitals with those of some other cities in different parts of the world. A contrast of this kind will, in my opinion, help to a truer understanding of the climate of these capitals, than any other. Accordingly I made a successful application to Mr. H.C. Russell, for the corresponding temperatures of the following cities: London, Edinburgh, Dublin; Marseilles, Naples, Messina; New York, San Francisco, New Orleans; Bombay, Calcutta, and Madras.

TABLE showing the Mean Annual Temperature, as well as the Mean Summer and Winter Temperatures, in twelve different cities.

City.	Mean Annual Temp.	Mean Summer Temp.	Mean Winter Temp.
UNITED KINGDOM			
London	50.8	62.9	39.5
Edinburgh	47.5	58	38
Dublin	50	61.1	40.7
. . . .			
SOUTHERN EUROPE			
Marseilles (France)	58.3	72.9	45.2
Naples (Italy)	62	74.4	47.6
Messina (Sicily)	65.8	77.2	55
. . . .			
UNITED STATES OF AMERICA			
New York	53.2	70.9	30.1
San Francisco	56.2	60	51.6
New Orleans	69.8	82	55.8
. . . .			
INDIA			
Bombay	78.8	82.6	73.8
Calcutta	78.4	83.3	67.8
Madras	82	86.4	76.6

It has been said that Australia is practically Southern Europe, and to a very great extent this is perfectly true. It will be seen, however, on reference to the preceding tables, that the Australian climate is more equable than that of Southern Europe, for there is not such a marked difference between the hot and the cooler months. In the New

England States of North America, as exemplified by New York, there are intensely hot summers and extremely cold winters--to which fact attention has already been drawn. And lastly, in India, the thermometer stands at such a height, winter as well as summer, that we can only be thankful our lines are cast in more pleasant places.

Having thus compared the summer and winter temperatures of the Australian capitals with those of other cities in different parts of the world, it will be advisable to direct our attention to some details connected with the climate of these capitals, and of the corresponding colonies generally. Commencing with Sydney we find that the climate is characterized by the absence of very violent changes of temperature, owing in great measure to its proximity to the ocean, which in winter is about 10 degrees warmer than the air. Its summer climate is marked by the absence of hot winds, which do not come more than three or four times, and the are short-lived, seldom lasting more than five or six hours. For a short time in the midsummer of each year, Sydney is visited regularly by moist sea breezes, which are enervating to many persons. While these continue the temperature seldom rises to 80 degrees, but there is so much moisture that they are very oppressive. Otherwise the climate is one of the most enjoyable in the world. In other parts of New South Wales towns may be found varying in mean temperature from 45.8 degrees at Kiandra to 69.1 degrees at Bourke. Speaking generally it is a fact that for the same mean annual temperature in New South Wales the range between summer and winter temperature is less than it is in Europe.

The climate of Melbourne is characterized by a low average humidity, moderate rainfall, and moderate winds, strong gales being of her rare occurrence. The most marked feature is the summer hot wind. A hot wind is always a northerly wind, and the highest temperature generally occurs a little before the win changes to west or south-west. When this takes place a sudden drop to a comparatively low temperature sometimes follows within a few minutes. These hot winds, however, are not frequent, only averaging eight or nine per annum. These characteristics will apply to all Victoria except the mountain ranges, where all the climatic elements vary with the altitude.

The climate of Adelaide is certainly healthy, and, with the exception of the extreme heat occasionally experienced in summer, the weather may be described as enjoyable. It must be remembered, however, that these high temperatures are always accompanied by extreme dryness, the wet bulb thermometer usually reading at such times from 30 to 35 degrees, or even more, below the temperature of the air. The heat is, therefore, more bearable than if it was combined with the humid atmosphere. When the thermometer stands perhaps at something over 100 degrees, the wet bulb thermometer will show 65 degrees, and it is this which enables persons to bear the heat of the summer and carry on their usual pursuits with less inconvenience and discomfort than is felt in tropical and damp climates, though the temperature may be 15 or 20 degrees lower, but nearly saturated with aqueous vapour, as at Port Darwin, where during the rainy season of the north-west monsoon the thermometer may stand at only 88 degrees, whilst the wet bulb at the same time indicates 86 degrees. Such an atmosphere, it need hardly be said, is far more enervating than the hot and dry air of the Adelaide plains. The summer, which may be termed warm and dry, usually extends over, say, five months; and during the remainder of the year the climate is simply perfect. The temperature in mid-winter over the Adelaide plains rarely, if ever, reaches the freezing point, although there may be sharp frosts, and on still clear nights, so frequently experienced, copious dews. On the ranges, and on the high lying plains 150 miles north of Adelaide, lower temperatures are reached, indeed in some years there have been falls of snow.

The climatic features of Brisbane are, as a mean expression, decidedly semi-tropical. The months from October to March may be classed as tropic when vegetation makes luxuriant growth, especially if the rainfall prove abundant. The rest of the year, from April to September, is marked by a dry, bracing, "continental" climate, during which the westerly wind often proves very cold, bleaching, and searching accompanied by great dryness accumulated during the passage of this current from southern-central Australia. Many settlers affirm that they feel the peculiar searching character of the dry cold "westerlies" more keenly than the more "honest" frost of the old country. Yet vigorous constitutions thoroughly enjoy the bracing nature of the westerly weather of winter. Hard ground frosts not unfrequently occur in the Darling Downs and Maranoa districts, especially during May, June, and July, in connection with the westerly type of climate; and, moreover, ice has at times been observed in the water-jugs of bedrooms, &c. As before intimated, the westerly winds are marked by great dryness, so that (saturation= 100) a percentage of relative humidity below 33 per cent. may occur during the prevalence of such phenomena, not only in Brisbane, but especially in the more western districts above mentioned. Such conditions are characterized by great diathermancy of atmosphere, and hence are frequently followed by days of considerable heat. Even in the tropics, in inland districts, ground frosts are known to have occurred owing to this extreme diathermancy of the atmosphere far from the coast, and the consequent attendant factor of active terrestrial radiation. In coast districts, or that fringe of country bordering the ocean north from Rockhampton, frost is of very rare occurrence, and the prevailing winds are between south-east and east-north-east, with a rainfall far more abundant than that obtaining in other parts of Queensland. The climate of the country surrounding the southern end of the Gulf of Carpentaria is very hot and trying from November to March, but genial thenceforward. It is certainly not unhealthy, and the fevers suffered from in the northern and gulf districts of Queensland are largely brought on by reckless or needless exposure.

In addition to the foregoing, which has been obtained from head-quarters, certain questions were submitted by me as to the climatology of the different colonies. As it will be seen, these interrogations are somewhat extensive in their scope, and supply knowledge upon points, which is not ordinarily met with in my descriptions of Australian climate. In drafting them everything which had a bearing on health was included as far as possible, and consequently in a work of this kind they unquestionably deserve a prominent place. In arranging them I purpose placing the different replies after each question in the following order, namely, New South Wales, Victoria, South Australia, and Queensland. And in the different answers it should be borne in mind that Mr. H.C. Russell is responsible for New South Wales; Mr. R.L.J. Ellery for Victoria; Sir Charles Todd for South Australia; and Mr. Clement L. Wragge for Queensland.

IS IT NOT A FACT THAT THE TEMPERATURE AND BAROMETRIC PRES-SURE ARE
EXPOSED TO SUDDEN AND MARKED CHANGES? HAVE YOU KNOWN THE TEMPERATURE TO
FALL, SAY, AS MUCH AS 22 DEGREES IN 15 MINUTES?

New South Wales.--The temperature sometimes changes rapidly in the summer, coming with a change from a hot wind to a cold southerly, although the instances are rare. Once in 30 years I have known such a change to amount to 20 degrees in 15 minutes. Under ordinary circumstances the change in temperature from hot to cold wind takes several hours to amount to 20 degrees. The fluctuations of barometric pressure are moderate, seldom amounting to half an inch in a day, or an inch in a week. In England, on the other hand, the pressure sometimes varies quickly to the extent of two inches.

Victoria.--Yes; the temperature much more so than the barometric pressure; it has fallen from a high temperature to 20 and even 30 degrees sometimes in as many minutes, when a hot north wind has suddenly changed to a cold southerly one. But such sudden and great changes occur very seldom, and then only in the hot summer months, and are known as "the change." On several occasions in the last 30 years it has fallen from 105 degrees in the shade to 70 degrees and 65 degrees in the shade in less than an hour.

South Australia.--Yes, in the summer; but, especially as regards temperature, rarely in the winter. One notable example occurred on February 9th, 1887, when during a heavy thunder-storm the temperature fell 25 degrees in 10 or 15 minutes, followed by a rising temperature. In other instances the fall of temperature has been almost equally rapid. From this it will be seen that we are subject to large and quick falls of temperature following extreme heat. The approach of hot weather is usually gradual, and the fall abrupt. The barometer has been known to show a rise of 6/10 of an inch in 24 hours; this, however, is exceptional.

Queensland.--There is no record of a fall of as much as 22 degrees in 15 minutes. But, on the other hand, a rise of 30 degrees in three hours is a common feature over the Darling Downs after sunrise. Owing to the diathermancy of the atmosphere already referred to, it is a fact, nevertheless, that in the "continental" or inland districts of Southern Queensland the temperature in winter is subject to sudden and marked changes. Barometric pressure, owing to the comparatively low latitude, is not exposed to sudden and marked changes, except during hurricane conditions, which usually affect the central coast-line in February and March.

AS A COROLLARY TO THE PRECEDING, WOULD YOU SAY THAT THE CLIMATE IS MARKED BY GREAT VARIABILITY?

New South Wales.--No; just the opposite. Indeed, as regards Sydney itself. there are few cities in which so much uniformity of temperature and slow changes, are to be found. The cause of any great change is the hot wind, and as that seldom comes more than three or four times in the year, great changes are infrequent. The mean diurnal range in Sydney is 11 1/2 degrees, and taking a series of years it is very unusual for the range on any day to reach 25 degrees.

Victoria.--No; because these are exceptional phenomena. In the late Spring and during early summer the climate may be said to be occasionally subject to sharp and sudden changes, which give it the character of variability. But the deviations from mean temperature, except for short periods, are not remarkable.

South Australia.--Yes, in summer; but not in winter.

Queensland.--Certainly not; with the exception of the wide diurnal range of temperature in winter in the southern "continental" districts, as at Cambooya and Thargomindah. The changes are, according to my knowledge, far more sudden and marked in the southern colonies (as during a "shift" from N.E. by W., to S.W. for instance, at Melbourne, and especially at Adelaide) than in Queensland and its coastal districts.

WITH REGARD TO SUSTAINED, PROLONGED, OR CONTINUED HIGH TEM-
PERATURES
DURING THE SUMMER MONTHS, FOR HOW MANY DAYS HAVE YOU
KNOWN THE
TEMPERATURE REMAIN CONTINUOUSLY AT A HIGH LEVEL? THIS IS A
VERY
IMPORTANT QUESTION, AS IT CONCERNS INFANTILE MORTALITY IN NO
SMALL
DEGREE; I SHALL BE GRATEFUL FOR YOUR EXPERIENCE?

New South Wales.--Much depends upon what temperature is deemed a "high level." If we assume that 90 degrees and upwards is a high level, then such periods are very rare in Sydney; in fact during the past 24 years there have only been three. In 1868 there were three consecutive hot days of which the mean temperature was 91.8 degrees; in 1870 a period of four days with a mean temperature of 91.3 degrees; and in 1874 a period of four days with a mean temperature of 90.2 degrees. Since then, although sometimes near it, the temperature has never been for three days over 90 degrees. Taking a lower level, we have one period of nine days in 1870, the longest on record, during which the mean temperature was 82.6 degrees. It must, however, be distinctly understood that what is here taken is not the mean temperature of each 24 hours, but the highest temperature reached during the day, and which would not as a rule last more than three or four hours, if so much. If the mean temperature of the day were taken these temperatures, as given, would have to be reduced at least 10 per cent.

Victoria.--It is very unusual to have a hot period lasting more than three days; when it does happen it is generally in February or March. In the majority of cases high temperatures (over 90 degrees) do not last more than one or two days. The exceptions generally occur in February or March, and have sometimes extended to four or five days hot weather, with a temperature of over 80 degrees with a maximum of about 90 degrees, has on a few occasions during the last 30 years extended from five to ten days; and in 1890, a memorable instance, to 12 days (the only case for 37 years).

South Australia.--The longest stretch of continuous heat noted was in January and February 1857. On January 28th, 29th, and 30th, the temperature exceeded 100 degrees, and during the whole of February it was over 90 degrees on 25 days, and above 100 degrees on 12 days, the mean being 107 degrees. In January 1858 there were 10 consecutive days over 90 degrees, of which eight consecutive days were over 100 degrees. In January

1860 there were in the beginning of the month seven consecutive days, above 100 degrees (maximum 107.5 degrees). In the middle of the same month, seven days were over 90 degrees, of which five exceeded 100 degrees, two days reaching 113.7 degrees. These are, however, exceptions to our usual experience. Although there are several other instances of great heat, yet the foregoing will suffice to show what we occasionally suffer without much harm being done.

Queensland.--During the period February 17th to February 23rd, 1891, the shade temperature at Townsville ranged between 81 degrees and 62 degrees, but at Cairns a range between 82 degrees and 70 degrees is of frequent occurrence, within at least fortnightly periods.

ANY INFORMATION WITH REGARD TO HUMIDITY OF THE ATMOSPHERE ALSO, WILL BE
OF GREAT VALUE. ALL PHYSICIANS ARE OF OPINION THAT A HIGH TEM-
PERATURE,
COMBINED WITH MOISTURE, IS VERY IRRITATING TO THE LUNGS OF THOSE
AFFECTED WITH PULMONARY DISEASE.

Before setting forth the different answers in response to this, it will be desirable to refer briefly to the term "humidity." The humidity of the atmosphere is defined as the degree of its approach to saturation. Air completely saturated is represented by 100, and that absolutely free of vapour by 0. As a matter of fact, however, the latter never occurs; even in the driest regions of Arabia a humidity of 10 per cent. is almost unknown. For its estimation the Wet and Dry Bulb thermometers are employed. These consist of two ordinary thermometers. One has its bulb exposed so as to register the temperature of the air. The bulb of the other is covered with muslin; this latter material being kept wet through its connection with a cotton wick dipping into a vessel of water. The water ascends from this vessel by capillary attraction, spreads over the muslin, and evaporates quickly or slowly, according to the dryness or moistness of the atmosphere. Thus when the air is driest the difference between the two thermometers will be greatest, and, on the contrary, when it is completely saturated with moisture the two readings will be almost identical.

New South Wales.--A considerable part of the colony, forming the western plains, is subject to great heat, caused, no doubt, by the sun's great power on treeless plains, and the almost total absence of cooling winds; yet, although in summer the temperature here frequently rises over 100 degrees, and sometimes up to 120 degrees, owing to the cold at night and in winter the mean temperatures are not greater than those of corresponding latitudes in the northern hemisphere. This region of the colony is remarkably dry, and stock of all kinds thrive well and are very free from disease. At Bourke, the driest place in the colony, the humidity for a long series of years is--in the spring 51 degrees, in the summer 49 degrees, in the autumn 61 degrees, and in the winter 74 degrees. At Sydney the humidity in the Spring is 69 degrees, in the summer 70 degrees, in the autumn 79 degrees, and in the winter 79 degrees.

Victoria.--The humidity of the air of Melbourne is low, the average being 71 per cent. In the summer it falls to 65, and on hot days is generally very low. The characteristic of our hot weather is that it is usually extremely dry; the exceptions are very few, and occur in the late Spring and early autumn during thundery, muggy weather. On the hottest days, with north winds, the dryness makes the heat much more endurable, and the humidity frequently falls to between 30 and 40 per cent.

South Australia.--Attention has already been drawn to the fact that the hot, dry air met with on the Adelaide plains is far more endurable than a lower temperature in which the atmosphere is surcharged with aqueous vapour. A damp atmosphere is a rare thing in South

Australia during the summer, though in March there are at times some warm and humid days. In the winter the air for the most part is dry, although the nights are often damp. The Mount Lofty Ranges, close to Adelaide, afford a cool retreat; they have a very large rainfall, in some years over 50 inches. The climate at Mount Gambier, in the south-eastern part of the colony, is cooler and damper; it has also a much heavier rainfall than the Adelaide plains.

OF WHAT DURATION ARE THE DIFFERENT SEASONS, AND TO WHAT MONTHS WOULD YOU APPORTION EACH SEASON?

New South Wales and Victoria.--Spring--September, October, November; Summer--December, January, February; Autumn--March, April, May; Winter--June, July, August.

South Australia.--Spring--September, October; Summer comprises the five months from November to March inclusive; Autumn--April, May; Winter--June, July, August. Practically, in South Australia the year may be divided into two seasons, namely, Spring, the seven months from April to October inclusive; and Summer, the five months from November to March inclusive.

Queensland.--With regard to Southern Queensland, the seasons may be provisionally apportioned as follows: Spring--August, September, October; Summer--November, December, January, February, Autumn--March, April, May; Winter--June, July.

WHAT ARE THE PREVAILING WINDS, AND WHAT PARTICULAR ROLE DO THE HOT WINDS PLAY?

New South Wales.--A general statement is not sufficient, for the winds

vary much at different places; but taking the colony as a whole, its prevailing winds come from some point between north-west and south-west, and hence the dry climate. In Sydney no less than 39.6 per cent. of the wind comes from this quarter. The winds known as southerly bursters are generally to be expected from November to the end of February; they are always attended with strong electrical excitement, a stream of sparks being sometimes produced for an hour at the electrometer. The approach of the true burster is indicated by a peculiar roll of clouds, which, when once seen, cannot be mistaken. It is just above the South horizon, and extends on either side of it 15 degrees or 20 degrees, and looks as if a thin sheet of cloud were being rolled up like a scroll by the advancing wind. The change of wind is sometimes very sudden; it may be fresh N.E. and in ten minutes a gale from S. Hence vessels not on the look-out are sometimes caught unprepared, and suffer accordingly. When a southerly wind commences anywhere south of
Sydney it is at once telegraphed to its principal coast towns, and a signal put up indicating its approach. As to the hot winds, they are so insignificant in number that it cannot be said they play any particular ROLE. Their effect is to raise the temperature, because they flow from the heated interior of Australia; but they do not last long. and for the majority of people are dry, healthy winds. Indeed, they are by no means so oppressive as the warm north-east wind, so charged with moisture, which comes in the summer.

Victoria.--In summer the N. winds blow to the extent of 8 per cent., the S.W. winds 24.1 per cent., and the S. winds 201 per cent. Northerly, or warm-quarter winds, in summer are 20 per cent., and southerly, or cool-quarter winds, 64 per cent. The northerly winds in winter, however, are bleak and cold, like easterly winds in England. The particular ROLE played by the hot wind is to precede a cyclonic movement, and is always in front of a low pressure area or V-shaped depression. It is frequently followed by thunderstorms and rain of short duration. It dries the surface and raises dust storms when strong. So far as its effects on the people are concerned, it does not appear to hinder the ordinary occupations of life. Some invalids are better during its continuance, some worse; but all weakly people feel some depression after "the change" comes. The aged are generally better in hot winds, unless they suffer from disease.

South Australia.--As far as the southern regions of the colony are concerned, we may say, speaking generally, that light winds and calms are a very distinctive characteristic. The prevailing wind in the summer is the S.E., varied by sea-breezes during the day. In the winter there are mostly dry, cold N.E. winds, broken at intervals by westerly and S.W. gales of moderate strength, squalls, and rain. The best and heaviest rainfalls are those which set in with the surface winds at N.E., the rain increasing in intensity as the wind veers to N.W., and breaking up into showers and squalls as it veers to S.W. In the interior, north of, say, latitude 30 degrees to about 18 degreess., the prevailing wind all the year is the S.E. North of latitude 18 degrees to the north coast the country is well within the influence of the north-nest monsoon during the summer months, with frequent thunderstorms and heavy
rains; and during, the winter dry S.E. winds prevail.

Queensland.--Eastern Queensland (or rather the Pacific Slope) is very seldom troubled with hot winds. The hot winds of "continental" Queensland are always very dry, and are usually accompanied by dust storms.

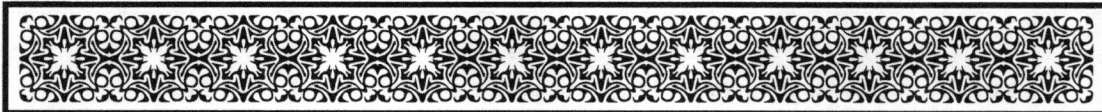

CHAPTER II.
THE ALPHABETICAL PENTAGON OF HEALTH FOR AUSTRALIA.

A few introductory remarks on this subject will serve a useful purpose. It will be seen that I have referred to the alphabetical pentagon of health--which is purely a provisional arrangement of my own. It consists of five headings, which fall naturally into alphabetical order. They are best considered, therefore, in the following way, namely:

* (a) Ablution--the Skin and the Bath.
*

* (b) Bedroom Ventilation.
*

* (c) Clothing.
*

* (d) Diet.
*

* (e) Exercise.
*

This is a convenient method of remembering the five great fundamental principles concerned in the preservation of health. It will serve, moreover, as a means of impressing them upon the memory, superior to any other with which I am acquainted.

This very number five, indeed, has a more than ordinary significance belonging to itself. It has been termed a mystical number. "Five," says Pythagoras, "has peculiar force in expiations. It is everything. It stops the power of poisons and is redoubted by evil spirits." According to the Pythagorean school of philosophy, the world is a piece of harmony and man the full chord. The major chord consists of a fundamental or tonic, its major third and its just fifth. The eighth note, or complement of the octave, is the diapason of man. These are of course very highly imaginative speculations. It is interesting to remember, however, that the system of astronomy first taught by Pythagoras was afterwards developed into the solar system by Copernicus, and is now received as the Copernican system. But, turning from grave to gay, we find that five wits have been described, viz., common sense, imagination, fantasy, estimation, and memory. Of these, common sense passes judgment on all things; imagination brings the mind to realise what comes before it; fantasy stimulates the mind to act; estimation has to do with all that pertains to time, space, locality, etc.; and memory is "the warder of the brain." Then again, have we not also the five senses of seeing, hearing, feeling, smelling, and tasting? Have we not likewise five fingers and five toes on either hand and foot? Moreover, is not fives an ancient and hollowed game, still popular wherever the English language is spoken, and is not its name derived from its being played with the "bunch of FIVES," namely the hand? And further, there must be numbers of Australians who know well what "five-corners" are. In addition to the foregoing, the number five has an important historical and legal association in connection with the Code Napoleon. Prior to Napoleon's time, different ways and customs prevailed in different parts of France, and altogether legal matters were in a chaotic state. It was greatly to his credit, therefore that he recognised the necessity for the entire alteration and remodelling of the whole system. But what was more striking than the recognition of the existing, defects was the speediness with which they were rectified, for the CODE NAPOLEON was devised and actually in operation between 1804 and 1810.

It consisted of FIVE parts, namely the "Code Civil," dealing with the main body of the private law; the "Code de Procedure Civile"; the "Code de Commerce," dealing with the laws relating to commercial affairs; the "Code d'Instruction Criminelle "; and finally, the "Code Penal." It is recorded that Napoleon was prouder of this than of his victories. "I shall go down to posterity," he said, "with my Code in my hand." The best proof of its excellence is that to-day it remains in force as the law of France (though it has been re-christened the "Code Civil" under the Republic), and that it has been the model for many Continental Codes, notably Belgium, Italy, and Greece.

But, leaving, these references to the many associations attached to the number five, it must not be supposed that my desire is to make people unnecessarily timorous about themselves on the score of health. This is certainly not my intention, for such a frame of mind would defeat the very object I have in view. Yet there still remains the fact that a little rational attention is indispensable if the vigour of the body is to be maintained at its best. There is a very great difference between carefulness carried to extremes in this respect, on the one head, and a heedlessness and total disregard of personal health, on the other. The golden mean between these two is the proper knowledge of what is required for the preservation of health, and so much conformity thereto as will give the best results. And yet it must be remembered that no cast-iron code can be laid down which would be applicable to one and all. No; idiosyncrasy, that personal peculiarity which makes each individual different from every one else, is too potent a factor to be ignored. In matters of this kind, each one, to a certain extent, is a law unto himself, and, consequently, what agrees and what disagrees is only discoverable by the individual concerned. In what follows, therefore, I have endeavoured to lay down rules for guidance which will be beneficial to by far the greatest number; although this element of the EGO must never be forgotten.

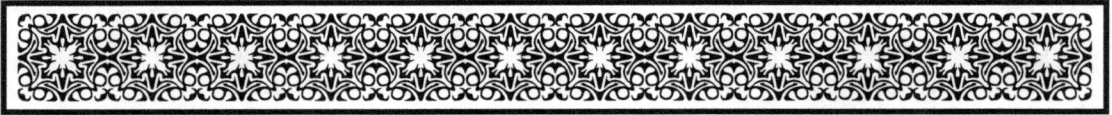

CHAPTER III.
ABLUTION--THE SKIN AND THE BATH.

It has been estimated that the external skin of an ordinary adult is equal to an area of about twelve square feet, and that in a tall man it may be as much as eighteen square feet. There is a considerable difference between twelve square feet and twelve feet square, and it is well to mention the fact in order that there may be no confusion. From this large surface alone, therefore, it is quite easy to see that the skin requires to have some attention paid to it. But it is really far more important than even its extensive surface would be likely to indicate, for it fulfils no less than seven different duties. In the first place it serves as an external covering to the body, and, as we shall see also, the internal skin acts as a support to the internal organs. Secondly, it is endowed with an extensive system of nerves, which give rise to the sensations of touch, of temperature, of pressure, and of pain. In this way we can tell whether a substance is rough or smooth, and whether it is hot or cold; we recognise, moreover, the difference between a gentle pressure of the hand and one so forcible as to cause pain. Thirdly, the skin, as we shall find farther on, contains thousands of small tubes for the purposes of perspiration, and besides this, there are other tubes secreting, an oily substance. Fourthly, the skin plays an important part in regulating the temperature of the body. Thus in a warm atmosphere the skin becomes reddened and moist, and much heat is lost; on the other hand, when the air is colder the skin becomes pale, cool, and dry, thus conserving the body heat. Fifthly, the respiratory action of the skin must not be forgotten, although it is nothing like so great as that of the lungs. Nevertheless quite an appreciable amount of oxygen is absorbed through the skin, and beyond all question carbonic acid is exhaled from it. Sixthly, it is an absorbent; that is to say, the skin is capable of absorbing into the body certain substances applied to it. In this way remedies are often introduced into the system by what is known as inunction. And lastly, the skin is a great emunctory, and carries off waste matters from the body. Accordingly it acts as a purifier of the blood, in which it assists the kidneys, intestines, and the lungs. And more than this, it often happens that the turning point in any disease is announced by a sudden, profuse, and markedly offensive perspiration, as if a considerable amount of deleterious and noxious matter has suddenly expelled from the system.

From the foregoing it is evident that the skin has many varied and important duties to perform. As we might expect, moreover, an organ with such functions is of complicated structure. Its component parts, therefore, deserve to have some little attention paid to them, since the importance of the skin from a health point of view will then be all the more appreciated. The skin is most conveniently considered under three divisions--the skin itself; the glands, producing perspiration, oil, and hair, which are found within it; and the appendages belonging to it, the hair and the nails. The skin itself may be described as the soft and elastic tissue which invests the whole of the surface of the body, and consists of two layers, the outer or scarf skin, and the deeper or true skin. The interior of the body is likewise lined with a covering, which is termed mucous membrane, from the fact that from its surface, or from certain special glands within it, or from both, there is constantly being secreted a thin semi-transparent fluid called mucus. At the various openings of the body, as the mouth, the nostrils, and other parts, the external and internal skins are continuous with one another. Indeed, at these apertures the mucous membrane, or internal skin, takes leave of absence from the world to line the cavities within the body. So that, as Professor Huxley expresses it, "every part of the body might be said to be contained within the walls of a double bag, formed by the skin which invests the outside of the body, and the mucous membrane, its continuation, which lines the internal cavities."

The use of the scarf skin is manifestly to protect the more delicate true skin, while at the same time it allows the waste products and used-up material to escape from the body. In the substance of the true skin are thousands of minute little bodies called papillae, which are specially concerned in the sense of touch, for the vast majority of these papillae contain the end of a small nerve. The numberless fine ridges seen on the palmar surface of the hands and fingers, and on the soles of the feet, are really rows of these papillae, covered of course by the layers of the outer skin. The supply of blood to the skin is also very plenteous, each of its innumerable papillae being abundantly supplied in this respect. As a proof of the amount of blood circulating within the skin, and of its extensive nerve supply, it is only necessary to mention the fact that the finest needle cannot be passed into it without drawing blood and inflicting-pain. In addition to the foregoing the skin also contains a countless number of very fine tubes, which penetrate through its layers and open on its surfaces by minute openings called pores. There are altogether three different varieties of these tubes distributed throughout the skin, namely, those intended for perspiration; secondly, those which lead from the oil glands; and lastly, those which enclose each hair of the body. The first of these, which carry away the perspiration from the body, are very fine, the end away from the surface being coiled up in such a way as to form a ball or oval-shaped body, constituting the perspiration gland. The tube itself is also twisted like a corkscrew, and widens at its mouth. It is estimated that there are between 2,000 and 3,000 of these perspiration tubes in every square inch of the skin. Now, as we have already seen, the external skin of an ordinary adult is equal to an area of about twelve square feet, and in a tall person it may be as much as eighteen square feet. The number of these tubes, therefore, in the whole body will be many hundreds of thousands, so that it will readily be seen how exceedingly important it is that they should be kept in thorough working order by cleanliness. The two great purposes fulfilled by the perspiration are the removal by its means of worn-out or effete material which is injurious to the system, and the regulation of the heat of the body by its influence. When it is stopped by any reason, such as catarrh or disease, the skin fails in its work, and the noxious matters, instead of being expelled from the body, are thrown back into the system. Hence there is a good deal of truth in the belief that a freely acting skin is always a safeguard against disease.

The second variety of tubes, those which furnish an oily-like fluid to the skin, resemble in--great part those which serve for the office of perspiration. At the extremity away from the surface of the body, each one has a gland, the oil gland, which secretes the oily material. The pores or outlets which open on the skin, however, are a good deal larger than the similar orifices of the perspiratory tubes, but they are not distributed so equally throughout the body. In certain parts of the skin they are especially numerous, as on the nose, head, ears, and back of the shoulders. The unctuous matter which is secreted by these oil glands is intended to keep the skin moist and pliant, to prevent the too rapid evaporation of moisture from the surface, and to act as a lubricant where the folds of the skin are in contact with each other. At times in these oil tubes the contents extend to the opening on its surface; the part in contact with the air then becomes darkened, and forms the little black spots so frequently seen on the face of some persons. The white, greasy matter which is thus contained within the tubes can often be squeezed out with the fingers or a watch key, and on account of its shape and black end is popularly supposed to be a grub or maggot.

The tube into which each hair of the body is inserted differs materially from the two preceding, in that its function is more restricted. It serves to form a sort of sheath which contains each hair, and is called the hair follicle. Usually one of the last described ducts opens directly on the side of the hair follicle, and its secretion serves the purpose of keeping the hair pliant. It will be more convenient, however, to enter into a fuller description of the hair and hair follicle when be come to speak of the hair, the nails, and the teeth.

Having thus gained some knowledge of the structure of the skin, and of its delicate formation, it will be the more readily understood why strict attention to the bath is necessary to produce a healthy frame. There is a continual new growth of scarf skin going on, and there are likewise the secretions from the perspiration ducts and oil tubes being poured forth. The outer skin which has served its purpose is being incessantly cast off in the--form of whitish looking powder, but instead of being thrown clear from the body it clings to it and becomes entangled with the perspiration and oily material, thus forming an impediment to the free action of the skin. If the pores of the latter be obstructed and occluded in this manner, the impurities which should be removed from the system cannot escape, and have therefore to be expelled by some other channel. Hence the work of removing this impure and deleterious material is thrown upon the liver, bowels, or kidneys, and often results in their disease. In our warm climate, where the skin acts more freely than it does in colder latitudes, the use of the bath is certainly indispensable, if the health of the body is to be maintained at all.

The cold bath, at any rate during the summer months, should always be there before breakfast, but in the cooler part of the year the shock may be lessened, if it be desirable, by using tepid water instead of cold. And since there is, as we have seen, a good deal of oily matter excreted by the skin, it becomes necessary to use something in addition to water for cleansing purposes, for the latter is unable to displace the greasy collection by itself. The only thing which will render it easy of removal is soap, as by its action it softens the oily material and dislodges it from the skin. Soap has acquired an evil reputation which it certainly does not deserve, and if it disagrees it is either due to the fact of its being an inferior article, or else the skin itself must be at fault. The best soap to use is the white, not the mottled, Castile, as it is made from pure olive oil. By the proper and judicious use of soap the skin is kept soft and natural, and the complexion is maintained in the hue of health.

Even in the matter of washing the face, there is a right way and a wrong way of doing it. The basin should be moderately filled with water and the face dipped into it, and then the hands. The latter are to be next well lathered with soap, and gently rubbed all over the face, following into the different depressions, such as the inner corners of the eyes and behind the ears. It is quite a mistake, however, to apply the lather to the inside of the ears, as it seems to favour the formation of wax; the different depressions and canal of the ears can be very well cleaned by means of the finger tips moistened with water. The face is then to be dipped into the water a second time and thoroughly rinsed, but it is better to pour away the soapy water for the rinsing. Many people apply the soap to the face by means of a sponge or bit of flannel, and do not wash the soap thoroughly off with fresh water before drying with a towel. The hands unquestionably make the softest and most delicate means of bringing the lather completely into contact with the surface of the skin and, besides this, the amount of pressure to be applied can also be regulated to a nicety. The face and neck should always be carefully and thoroughly dried by means of a suitable towel. But for the ears something of a softer material, such as a clean handkerchief, is more convenient in following out the various hollows and the canal itself.

Many houses, and fairly sized houses too, are destitute of a bath, and if there is no room for the erection of one, or if the means for having it built are not forthcoming, it becomes necessary to see what cheap and efficient substitute can be made. A sponge bath, or large tub, with a bucket of water and a good-sized sponge, can readily be obtained, even in the most humble dwelling, and answers as well as can be wished. When the body is simply sponged over with tepid water it makes one of the mildest baths that can be taken; but those who are in ordinary health can well lather them selves over with soap and cold water, and then wash it off with some squeezes of the sponge copiously wetted with the water.

Next in order to the sponge bath comes the plunge bath, and with either of them the face should always be washed first, in the manner previously directed, so as to prevent a rush of blood to the head. In taking a bath, whether it be the sponge or the plunge bath, plenty of water should always be dashed over the front of the chest, for it makes one hardier and less susceptible to the effects of cold. In fact, besides acting as a preventive to attacks of common cold, it really strengthens the lungs, and renders the body more capable of resisting disease. If in addition a little cold water is habitually sniffed up the nostrils at the time of taking the bath it will have many a cold in the head. After coming out of the bath the towels should always be used to thoroughly dry the body, and it is certainly better to have two for the purpose. The two towels should be sufficiently large in size, at least five feet in length and of ample width; anything smaller is altogether useless. One of them should be of some soft absorbing material so as to thoroughly dry the body, while the other should be rougher, to use with friction to the skin. In fact, this rubbing down with the rougher towel is in some respects the most important part of the bath, and there should always be enough friction to get the skin into a glow. If there is not this feeling of reaction, but a decided chilliness, it is a sure sign that the bath is not agreeing, and one with tepid water must be substituted, or else it will have to be stopped altogether for a time.

But although there may be a certain proportion of people whom the cold bath does not benefit, yet I am fully convinced that the number is comparatively speaking small. A good many make the excuse that they cannot take it, while all the time laziness is the real trouble. Once the advantages derived from the cold bath are experienced, all the objections raised vanish into thin air. Not only is there that feeling of exhilaration which abides with those who habitually employ it, but it is to be remembered that its greatest value consists in the immunity which it confers against diseases of the catarrhal type. The effect of the cold bath is to give tone to the whole system, and to brace up the body. But it does more than this; by maintaining the functional activity of the skin, the liability to catch cold is greatly lessened. There are many explanations given of the phenomena which occur in "taking cold." They are believed, however, to arise from a disturbance of the heat-producing forces of the body. As it has been already pointed out, the skin is the great temperature-regulator of the body. Accordingly this latter all-important duty is best promoted by keeping the functional activity of the skin in full swing. The prevention of catarrh means, therefore, a healthy action of the skin, and for this nothing is so good as the daily cold bath. The praises of the latter are well sung in the following extract: "Those who desire to pass the short time of life in good health ought often to use cold bathing, for I call scarce express in words how much benefit may be had by cold baths; for they who use them, although almost spent with old age, have a strong and compact pulse and a florid colour in their face, they are very active and strong, their appetite and digestion are vigorous, their senses are perfect and exact, and, in one word, they have all their natural actions well performed."

The beneficial effects which follow the daily cold bath have been thus dwelt upon because I believe that in Australia the greatest good to the greatest number would follow its use. At the same time, however, it is necessary to remember that there are some persons, and some even apparently robust persons, who can never take them. Such baths, also, are injurious to those who are pale and bloodless, or those who suffer from a tendency to congestion of the internal organs--excepting under medical advice. And, in addition, it must also be remembered that warm baths have claims for consideration from a cleansing point of view, and a few words upon them in this respect will not be thrown away. Now, the daily use of the cold bath, together with the assiduous application of soap, may be sufficient to keep the skin cleansed from impurities. Yet as a matter of fact this will the more certainly be ensured by a weekly --or, better still, bi-weekly--warm cleansing bath. The best time to take it is before bedtime, so that there is no risk of taking a chill afterwards. After the body has been well lathered over with soap, and this has been thoroughly washed off, the cleansing process may be then considered as completed. It is next recommended that two handsful of common salt should be added to the warm water, and the body steeped therein for a minute or two. The particles of salt pass into the skin so firmly that they cannot be removed even by the most vigorous rubbing. In this way the functions of the skin are stimulated to a considerable degree; the process of nutrition throughout the body greatly promoted; and the liver roused to action. From this it is easy to understand why hot sea-water baths are so beneficial.

There is another effect of the warm bath which deserves to be well remembered, for it has an historical association. It is related of the great Napoleon, that after a day's fighting, instead of indulging in a night's rest, he would take a warm bath. It was so efficacious that he was enabled to begin his exertions almost immediately. The explanation of this lies in the fact that when the mascles are tired out and the vigour of the body diminished, the hot bath rouses the circulation and renews the worn-out tissues. In the same way, after a night's dancing, twenty minutes or so in a warm bath, and a couple of hours' sleep, will be almost as good as a whole night's rest. In addition to the foregoing, however, it must not be forgotten that the warm bath, or to speak more correctly the hot bath, is a true medicinal agent. It is used in many cases of disease, especially those in which the skin is inactive. A feverish cold is often nipped in the bud by a hot bath at bedtime; a free perspiration usually follows, and thus relief is obtained. In some forms of rheumatism and gout, too, the hot bath is of signal benefit. There are many cases of a spasmodic nature, also, in which it is of great value. At the same time it must be borne in mind that the hot bath, when used to an excess, tends to induce a debilitated condition.

THE HAIR.

The loss of hair is so frequent in Australia, at least amongst the male population, that it requires a little consideration; and apart altogether from this, the whole subject is one of extreme interest, so that some reference to the actual structure of the hair and the hair-follicles is called for. The roots of the hair are formed in the hair-follicles, which may be described as little pear-shaped bags, formed either in the true skin or in the cellular tissue beneath it. Each hair-follicle, hair-sac, or hair-pit, as it is variously termed, bulges out at its deeper part, contracting to a long narrow neck as it passes to its skin. Near the surface of the latter the follicle widens out again, and it is from this part that the hair emerges. As it has been previously mentioned, a duct from one of the oil glands usually opens into each follicle. At its very bottom, also, is the papillae or little mound-like elevation. This protrudes into the follicle, and from it the hair is formed.

The blood supply for the hair is very abundant. There is a complete system of blood vessels encircling every one of the follicles, and besides this each papilla has a special distribution of blood to itself. That part of the hair lying within the hair-follicle is called the root. The lower end of the root, which swells out into a knob, named the bulb, is concave in shape underneath, so as to fit on top of the projecting papilla. The shaft is the long stem of the hair, while its extreme end is termed the point.

By the aid of the microscope it may be seen that the hair itself on the outside is covered by a layer of scales--the cuticle--overlapping one another like the tiles on the roof of a house. Beneath the cuticle is the fibrous part, consisting of many cells closely packed together. In many instances the fibrous part takes up the whole interior, but in the centre of the coarser hair there is the medulla or pith, composed of very minute cells. From this it follows that the hair is not a narrow tube, as is commonly supposed. This mistake has arisen from the fact that, when viewed transversely, the colour of the central and outer part of the hair is different.

Having in this way become acquainted with the actual structure of the hair and of the hair-follicles, it will be desirable to consider somewhat briefly the management of the former. We have already seen that the skin requires a good deal of attention in order to ensure the perfection of bodily health. And although the hair does not fulfil such an important function, yet, on the other hand, it must not be neglected. Even on the score of appearance alone, it has much claim for attention. Many people would be vastly improved in this way were they only to visit their hairdresser more frequently. It is very unsightly, to say the least of it, to see the hair straggling all over the back and sides of the neck, and the beard (if a beard be worn) with a wild, untidy look. Besides this, in our semi-tropical climate, a little more care in this respect would be certainly conducive to coolness and comfort.

But in addition to these considerations, there is another very cogent reason why the hair should be more often attended to; and it is the fact that if it be kept of an ordinary length, somewhat frequent cutting promotes its growth. There is more than one reason given as an explanation of this; indeed, there are at least three. In the first place, the shorter the hair the less it is dragged on in its roots; secondly, its roots are prevented from becoming blocked at the mouth of the hair-follicles--and lastly, the weight of the hair is considerably lessened. From this it will be obvious that it is not the actual cutting of the hair in itself which is so beneficial in invigorating its growth, but that, by reason of the cutting, certain results follow which strengthen it greatly.

We have just seen that the accumulations of DEBRIS and other material at the roots of the hair are prejudicial to its growth. It must not be inferred from this, however, that incessant washing of the scalp, by removing these collections, is a good thing. Now, it is advised by some that the hair should be wetted daily at the same time the bath is taken. But as a general rule this is a mistake; only those who have a superabundance of natural oil can afford to carry out such a practice. With the great majority of people it is absolutely detrimental to the growth of the hair to wash it oftener than once a week. After washing the head, the hair should be thoroughly dried. Many attacks of neuralgia, especially in the fair sex, are due to the effect of getting into a draught while the hair is still wet.

There are several points to be borne in mind in connection with the growth and preservation of the hair. With many persons the scalp is very tender and will not tolerate vigorous brushing. In such instances the brush should always be a soft one; indeed, a hard brush cannot be recommended under any circumstances. The teeth of the comb, also, should never be so sharp as to irritate the scalp, nor should they be set too closely together. A certain amount of brushing is necessary to keep the scalp and hair in healthy action, but it must never be carried to excess. Singeing the hair is greatly believed in by a number of people, and in some cases it appears to be of benefit. Many believe that singeing seals up the cut ends of the hair, which they affirm bleed when cut. This has no foundation in fact, however, for, as it has already been explained, the hair is not a tube. A hard, unyielding covering for the head is not at all suitable; the lighter and more ventilated the head-gear the better. But, the truth is, a sensible and suitable head-covering for Australian use has yet to be devised. Thinning of the hair, and even actual baldness, are not unfrequently started by the hard rim of the hat employed. This mechanically interferes with the supply of blood to the scalp, and thus it is that the crown suffers most in this respect, since it is the more starved of blood.

As I have previously shown, the hair often suffers from want of natural oil. The investigations of Liebreich have shown that this is closely allied to lanolin, which is the purified fat of sheep's wool. Moreover, it has been found that this lanolin is the very best substitute for the former. It is, however, too sticky to be used alone as a pomade. Accordingly, Dr. Allan Jamieson, of Edinburgh, a very high authority on diseases of the skin and hair, advises that it should be mixed with oil of sesame in the following proportions:

Oil of sesame....1 drachm.

Lanolin..............2 ounces.

This may be conveniently perfumed with a few drops of oil of bergamot, oil of orange blossom, or oil of rosemary. For the preservation of the hair, therefore, it should be trimmed short; the scalp kept clean, but not overwashed; and the hair, if naturally dry, lubricated by the foregoing pomade. These must be supplemented, also, by taking care that the head-covering is not too heating, that the rim of the hat is not too hard, and that irritation of the scalp by hard brushes and fine combs is strictly avoided.

If the thinning of the hair has progressed to a more advanced stage, other measures will have to be adopted. The most useful application which I know of to restore growth is the following. It is a formula given by Messrs. Squire, the well-known chemists of London, and has had an immense sale extending over many years.

Cantharidine (the best) 1 grain.

Acetic ether   6 drachms.

These are to be dissolved together; then add;

Rectified spirit   3 ounces.

Castor oil   1 ounce.

As with the pomade, this is best perfumed by the addition of about 20 or 30 drops of oil of bergamot, oil of lavender, oil of orange flower, or oil of rosemary, as fancy dictates. The bottle should be kept tightly corked, and a little of the preparation rubbed well into the hair-roots daily. If it create any irritation after two or three days' use, it is best to wash the scalp with a little warm water and soap. The pomade which has been recommended may be afterwards employed for two or three days till the irritation has subsided, when the application may be renewed. A better plan still is, from the first, to use the hair restorer on one day, and the pomade on the next, alternately. This foregoing application is of course not infallible, but it will be found to do more good in a greater number of cases than any known preparation.

THE NAILS

From the fact that the nails are in reality appendages of the skin, they are naturally entitled to some brief consideration. Beneath the nail is the matrix, that part of the true skin from which the nail is formed. The matrix has not a perfectly smooth surface, but is arranged in 8 scries of parallel ridges with alternating grooves. The nail is of a rosy pink colour, because it is transparent enough to let the blood, circulating beneath, be seen through it. Near the root is a little crescentric-shaped white portion called the lunula. The growth of the nail takes place from below. It cannot grow backwards, since it is confined in a groove. But as the fresh cells form they gradually thrust the whole nail forward, till at last it requires paring. As a matter of fact, however, the nails really require more attention than they usually receive. The finger nails should be trimmed into a bow shape, and the corners rounded off, while the skin near the root of the nail, which tends to grow over the lunula, should be repressed into position by means of any suitable appliance. On the contrary, those of the feet should be cut squarish in shape, with a hollowed-out centre, so as to prevent the nail from ingrowing.

THE TEETH

It is not my purpose to enter fully into all the details concerning the teeth, but there are one or two matters of great importance connected with them which require a few words. There are many people, beginning to get on in years, perhaps, who have had the misfortune to lose many of their teeth. The first thing that happens is an inability to masticate their food; and, before long, indigestion sets in, with all the evils attendant on its train. These unfortunates know that they have indigestion; the pain and discomfort after food tell them that. They do not know, however, that all their sufferings arise solely from their want of teeth. They begin to lose flesh, and get altogether in a bad way. But if they can be induced to apply to a competent and skilful dental surgeon, they are properly fitted with what they require, and the consequence is their sufferings almost immediately cease. They begin to enjoy their food, and before long their whole appearance is transformed into one of health. In the opinion of all dental authorities, when the natural teeth are lost, artificial substitutes unquestionably conduce to health and comfort.

It is quite deplorable to see what little interest people take in the preservation of their teeth; even those who should know better are in too many instances quite as neglectful. But the teeth play a very important part in the thorough division of food, and if this be not ensured the health is bound to suffer. They should be kept scrupulously clean, therefore, and the formation of tartar prevented.

These two objects are best accomplished by their thorough cleansing with a moderately stiff brush. Too soft a brush is insufficient for the purposes of removing the accumulations which collect upon the teeth. A tooth-powder or dentifrice of some kind will also be required. One of the simplest, and possibly also one of the very best, is composed of the following:

Powdered borax	1/2 an ounce.
Powdered orris root	1 ounce.
Powdered white Castile soap	1/4 of an ounce.
Precipitated chalk	3 ounces.
Oil of cloves	2 drops.
Oil of winter green	1/2 an ounce.

This leaves nothing to be desired, and will be found satisfactory in every respect.

It is customary to dip the tooth-brush into water, so as the better to enable it to take up the dentifrice. But it will be found an advantage if, after dipping the brush into water, it then be rubbed once or twice over a piece of white Castile soap. It will by this means pick up a larger amount of the powder. The teeth should be attended to after each meal, although cleansing them the last thing at night is an important duty, never on any account to be neglected. It must not be imagined, however, that even the foregoing is sufficient. Particles of food, which the brush fails to remove, collect between the teeth, and, if allowed to remain, ultimately lead on to decay. This is most likely to occur when the teeth are crowded close together in the jaw. But under all circumstances, whether the teeth be closely set together, or whether they be more widely apart, a piece of floss silk should be passed between them daily, so as to remove any adherent particles, and at the same time to thoroughly cleanse the sides of the teeth.

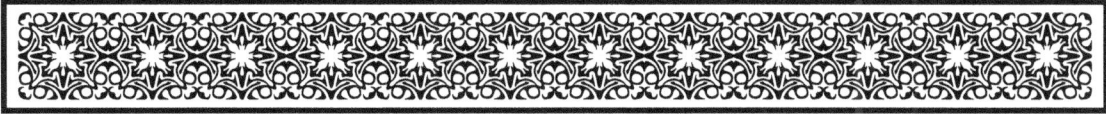

CHAPTER IV.
BEDROOM VENTILATION

Now, if all houses were built in accordance with the requirements of modern sanitary ideas, there would be but little difficulty in grappling with the problem of bedroom ventilation, for the sleeping apartment would be a well ventilated room, with all the latest contrivances, such as Tobin's ventilators, for the admission of fresh air. But as the greater number of people have to live in rented dwellings in which the rooms are very small, it becomes necessary to know what can be done to remedy existing defects. In the first place the bedroom should always be upstairs if possible; it is decidedly healthier, and there is a better chance for the supply of fresh air. The very worst room in the house that could be chosen for a sleeping apartment would be one on the basement. Then again, a fireplace in the bedroom is a priceless boon, and it is almost impossible to rectify such a deficiency. But as too many rooms are built without it, we are compelled to look to the window for our air supply. It is estimated that nearly one-third of every person's life is devoted to sleep; that is to say, about one-third of it is spent in the sleeping apartment. It is only natural, then, that this room and its surroundings should merit some special attention. As a matter of fact, from a health point of view, it should receive more consideration than all the rest of the house put together, for during our waking hours; we are moving about and constantly changing our location; but during sleep, when life is in abeyance to a certain extent, the system has passively to receive and be supported by whatever pure air the bedroom happens to possess. If, as too often is the case, that chamber is looked upon as a sort of cupboard, where, amongst other things, there is room for a bed, so much the worse for any one who has to sleep there. If the sleeper arises in the morning in a dazed and semi-suffocated state and quite unfitted for the day's work before him, instead of feeling refreshed, there is no occasion to seek far for the cause. For the mental toiler, also, it is equally important that the period devoted to the restoration of brain material and the imbibition of a fresh supply of nerve power for the ensuing day's requirements should be passed under circumstances the most favourable for bestowing them.

From this we see that a due amount of sleep, under favourable circumstances as regards ventilation, is necessary both for brain and muscle; and that, in fact, unless it be forthcoming, there will be an inability for either brain worker or muscle user to properly fulfil his duties next day. But in addition to this there is still the fact that we have to do with the semi-tropical climate of Australia. It will be as well, therefore, to make reference to what has been said on the subject as far as India is concerned. Sir Joseph Fayrer, whose opinion on such matters must always carry respect, in the course of an address on the preservation of health in that country, went on to say: "It is very important that you have good sleep, for nothing in the hot weather more refreshes or invigorates you. Early rising is the rule in India, and I advise you to conform to the usual practice."

Sir James Ranald Martin, another authority on Indian affairs, in commenting on the prevention of disease, also calls attention to the need for extra sleep, which is always required in hot climates. He points out that by giving the frame a thorough and complete rest from the great stimulus of heat, both tone and vigour are imparted-- providing for the requirements of the coming day, as well as repairing those of the preceding. The general truths contained in the foregoing apply equally to Australia, and during the hot summer months, therefore, it must not be forgotten that an extra allowance of sleep is quite indispensable.

In a great many cases the space under the bed is regarded as an admirable receptacle for a collection of boxes, parcels, hat-boxes, old boots, and other interesting relics, while they are effectually concealed from view by a species of curtain reaching from the bed to the floor. The drapery which thus hangs down is dignified by the name of a "valance," and though originally intended for the purpose of embellishment and ornamentation, it is better that decorative art should be more limited in its application, so as not to interfere with the free circulation of air throughout the room. The sleeping apartment is also considered as being particularly well adapted for the storage of old clothes, and consequently garments of this description are not hidden away, nor furtively concealed, but are triumphantly exposed to gaze in various parts of the room. Indeed, the more obtrusive they are, the better the purpose of the bedroom is believed to be served. If it could be only understood how these unnecessarily occupy the air space of the room, and interfere with its ventilation, this sort of thing would never be tolerated for a moment.

And while on the subject of the accumulation of useless articles in a bedroom, it seems fitting here to devote a few words to another kindred matter, namely, the hoarding up throughout the house of what may literally be designated as lumber. It is astonishing what a number of utterly valueless things are allowed to remain in nearly every household, and it is well remarked that no one ever knows what a collection of rubbish he possesses till he has occasion to remove. There may not be much to be ashamed of in the first load or two of furniture, but at the latter end there is a strong feeling that a dark night would be more adapted for moving--the darker the better. At least every twelve months there should be a regular clearance of worn-out articles, and that miscellaneous collection of odds and ends which can be of no earthly value to anybody, unless he be an antiquary.

Let us now go on to consider what ill effects result from the breathing of vitiated air. In his work, A Manual of Practical Hygiene, Professor Edmund A. Parkes has pointed out: "When air moderately vitiated by respiration is breathed for any period and continuously, its effects become complicated with those of other conditions. But allowing the fullest effect to all other agencies, there is no doubt that the breathing of the vitiated atmosphere of respiration has a most injurious result on the health. The aeration and nutrition of the blood seems to be interfered with, and the general tone of the system falls below par. Of special diseases it appears pretty clear that affections of the lungs are more common." The volume of air inhaled and exhaled by the adult in the twenty-four hours averages 360 cubic feet, or 2,000 gallons, while the amount we take in the shape of liquid or solid food does not amount probably to more than 5 1/2 pints, which is equal to only 1-3000th part of the volume of air passed through the lungs. From this it will be seen how necessary it is that such a large amount of air should be perfectly fresh and wholesome, for the lungs act as a pair of immense sponges or absorbers. When the ventilation does not allow of a continuous supply of fresh air it smells close, and is surcharged with an increased amount of carbonic acid, while the noxious exhalations from the breath and lungs deposit themselves throughout the room. Nor are the ill-effects of impure air confined to man alone, for it is well known that cows, horses, sheep, and other animals, when penned up in close quarters, show an increased death-rate from many diseases.

But though it is perfectly plain that badly ventilated sleeping apartments tend greatly to the production of diseases of the lungs, it is not generally understood by the greater number of persons that diseases of the heart are brought on by similar conditions, and there is without doubt a great increase of heart diseases at the present time. It is estimated that upwards of 10,000 people in England alone die yearly from affections of the heart; yet, taking into consideration the ceaseless work of that organ (in the words of the motto upon Goethe's ring, "Ohne Rast"--without rest), it is wonderful that it is not more frequently diseased. It is said that "the heart is a small muscular organ weighing only a few ounces, beating perpetually day and night, morning and evening, summer and winter; and yet often an old man's heart nearly a hundred years of age is as perfect and complete as when he was a young man of twenty" (Haughton).

The effect of impure air in its action on the heart is thus spoken of by Dr. Cornelius Black: "I showed the effect of impure air in promoting the degenerative tendency in the structures of the heart, and especially those of the right side of the heart, after the age of forty. I was then led to a passing consideration of the baneful influence produced upon the heart by badly-ventilated houses, schools, manufactories, pits, theatres, underground railways, and all places of a similar character." "The impure atmosphere of the bedrooms of the poor, and indeed of many of the middle class, caused by deficient ventilation, proves a sharp spur to the degenerative tendency manifested by the heart, and especially by the right side of the heart, after the age of forty." "I hold that the breathing of impure air is a fruitful source of disease of the right side of the heart occurring after middle age. How many people ignorantly favour its occurrence by confining themselves to closely shut, non-ventilated, stuffy, sitting rooms, in which the carbonic acid has accumulated to a poisonous degree in the air they respire! How are these evil results to be prevented? The simple answer is, let the rooms in which you live be effectively ventilated by an incoming current of fresh air, and so arranged that no draught shall be felt."

Sanitarians who have devoted a good deal of time and study to the working out of questions relating to the amount of fresh air in bedrooms have decided that each person should, if possible, have at least 1,000 cubic feet of space, or in other words, the same amount contained in a room 10 feet long, 10 feet wide, and 10 feet high. It is also estimated that the amount of fresh air entering into a room of this size should be 3,000 cubic feet per hour, that is, the air in each room should be completely changed three times every hour. These observations of course apply only to the least amount of air which every sleeper is strictly entitled to. As a matter of fact, however, any more than this is simply of distinct advantage as far as health is concerned. The bedroom, instead of being the smallest room in the house, as it too often is, should be really the very largest. Now it has been previously stated that foul or vitiated air collects in a sleeping apartment unless there be a continuous circulation of fresh air; and that the noxious exhalations from the breath and skin constitute the chief sources of air pollution. The practical point to discover is how to have this continuous circulation of fresh air throughout the room without causing a draught. Before considering this, a few words on the position of the bed itself will possibly be appropriate. It is always better to have it standing more in the centre of the room with its head against the wall, than to have it jammed alongside the latter. And it certainly should have placed north and south if the shape of the room admits of it. The wire-wove mattress is of great advantage both for comfort and for coolness; and here in Australia, during the summer months, proper mosquito nettings are as necessary as the bed itself. If the bed is provided with a head-piece, as it should be, there is no difficulty in fitting on the netting.

Every bedroom window should be made to open freely, and what other defects exist--such as the smallness of the apartment, or the absence of a fireplace--can be remedied to a great extent by means of the window. In many instances the bed is placed so near the latter that when it is open there is a strong draught playing directly on the bed, and this is an evil which must be avoided. In such case, to rectify matters, raise the bottom window a few inches, and have a piece of board made to fit in under it, so as to support the sash and fill in the space between it and the sill. The air freely enters the room between the two sashes, because the top of the lower sash is by this contrivance raised above the lower part of the upper one. Another great advantage is that the air is directed upwards to the ceiling by having to come in over the lower sash, and thus a gentle current of fresh air is constantly being circulated throughout the room without creating any draught. There are other devices to attain the same end, such as having apertures cut in the glass of the windows, but they are not so effective, so inexpensive, nor so simple as the preceding. In bedrooms there are the long French windows leading on to a balcony, and where such is the case the air current can be regulated to a nicety by having only one of the window-doors open, and directing the ventilation away from the bed. Many people prefer to sleep with the door itself open, and by having a PORTIERE or certain suspended outside, privacy can be ensured, while an upright screen standing at the head of the bed will effectually ward off any cold currents of air. In our summer weather there is but little difficulty experienced in regulating the air supply, for there is generally a desire to have as much fresh air as possible. Far too many people, however, look upon the bedroom in the light of an oven, where they are to be baked during the hours of repose, and this is the case even during the summer. In the cooler parts of the year they are apt to forget there is just as much necessity for fresh air as in the warm months.

Soiled or dirty clothes should not on any account be allowed to remain in the sleeping apartments, as they are a constant source of foulness to the air. All unclean linen ready for the wash had better be kept away from the bedroom in one of those long baskets which stand upright and are furnished with a lid. They are admirably adapted for the purpose, and may be obtained for a few shillings from any of the institutions for the blind, where they are made by the inmates. A word of advice, by the way, to those about to travel on a long voyage, is never to forget one of those canvas bags for the soiled clothes: they are invaluable at sea.

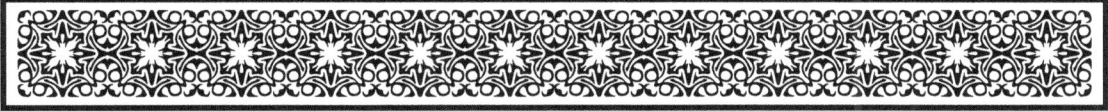

CHAPTER V.
CLOTHING, AND WHAT TO WEAR.

It is worth considering somewhat minutely what are the requisites of
perfect clothing, and what properties our different kinds of wearing
apparel possess. Without doubt any reflection on the question of what
is usually worn and what ought to be worn is not only of considerable
interest generally, but of great moment likewise from a health point of
view. It cannot be maintained too strongly that the question of the
proper material for a suitable covering for the body takes a footing
nearly equal to the very important one of diet itself. Now, there is no
form of clothing which on its own account creates heat, or has the
property of bestowing warmth upon the body, but the difference in it
consists in its power of preventing the escape of the body heat. These
qualities in the different varieties of wearing apparel will depend to
a great extent upon the thickness of the materials, and also upon the
varying power which they possess in detaining air within their meshes.
It is this latter property of retaining the air, which is warmed by
contact with the body, in their interstices, which constitutes the
great difference in the various clothing materials. This is also an
explanation of the well-known fact that loose garments are always
warmer than tightly fitting ones, for in the former there is the layer
of warm air in contact with the body, which has no opportunity for
existing in the latter. In the same way two or three layers of
under-garments will always be warmer than a single one, equal to their
combined thickness, since there is a separate layer of air between each

of the thinner ones.

All the differences in the various fabrics are due in chief part to the properties of heat. The ordinary or normal temperature of the human body is between 98 degrees and 99 degrees Fahrenheit, while that of the air will vary considerably, according to the climate and locality. Each individual, therefore, must be regarded as a material, though living, object which is enveloped in a surrounding atmosphere. As such, heat will conform to certain fixed laws in its relations to the two bodies. It is always a definite fact that when two bodies in contact with each other are of different temperatures, they tend to become of equal temperature. The warmer will part with its heat to the cooler, and the latter will in like manner reduce the temperature of the former. By covering, then, the surface of the body, it is prevented from giving its heat directly to the air, for the clothes intercept it by absorbing the heat themselves.

In the second place the clothes prevent a too rapid escape of heat from the body, and by keeping a layer of warm air in contact with the skin, they preserve the body heat. Again, the various materials used to clothe the body vary much as to the readiness with which they conduct heat; accordingly we speak of good and bad conductors of heat. A bad conductor, such as wool, will keep the heat of the body from escaping to the sir, and thus forms warm clothing, while a good conductor like cotton will lead away the heat quickly and prove cooler.

As said before, the texture of the material--that is, the size of its meshes--which allows air to pass more or less freely through it, also exercises a greater effect upon clothing. No healthy clothing is absolutely air-proof, the access of the air through it being necessary to our health and comfort. Thus oil-skin and mackintosh, which are air-tight as well as water-tight, make most people feel very uncomfortable.

In addition to their texture or permeability to air, and to
their conducting or non-contracting powers, fabrics also vary according
to their hygroscopic qualities. By hygroscopic is meant the power of
absorbing moisture; thus a thin flannel is one of the coolest materials
we can have, for it absorbs perspiration; while linen, which is
non-hydroscopic, when moist allows the fluid to evaporate rapidly, and
thus cools the body too quickly, and therefore dangerously. Hence flannel
is a most suitable fabric in which to take exercise, as there is less
danger of taking a chill.

There are four chief materials to be considered in connection with
clothing, namely--cotton and linen, which belong to the vegetable
kingdom, and silk and wool, which are obtained from the animal world.
These four, either in their own form or else in combination with each
other, such as merino, constitute most of our wearing apparel. Cotton
is the fine, soft, downy material of a hairy nature which is found on
the seeds of a certain plant, the cotton plant, which belongs to the
mallow family. Its fibres are flattened in shape, and are twisted at
intervals. The form of the fibres has an important effect in the action
of cotton material on the skin. Being of a flattened shape, they have
sharp edges, which in delicate skins are apt to cause irritation.
Cotton wears well, it is not absorbent of moisture nearly to the same
extent as linen, nor does it conduct away the heat of the body so
quickly as the latter, hence it is a warmer material than linen. On the
other hand, it does not retain the heat against the body like wool, and
is an appropriate material for dress in hot climates. In merino there
is a mixture of about one-fifth to one-half part of wool with cotton.

Linen, the other product of the vegetable kingdom, is obtained from the
fibres of the common flax. Its fibres, unlike those of other
fabrics, are distinguished by their roundness and their freedom from
stiffness. These properties give to it that peculiar softness which

makes it so agreeable to the feel, and comforting and soothing to the skin. But, on the other hand, it has certain characters which are a drawback. As was stated before, it differs from cotton in that it is cooler, but unfortunately it absorbs moisture from the body quickly, and becomes saturated with perspiration. This is removed so quickly by the action of the external air, causing rapid evaporation, that there is great danger of a chill.

The next material in alphabetical order is silk, and it is also the first product of the animal world to be considered. As is well known, it is obtained from the cocoon of the silk-worm. The fibres of this material are round in shape like those of linen, and they are even softer than the latter. On this account the phrase "as soft as silk" has passed into a saying. It is softer to the feel than either cotton or linen, and is a bad conductor of heat, as it has little tendency to remove the heat from the body. It is therefore a warmer material than either of them; but, on the other hand, from some peculiar action caused by the slightest friction against the skin, it seems at times to cause irritation, and draw the blood to the surface. In many instances the flow of blood is 80 severe as to set up an eruption of the skin, and there is often so much irritation and intolerable itching produced, that the garment has to be left off.

Last, but not least, of the quartette under consideration comes wool, and it is just one of those materials whose place it would be almost impossible to fill. It is obtained from the sheep, and is one of our chief productions in Australia. Unfortunately it is somewhat irritating to some skins, and many persons will declare that they cannot bear the feeling of anything woollen. Another objection may be taken to it on cosmetic grounds, and it certainly is difficult to make a flannel garment look attractive; but still, with a little taste in the way of bordering, this may be overcome to a great extent. On the other hand, it has great advantages which none of the foregoing fabrics possess, and which have been already referred to.

Having thus minutely and scientifically examined into the properties of the various clothing materials, it will clearly be seen that the one which possesses the greatest advantages with the least possible disadvantages is wool. Hence it is to be chosen in preference to all other fabrics for wearing next the skin, because it wards off all risk of a chill striking the body. Its disadvantages, as said before, are mainly two, the first being that some declare it is impossible to wear it next the skin on account of its causing irritation; this, however, can only apply to new flannel, since after two or three washings it feels as smooth as the most fastidious skin could desire. The next objection, that it cannot be made to look attractive or ornamental, is to a certain extent true; but if it is simply a question of health VERSUS appearance, those who would sacrifice the former deserve to suffer. In this matter we may learn a wrinkle from a practical class of men, namely, sailors. One will find many of them pin their faith on the virtues of an abdominal flannel bandage, reaching from the lower part of the chest well down to the hips. It thus covers the loins and abdomen, and for warding off attacks of lumbago and muscular rheumatism, and for protecting the kidneys, it certainly is valuable.

A flannel under-garment reaching from the neck well down to the hips should always be worn, and in summer it may be of a thinner material than in the cooler weather. It is better to have four made, so that two can be washed at a time. In this way two can be in use every week, changing them day by day, so that one is getting thoroughly aired while the other is being worn. The one which is being aired should be turned inside out, so that the part which has been in contact with the skin becomes thoroughly purified. It must be remembered, however, that flannel is very liable to shrink from repeated washings. This may be provided for by taking care that the under-garment, when first obtained, is several sizes too large. In fact, it can hardly be too large at first, especially in the case of the thicker one for the cooler months, which shrinks much more proportionately than does the thinner one for the hot season. This shrinking, however, can to a great extent be presented by paying attention to the following points: These woollen under-garments should be washed by themselves not with any other clothes, in only moderately hot water. Next, while they are still damp, and before becoming dry, they should be thoroughly stretched upon a table and then well ironed out.

With regard to the sleeping apparel, there is no doubt the modern pyjamas are a great improvement on the old-fashioned bedgown. They are more thoroughly protective to the skin, and keep the extremities uniformly warm, which the latter fails to do. They are better made of flannel, thin in summer and thicker in winter. Persons who are in the habit of wearing woollen material next the skin during the day should certainly keep to the same at night, otherwise the change is too great, and there is thus great risk of taking a chill. The flannel under-garment which has been worn during the day can then be taken off at night without any danger, and has the opportunity of being aired. It might hardly seem necessary to refer to this fact, namely, that the under-garment which has been worn during the day should be taken off at night. Yet I can only say that instances in which this particular garment is never taken off at all, but is worn continuously both night and day, perhaps for a whole week at a time, are not altogether so rare as they might be.

In conclusion reference may be briefly made to a subject which is probably within the experience of everyone. There ale many people who pride themselves on not requiring any extra clothing during the colder months, and evidently look upon this fact as a proof that they possess Spartan powers of endurance, and that cold is a matter of perfect indifference to them. Now, it may be that a few individuals differ essentially from the rest of humanity, and do not require any change of clothing all the year round. But the majority of people who profess this disregard to climate certainly appear as if they would be all the better for warmer material, for their faces look pinched and their hands seem nearly frozen with the cold. But the fact is that even if the want of thicker clothing is not particularly felt during the cold weather, it is always wiser to wear an extra allowance, for the heat of summer can be endured better if this principle is carried out. If a common-sense view of the matter is taken, then it will be readily apparent why it is desirable to wear plenty of warm clothing during the colder months.

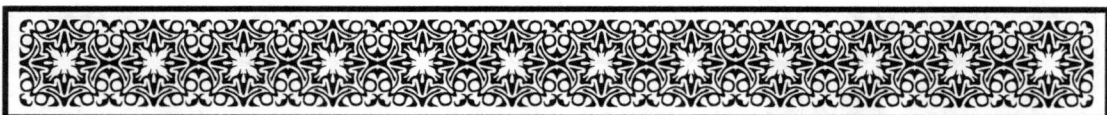

CHAPTER VI.
DIET

The larger part of this work is taken up with a consideration of the most suitable diet for those living in Australia. In this way a greater restriction in the amount of butcher's meat is counselled, while a more widely extended use of fish, vegetables, and salad plants is advocated. And as far as beverages are concerned, Australian wine of a low alcoholic strength is recommended as being the most natural beverage for every-day use. But there are a few other matters connected with food, and drink, and daily habits which will deserve some little reference, and accordingly they will be dealt with. These are fruit, tea, coffee, iced drinks, and the use of tobacco. All these are important enough to merit notice; indeed, they are subjects possessing more than usual interest.

Before proceeding to give attention to these, however, it will be most convenient, at this stage, to make some remarks upon the vital topic of the first meal of the day. With the great bulk of our population sufficient heed is never given it, and yet it is of infinite consequence. By far the greater number of people dawdle in bed till the last possible moment, when all at once they jump into their bath--that is, if they take a bath--swallow a hasty breakfast, and make a frantic rush for their steamer, train, or tram, in order to begin their daily work. How very much better than all this bustle, hurry, and scuttle an hour's earlier rising would be! It would afford ample time for the bath, which should be a bath in the truest sense of the term; it would, above all, give a proper opportunity for a leisurely breakfast, which is in every respect the most important meal of the day; and lastly, it would save that wild dash at the last, which is so fatal to proper digestion and well-being.

But it is a sad fact that, in most cases, even when there is due time given to it, the monotony of the ordinary breakfast is almost proverbial. With regard to the average household it is a matter of deep conjecture as to what most people would do if a prohibition were placed upon chops, steak, and sausages for breakfast. If such an awful calamity happened, many the father of a family would have to put up with scanty fare. It is very much to be feared that the inability to conceive of something more original for the morning meal than the eternal trio referred to is a melancholy reproach to the housekeeping capabilities of many. To read an account of a highland breakfast, in contradistinction to this paucity of comestibles, is to make one almost pensive. The description of the snowy tablecloth, the generously loaded table, the delicious smell of the scones and honey, the marmalade, the different cakes, the fish, the bacon, and the toast, is enough to create a desire to dwell there for a very prolonged period. However, REVENONS A NOS MOUTONS; this has been adverted to, not so much with the idea of urging people to copy such an example, because expense would render it an impossibility, but to try and awaken a determination to make more variety at the breakfast table. It is to be hoped that some of the recipes at the end of the volume will serve as a means of initiating a reform in this respect.

But under all circumstances, whether brain or muscle be employed by the bread-winner, a substantial breakfast is of first-rate importance. There is one form of food which it is especially necessary should constitute part of the meal, and which must be referred to. This is that variety known as the hydro-carbons or fats. The value of fat, in any of its many forms, in promoting the health of the body and preventing the onset of wasting diseases is hardly appreciated, and besides this action it markedly serves to nourish the brain and nervous system. Dr. Murchison, the late eminent physician, was wont to declare that bacon fat or ham fat was worth a guinea an ounce in the treatment of wasting diseases. Cod liver oil, also, has a wide repute in the treatment of the same class of maladies. Indeed, it is related of an eminent barrister that he used to take a full dose of cod liver oil some time before going to plead an important case, for he found it better brain food than anything else.

In our semi-tropical climate, however, a dislike is often taken to butter when it is presented at breakfast in the form of semi-liquid grease. It would require a person with the stomach of an ostrich to digest, to say nothing of relish, such an oleaginous compound during our hot months. But if this necessary and all-important article of diet can be presented in an appetising shape, what a desirable result is achieved I The mass of the people--I am not referring to those who are well endowed with worldly gifts--are apt to look upon the ice chest as a luxury which is altogether beyond their means. But, as I have said elsewhere, I am firmly persuaded that if the price of ice were brought down to one-halfpenny per pound, and if a company were formed to deliver such a small quantity as six pounds per day, or every second day, it would be a great boon, and moreover a wonderfully profitable speculation. A very small and suitable ice chest could be constructed, to sell at a few shillings, solely to preserve the butter in a congealed, and therefore palatable, state, for children as well as for adults. The former would take it with great avidity, and the benefit to health resulting therefrom would be incalculable. Even in some of the better-class houses ice is looked upon too much as a luxury, and not, as it should be, a necessity; indeed, the money saved from gas during the summer months might well be expended in ice.

Not only is this fatty breakfast a necessary feature in the diet of everybody, particularly of the young and growing population, but it is likewise a most important matter with all brain workers. If the business or professional man can put in a liberal breakfast, consisting largely of butter, fat bacon or ham, he can go on all day with a feeling of energy and buoyancy. It is in this aversion to fatty matter, in any shape or form, that the bilious and dyspeptic are so fearfully handicapped. And not only is it necessary for an active mental worker to be supplied with a good proportion of fatty material, but, as I have just said, it is essential that his breakfast should be a substantial one, in which his food is not stinted in any way. As Dr. Milner Fothergill said: "I would always back a good breakfaster, from a boy to a game cockerel; a good meal to begin the day is a good foundation." So, too, Mr. Christopher Heath, the well-known London surgeon, in his advice to house surgeons and other medical officers living in hospitals, says, "the first symptom of \\`knocking up,/' is an inability to eat breakfast," and goes on to point out how important a meal it is, and that it should be taken deliberately and without undue haste.

FRUIT

It is undoubtedly a most fortunate thing for us in Australia that fruit is so abundant, and that it is easily within the reach of all. There is something wonderfully attractive about it; its colouring in particular appeals so to the eye that a good show of well-assorted fruit is always certain to ensure attention. Many fruits, moreover, have a magnificent fragrance which lends to their agreeable taste. It is somewhat of a pity that fruit is not more ordinarily eaten at meals, particularly with the breakfast. There is an old proverb that fruit is gold in the morning, silver at noon, and lead at night; and it is undoubtedly a fact that it is especially beneficial when eaten early in the day. In France, fruit is a constant part of every meal, and there is no question but that such a proceeding is desirable. It was formerly the custom with English people at regular dinners to have dessert on the table all through the courses, but it is now more customary to present it at the termination of the repast, so that it is quite fresh and not saturated with odours absorbed from the soup, fish, etc.

The agreeable qualities of fruits may be said to reside in three different factors. First, there is the proportion of sugar, gum, pectin, etc., to free acid; next, the proportion of soluble to insoluble matters; and thirdly, the aroma, which, indeed, is no inconsiderable element therein. This latter quality--the aroma, fragrance, or perfume of fruit--is due to the existence of delicate and exquisite ethers. These subtle ethers Are often accompanied by essential oils, which may render the aroma more penetrating and continued. Those fruits like the peach, greengage, and mulberry, which almost melt in the mouth, contain a very large amount of soluble substances. Some fruits, like the peach and apricot, carry but a small amount of sugar as compared with the free acid they contain. Yet the free acid is not distinctly perceptible, because its taste is covered by a larger proportion of gum, pectin, and other gelatinous substances. There are other fruits again, such as the currant and gooseberry, which are markedly acid, because there is only a small amount of gum and pectin, and a relatively larger amount of free acid.

With regard to fruit when eaten in its raw state, the question of ripeness is a most important ones and is always to be considered; so that whatever views may be entertained as to the dietetic value of ripe fruit, there is a consensus of opinion on the fact that when unripe it is most injurious. Care must be taken, therefore, to see that it is perfectly ripe, and no considerations of economy must be allowed to over-ride the fact. At the same time, though ripeness is a necessary qualification of wholesomeness, yet fruit must not be over-ripe, as changes occur which render it undesirable for the system, and thus in avoiding Scylla we may fall into Charybdis. The skin of fruit should never be eaten, nor should the stones, pips, or seeds be swallowed, as there is a danger of their accumulating in a small pouch of the bowel known as the vermiform appendix. Their lodgment in this little pocket is a constant source of peril, and would soon set up an inflammation, which must always be attended with a considerable amount of danger.

As to the question of the unripeness or over-ripeness of fruit, the following remarks by Dr. F.W. Pavy, an acknowledged authority on all that relates to food, and worth recording:--"Fruit forms an agreeable and refreshing kind of food, and, eaten in moderate quantity, exerts a favourable influence as an article of diet. It is chiefly of service for the carbo-hydrates, vegetable acids, and alkaline salts it contains. It enjoys, too, in a high degree, the power of counteracting the unhealthy state found to be induced by too close a restriction to dried and salted provisions. Whilst advantageous when consumed in moderate quantity, fruit, on the other hand, proves injurious if eaten in excess. Of a highly succulent nature, and containing free acids and principles liable to undergo change, it is apt, when ingested out of due proportion to other food, to act as a disturbing element, and excite derangement of the alimentary canal. This is particularly likely to occur if eaten either in the unripe or over-ripe state; in the former case, from the quantity of acid present; in the latter, from its strong tendency to ferment and decompose within the digestive tract. The prevalence of stomach and bowel disorders, noticeable during the height of the fruit season, affords proof of the inconveniences that the too free use of fruit may give rise to."

The different forms of fruit, and also of vegetables, owe their great value to the fact that they possess powerful anti-scorbutic properties. It will be best and simplest to define the word "anti-scorbutic" as "good against the scurvy." This latter disease is notably dependent on a want of fresh fruit and vegetables in the dietary, and consequently is more often observed amongst sailors; and though accessory conditions, such as great privations, bad provisions, or unhealthy surroundings, may predispose to it, yet that which essentially produces it is the deficiency of the former articles from the food. At the present time it is not nearly so frequently seen, since, according to the mercantile marine regulations, subject to legislative enactments passed in 1867, in lieu of vegetables, one ounce of lime juice, sweetened with the same quantity of sugar, must be served out to each man daily.

In scurvy there is some great change effected in the blood, and it is as well to refer briefly to the characters possessed by the latter. The blood as it exists in the body is a red alkaline fluid, having a saltish taste and possessing quite a noticeable odour. It consists of minute bodies, the corpuscles, immersed in a liquid, the LIQUOR SANGUINIS. Salts also enter into its composition, and include the chlorides of potash and soda; the phosphates of lime, magnesia,-and soda; the sulphate of potash, and free soda. Of these the salts of soda predominate, and the chloride--that is, common salt--is usually in excess of all the others. The uses of these salts in the blood are to supply the different tissues with the salts they respectively require, to take part in maintaining the proper specific gravity and alkaline character of the blood, and to prevent any changes going on within it.

In scurvy, as mentioned before, the blood seems to undergo some great change, and there are accumulations of it beneath the skin. The gums become spongy, bleeding on the slightest touch, and the teeth frequently loosen. Blood often flows from the mouth and nose, or is vomited from the stomach, or is passed through the bowels. Dr. Garrod advanced the view that scurvy was dependent on a deficiency of potash in the stem, and that vegetables which contained potash supplied the want. It is questionable, however, whether the disease is due to this fact alone, since beef tea, which contains a good deal of potash, may be given freely to a scorbutic patient, yet he fails to recover till proper anti-scorbutic diet is supplied. Dr. Ralfe found by experiments that when acids are injected into the blood, or an excess of acid salts administered, the same changes occur in the blood as in scurvy. Hence he supposes that the latter disease is caused by a decrease in the alkalinity of the blood, which results from the absence of fruit and vegetables from the food.

Now, although characteristic cases of scurvy are as a rule to be met with chiefly in sailors, yet there is no doubt that an insufficiency of the preceding in the dietary brings about an unhealthy condition of the system. Many typical examples of this are frequently seen in the patients admitted into our hospitals. They have been living, perhaps, in isolated districts in the country, where their sole food was mutton and damper, with no restriction placed on tea and tobacco. As a rule their skin presents evidences of the need of proper diet, for it looks unhealthy and is often covered with boils. But apart from these cases, which so plainly indicate the origin of the poor condition of the blood, there are many instances in which, from the want of vegetable food and fruit, the system becomes greatly deranged. moreover, what is known as the blood being "out of order" is mostly due to an unsuitable diet, consisting of animal food in excess, and a corresponding deficiency of the other essentials.

The use of fruit, again, is especially indicated in persons disposed to the formation of uric acid in excess. When this actually occurs, the system becomes overloaded with deleterious matter, and the blood and body fluids are then saturated with a MATERIES MORBI. This morbific material is best understood by regarding it as being in an incomplete or half-way stage, in which form it is injurious. But, on the other hand, if it had proceeded to its final change, the completed product would have been harmless. Indeed, it is as the latter that it mostly leaves the body in ordinary conditions of health. Well then, the retention within the system of this incompletely transformed material gives rise to various symptoms. One of them is a bitter or "coppery" taste in the mouth, notably in the early morning. Oftentimes, too, patients will complain that they do not feel at all refreshed on rising, even when they have slept fairly well--which does not happen too frequently. There may be also a great tendency to drowsiness, accompanied by severe pains in the limbs, coming on about an hour after meals. Other symptoms which are commonly met with are great irritability of the temper and lowness of spirits. There is frequently a headache of a peculiar kind. It comes on generally in the morning, and may last all day, or even for several days. It is a dull, heavy pain, felt most often in the forehead. A curious feature of the affection which sometimes exists is an incontrollable desire to grind the teeth during the waking hours. There are other symptoms, also, characteristic of the same malady, namely, palpitation of the heart and intermittency of the pulse; a liability to colds on the chest; and perhaps repeated attacks of difficulty in breathing. From all this it follows that a more liberal supply of fruit for such individuals would be followed by the most beneficial results and their children might well be taught to follow their example. For it must be remembered that all fruits contain alkaline salts which are good for the blood. These alkaline vegetable salts become changed within the body, and converted into the carbonate of the alkali, in which latter form they pass out of the system.

But before finally closing this portion it is necessary to say a few words about olives, from which the famous olive oil is obtained, and indeed with regard to their virtues nearly a volume might be written. With many people the olive, like the tomato, is an acquired taste, and unfortunately too many fail to overcome their first impressions; but it is certainly worth acquiring, even if the process takes a long time and requires much perseverance, on account of its highly nutritive value. Children are often very fond of olives, and persistent efforts should be made to induce those who do not like them to overcome their aversion. We speak of "French olives" and "Spanish olives"; the former are gathered young, and are small and hard, while the latter are allowed to remain till a later period of growth, when they become softer and more pulpy. The French olives are more piquant in flavour than the larger kind. They are also better to eat as a fruit, though many prefer the Spanish, and are sometimes employed to clear the palate before drinking wines. The larger or Spanish olives are more adapted for cooking, as in the dish known as beef olives, and also for salads. There must be no misconception as to the name French or Spanish as applied to olives; it does not refer to the country from which they are derived, but simply serves to indicate that they are taken from the tree at a particular time in accordance with the habit observed in the respective countries. The mode of preparing the olives as they reach us is as follows: They have been gathered when green, and soaked first of all in strong lye--that is, water saturated with alkaline salt, obtained by steeping wood ashes in the former. They are next soaked in fresh water to remove the somewhat acrid and bitter taste, and are then bottled in a solution of salt and water. Ordinarily they are presented at table in a dish or other suitable vessel, with a little of the liquid in which they have been preserved. In conclusion it may be added that olives form an historical dish, for we are told that the supper of Milton the poet consisted usually of bread and butter and olives.

TEA

Tea, with which we are all so familiar, is in reality a number of dried rolled leaves of the tea plant, Camellia Thea, cultivated chiefly in China and the contiguous countries. It is used excessively throughout Australasia--for has it not been shown that our four million people use more of this beverage than the millions who inhabit Continental Europe, if Russia be excepted? This fact is much to be deplored, for when taken in excess it causes severe functional derangement of the digestive organs, and prejudicially affects the nervous system. The gentler sex are greatly given to extravagant tea-drinking, exceeding all bounds of moderation in this respect. Many of them, moreover, live absolutely on nothing else but tea and bread and butter. What wonder, then, that they grow pale and bloodless; that their muscles turn soft and flabby; that their nervous system becomes shattered; and that they suffer the agonies of indigestion? Their favourite time for a chat and the consumption of tea is at any period between ten o'clock in the morning and three in the afternoon. Now, if there is anything of which I am certain, it is that tea in the middle of the day, say from ten o'clock to three, is a deadly destructive fluid. And I am equally certain, too, that innumerable numbers of young girls employed in business do themselves an irreparable amount of injury by making their mid-day meal consist of nothing else but tea and a little bread and butter. There is no nourishment whatever in such fare, and it inevitably leads to the bad symptoms already detailed and general unhealthiness, if not to the onset of graver disease. No, they require something which is nutritious, such as a little warm soup of some kind, a modicum of bread, and say two different varieties of vegetables to follow. Of course this may be extended to include pudding, stewed fruit, &c., but the former is ample enough in many respects. This is a very important matter to which the attention of proprietors and managers of large establishments, factories, and other places employing many female hands might well be directed. And, moreover, if ever there was an opportunity for an active organization to achieve really valuable work, it would be in seeing that our city girls had something better to eat in the middle of the day than tea and bread and butter.

As in every other case, however, there is all the difference in the world between the use of anything and its abuse. It is wrong to assume that, because a great deal of something is injurious, a small quantity judiciously employed is equally pernicious. And so it is even in the case of tea, for it is not to be denied that a fragrant cup of tea is very agreeable. As Dr. Vivian Poore most appropriately remarked in reply to the argument that the lower animals did not require tea, coffee, &c.: "We are not lower animals; we have minds as well as bodies; and since these substances have the property of enabling us to bear our worries and fatigues, let us accept them, make rational use of them, and be thankful." Of course everything hinges upon the correct interpretation of the terms "small" quantity, and "judiciously" employed. It may be said, however, that the drinking of large cups of tea is never to be sanctioned under ally circumstances whatever. It should rather be looked upon as a delicate fluid to be imbibed only in very small quantities. It should certainly not be used in the middle of the day, between those hours which I have specified; nor should it be taken during the evening, for it almost always disturbs the night's rest.

There was a great controversy as to the proper way of making tea in the medical papers not very long ago. It is of course a perennial topic, and always excites considerable interest. This particular discussion began in this way. A new tea-pot, called the anti-tannic tea-pot, appeared on the scene, and was favoured with a long description by the BRITISH MEDICAL JOURNAL. It was claimed for this special model that it extracted only the theine, and not the tannin from the tea. Now, as a matter of fact, it is simply impossible to make tea, no matter how it is made, entirely free from tannin. It is quite true that many suppose by infusing the tea for a very brief period only--two or three minutes --the passage of the tannin into the beverage can be prevented, but, as Sir William Roberts has pointed out, this is quite a delusion. Tannin is one of the most soluble substances known, and melts in hot water just as sugar does. Tea made experimentally, by pouring boiling water on the dry leaves placed on filter paper, contains tannin. As Sir

William remarks, you can no more have tea without tannin, than you can have wine without alcohol.

Nevertheless, it is a fact that this anti-tannic tea-pot has many excellent points about it, and is sure to meet with favour. It is really an attempt to make tea by a more certain method than is generally employed; for I think it must be admitted that the present happy-go-lucky style has not much to recommend it. On one occasion the tea will be excellent--and on another either as weak as water, or with such a sharp acrid taste that it is almost undrinkable. In the latter case the tea has been allowed to soak so long that it has become a decoction instead of an infusion. The consequence of this prolonged action of the hot water on the tea is that it brings out the bitter extractive material of the plant, and it is this which proves so particularly pernicious. Tea at sea is proverbially unpalatable, and invariably disagrees, owing chiefly to the fact that it is a boiled decoction of tea leaves and nothing else.

COFFEE

Coffee is the roasted and ground product of the seeds found within the fruit of a tree, the Coffea Arabica. Originally a native of Abyssinia, it was transported into Arabia at the beginning of the fifteenth century. Since then it has been widely cultivated in the West Indies, in Ceylon, and in other warm countries. The fruit itself much resembles a small cherry in size and appearance, and usually contains two small seeds--the coffee beans themselves. The choicest coffee is the mocha or Arabian coffee, and the bean is very small. Of the West Indian varieties, the Jamaica and the Martinique coffee are the best. The exhilarating and agreeable properties of coffee are dependent in great part upon three active principles which it contains. The first of these is caffeine, which is almost identical in composition with, and practically the same as, the theine present in tea. Next there are the volatile oils, developed by roasting, from which coffee derives its aroma. Indeed, as far as they are concerned, there are many who believe that these ethereal oils have more to do with the characteristic properties of coffee than even the caffeine itself. And, lastly, there are the acids known as caffeo-tannic and caffeic acids, which are modified forms of tea tannin. They exist to a far less extent, however, than does the tannin in tea.

Coffee has a decidedly stimulating effect upon the nervous system; so much so that in France it has been called UNE BOISSON INTELLECTUELLE (an intellectual beverage), from its stimulating all the functions of the brain. Not so long ago a writer, Dr. J. N. Lane, in the BRITISH MEDICAL JOURNAL gave some interesting, information with respect to coffee and brain work. As the result of his own experience he recommended "a cup of strong coffee, without cream or sugar, preceded and followed by a glass of hot water every morning before breakfast. The various secretions are thus stimulated, the nerve force aroused, no matter how the duties of the preceding day and night may have drawn upon the system. Another cup at four in the afternoon is sufficient to sustain the energies for many hours." It is only fair to add, however, that the JOURNAL went on to remark that in this way some 50 grains of caffeine would be taken each week, and that very little more might develop injurious symptoms, so that the power of doing an illimitable amount of work would be obtained under somewhat risky conditions.

One of its most remarkable effects is that of relieving the feeling of fatigue or exhaustion, whether this be produced by brain work or bodily labour. It enables the system also to bear up under an empty stomach and when the supply of food is shortened. In this way it is of signal value to the soldier in the field. Professor E.A. Parkes, all admitted authority on these matters, bears testimony to the fact that in military service it invigorates the system and is almost equally

useful against both cold and heat--against cold by reason of its
warmth, and against heat by its action on the skin. It appears, also,
to do sway with the need for sleep, probably from its arousing the
mental faculties, and the effect of a strong cup of coffee in inducing
wakefulness is well known. Coffee has, moreover, a distinct action on
the heart, and tends to strengthen it. The Germans are great believers
in its virtues, and Vogel, one of the principal authorities on diseases
of children, recommends it for them, mixed with cream, both as a food
and as a tonic.

In addition to the foregoing, coffee is also employed by reason of its
important medicinal virtues. In malarious countries a cup of hot strong
coffee, in the early morning, is regarded as a preventive against fever
and ague. It is a valuable agent in many cases of heart disease,
particularly when associated with dropsy. In Bright's disease of the
kidneys, where dropsy is present, it is likewise given with benefit.
Strong coffee is also a well-known remedy in asthma, both in relieving
the actual attack and in acting as a restorative after it is over. It
frequently gives great relief in many forms of nervous headache,
particularly in that variety known as migraine, in which the pain is
generally limited to one side of the head. And, lastly, coffee is a
valuable remedy in opium poisoning, where there is such a tendency to a
fatal coma.

From the foregoing it must be evident that coffee occupies a very high
position as a beverage. All that concerns its preparation, therefore,
is of undoubted interest. In the first place, to obtain coffee in
perfection it is indispensable that the beans be roasted at home, and
not only should the roasting be done in the house, but the operation
ought really to be performed immediately before the coffee is made, and
the reasons thereof I shall give in speaking of the process of
roasting. Many people do not care sufficiently about the
perfection of coffee to go to this trouble, and are content with having

their roasted coffee beans sent to them daily from their grocer. The leading establishments roast their coffee beans daily, and from them the latter may be obtained and ground in the mill at home. This, of course, though not giving the real thing, is an immense improvement on the hallowed tradition, so dear to some, of purchasing their weekly supply of,,round coffee at a time and keeping it in a tin or vessel for use as required. But, as I said before, if perfection is aimed at, the roasting must be done at home.

In the selection of the green beans care should be taxiway to see that they are nearly all of the same size, for if some are small and others large, when it comes to roasting it will be found that the small ones are done to a cinder, while the larger beans are hardly touched. The beans, too, should be perfectly dry; if moist, they should be dried in a dish by the fire or in the oven before going into the roaster. On the coffee plantations the drying of the bean is considered a most important matter when preparing them for export.

In the process of roasting, a volatile oil which gives to coffee its unique fragrance is developed. It is somewhat curious that no amount of boiling could educe this from the raw bean. This oil is exceedingly volatile, and begins to disperse and evaporate the very moment it is born. Hence, to obtain the perfection of coffee, no time should be lost in grinding and making it directly it is roasted. When the fragrant vapour of the roasted bean is first given off, it is soon followed by a peculiar noise, caused by the splitting and crackling of the external silvery greenish covering of the raw beans. At this time, or very shortly afterwards, the latter are of a yellowish hue, but before long they change into that desirable lightish brown colour, when the peculiar volatile coffee oils are at their best.

The best mill for grinding the coffee, and one which may be obtained from any ironmonger, is that which can be screwed on the edge

of the kitchen table or dresser. It has a little contrivance to
regulate the size of the grains. and care must be taken not to grind
the coffee too fine; it should be in minute crumbs rather than in
powder.

As I have already said, the perfection of coffee is only to be obtained
under three conditions. These are, first, that the beans should be
roasted at home; that they should be ground without much delay; and,
thirdly, made into coffee as soon as possible. Many people are,
however, unable to carry out the first of these three requirements. The
next best substitute is to have the roasted coffee beans sent daily to
them by their grocer. This is a practice which might be followed more
frequently with a great deal of advantage, for all are able, at least,
to possess a mill and grind their own coffee at home.

The making of the coffee is quite as important as the preceding, and
the number of different models of coffee-makers is almost perplexing.
But of them all, the one which is simplest, and perhaps most effective,
is the ordinary CAFETIERS, or French coffee-pot. This has the advantage
of costing only a few shillings, and is readily obtainable from any
ironmonger. It consists of an upper compartment in which the coffee is
made, and a lower part--the coffee-pot itself--into which the coffee
descends. These two portions are quite separate, although the upper
fits on the lower. The floor--on which the coffee is placed--of the
upper part is perforated by a number of minute holes There is also a
movable strainer about an inch in depth, which fits on top of the upper
part; and a presser, consisting of a long rod with a circular plate at
its end, which for convenience passes through the centre of the
strainer, and rests on the perforated floor of the upper part.

There are one or two points to be borne in mind in the making of
coffee. As a rule English-speaking people do not allow enough coffee to
each cup. The almost universal fault of coffee, made elsewhere than on

the Continent, is its want of strength and flavour. With regard to the admixture of chicory, this is largely a question of taste, and the palate must be consulted in the matter. The great majority of people, however, cannot do without it, and it is quite (when genuine) a harmless addition. Madame Lebour-Fawssett recommends the following proportions: For making CAFE NOIR, or coffee after meals, there should be six teaspoonsful of coffee, heaped up, and a very small teaspoonful of chicory, or none at all, for one pint of water. The chicory must be left out altogether, and another teaspoonful of coffee substituted for those who object to chicory with their CAFE NOIR. For morning coffee or cafe au lait there should be ten or twelve teaspoonsful of coffee, with a sixth part of chicory, for each pint of water. As Madame Lebour-Fawssett remarks, CAFE AU LAIT is never complete without chicory, but care should be taken not to overdo it, since too much chicory renders the coffee quite undrinkable. Of course, if you do not require as much as a pint of coffee, the quantities may be reduced, still observing the same proportions. Before pouring out the coffee, the cup should first be half filled with hot milk, and then the coffee added.

Now, having seen what proportions of coffee and chicory are to be employed for CAFE NOIR and CAFE AU LAIT respectively, it will be better to describe the actual making of the coffee, since the CAFETIERE will then be more easily understood. We will suppose its upper part is fitted into its place on the top of the lower portion, and that the strainer and presser have been removed for the time being. Enough boiling water should first of all be poured in to fill both the upper and lower compartments, allowed to stand for a couple of minutes, and then poured away. This brings everything to a proper heat for receiving the coffee.

Next put the amount of coffee necessary upon the perforated floor of the upper part. The coffee should then be well pressed down with the presser, and the latter instrument next laid aside. After this the strainer should be replaced on top of the upper compartment, and the required amount of boiling water, a little at a time, poured in through it (the strainer). The object of pouring in the boiling water slowly is to give it time to percolate through the densely pressed coffee lying on the floor of the upper part. There is a little tin cover fitting over the spout of the lower compartment, which should be adjusted to keep in the steam. The whole may then be set aside for a few minutes, and when the coffee has passed into the lower part, it is ready for use. With a little practice, and by paying attention to these details, the most perfect coffee may be made.

ICED DRINKS

In Australia some reference to the subject of iced drinks is necessarily required, for they are in great request during the hot season. There is a considerable amount of diversity of opinion as to their good and bad effects, but it will be found that the experience of most medical men is that when used in moderation they greatly relieve thirst and are not injurious. This, indeed, is my own belief, and were it not for the abuse of iced drinks, the same opinion would be held almost universally. America is the country of countries in which the inordinate use of ice has gained for it a reputation which it has never deserved. Ice, says George Augustus Sala, is the alpha and omega of social life in the United States. At the hotels, first-class or otherwise, the beverage partaken of at dinner is mostly iced water. Every repast, in fact, begins and ends with a glass of iced water. When consumed in this way it is no wonder that it often disagrees, and that ice-water dyspepsia is a definite malady in America. And more than this, imagine carrying the employment of ice to such an extent that it culminates in that gastronomical curiosity, a BAKED ICE! The "Alaska" is a BAKED ICE, of which the interior is an ice cream. This latter is surrounded by an exterior of whipped cream, made warm by means of a Salamander. The transition from the hot outside envelope to the frozen inside is painfully sudden, and not likely to be attended with beneficial effect. But the abuse of a good thing is no argument whatever against its use in a moderate and rational manner.

It will be desirable, however, to see what is believed in India about iced drinks, for it will be something of a guide for us in Australia. There are two authorities in particular who have been already referred to, and who have written on this matter in its application to India. The first of these is Sir James Ranald Martin, who had twenty-two years experience there in different parts, and is therefore entitled to be listened to. He says that ice is a matter of necessity in the East, and quotes Dolomieu, who observes of iced drinks that "they revive the spirits, strengthen the body, and assist the digestion."

There is also that other great name, that of Sir Joseph Fayrer, who is most competent to speak on Indian matters. In setting forth rules for the guidance of those who purpose living in India, he remarks that iced water may be drunk with impunity there; that he has no recollection of seeing any one suffer from drinking iced water or iced soda water in a hot climate; and that in the great heat it is good, since it tends to keep down the body temperature. When the system is prostrated by the sun or extreme heat, or exhausted by physical or intellectual exertion in a hot and damp atmosphere, he believes that a glass of iced water slowly swallowed is far more refreshing than the iced brandy, or whisky peg, or draught of beer, too frequently indulged in under such circumstances.

The different writers on food and dietetics, who have given considerable attention to the same subject, are almost unanimous in their opinion to the same effect. There will be no occasion to refer to all of them, but three at least deserve a brief mention. Dr. Burney Yeo has recently observed that iced water, when taken in small quantities, is refreshing and cooling, and likewise stimulates the digestive functions. On the other hand, it is certainly injurious when taken in inordinate amount. According to Dr. T. King Chambers, cool drinks are beneficial to the stomach in hot weather, since they help to reduce the increased temperature to which the over-heated blood has brought it. Ice, moreover, is a valuable addition to the dietary both of the sick and of the healthy. There is one caution to be observed, however, and it is that ice is injurious when the system is exhausted after violent exercise. And lastly, Dr. Milner Fothergill believes the craving for cool drinks during the hot weather is such, that there is evidently some irrepressible desire to be satisfied. He even writes that in his opinion the dyspepsia of Americans is not entirely due to the free use of iced water, but that there are other causes which help to bring it about.

But while all this is greatly in favour of the moderate use of iced drinks, the purity of the source from which the ice is obtained is also a matter of the highest importance. Ice is not ice when the water from which it is derived is impure. There was an outbreak of sickness amongst the visitors at one of the large hotels at Rye Beach, a watering-place in America, one summer. The symptoms were an alarming disturbance of the with severe pain, great feverishness, and depression of spirits. It was found that the ice which occasioned this outbreak had been taken from a stagnant pond containing a large amount of decomposing matter. A portion of it was carefully melted, and was found to contain a considerable quantity of decaying vegetable matter. In the case of artificial ice, the question of purity is even more important. The reason for this is that the water used in the manufacture of artificial ice is usually frozen solid, and whatever substances, consequently, are dissolved in the water remain in the ice itself.

TOBACCO

Five out of every six male adults smoke, whether it be cigarette, cigar, or pipe. That is, in a gathering of, say, 600 men, 500 will be smokers and 100 non-smokers. At least, this is the estimated proportion in the old country. In Australia the ratio is about the same, but the average amount of tobacco used by every smoker is greater. According to Mr. T. A. Coghlan in his WEALTH AND PROGRESS OF NEW SOUTH WALES, the annual consumption of tobacco in Australia for each inhabitant is 3 lbs. all but a fraction. For the United Kingdom the corresponding amount is 1.41 lbs.; and for the United States of America, 4.40 lbs. Italy, it would seem, consumes in the same way 1.34 lbs.; France, 2.05 lbs.; Germany, 3 lbs.; Austria, 3.77 lbs.; Turkey, 4.37 lbs.; while Holland reaches the excessive amount of 6.92 lbs. Of the five colonies of Australia, namely, New South Wales, Victoria, South Australia, Queensland, and West Australia, the use of tobacco is greatest in the latter two; the figures for Queensland being 3.53 lbs., and for West Australia 4.11 lbs.

With regard to the effect of tobacco on the human system, it will perhaps be most convenient to make a division into the following three classes. In the first place there are a certain number of people upon whom tobacco in any shape or form has an absolutely poisonous influence. There must be some peculiar susceptibility of the system in their case which renders them especially vulnerable to its action. On this account, therefore, they are better without tobacco at all, and any attempt to habituate themselves to it must be attended with prejudice to health. Secondly, there are many other people who can only use tobacco in its very mildest forms. They may be able to smoke a few cigarettes daily, perhaps only three or four; if they indulge in a cigar, it must be one of the mildest; if a pipe, the tobacco will have to be the very lightest. Anything exceeding their allowance is an excess for which they are obliged to pay the penalty. Then, again, there is a third class who can enjoy tobacco in moderation. But these are the very people who are most apt to abuse their privilege. And although they do not recognise it at once, the effect of their excessive smoking is bound to assert itself at last, and compel them to curtail their allowance. If those in the second category, who can enjoy the mildest tobacco in the smallest quantities, and those in the third, who can smoke in moderation, were never to exceed their proper amount, no very great harm would follow. But it most frequently happens that both overstep their respective bounds, and the result is injury to health.

The tobacco plant, NICOTIANA TOBACUM, belongs to the order Solanaceae,
which also includes belladonna, capsicum, henbane, and likewise the common potato. Its active principle, an alkaloid--nicotine or nicotia --is combined with a vegetable acid. Some of the alkaloids, such as morphine, strychnine, &c., are crystalline in character, but this, along with a few others, is liquid. A single drop of it is fatal to the smaller animals, a cat or Even as it is, the first smoke usually produces characteristic results. There is generally pallor of the face, nausea, and vomiting. Usually a cold, clammy sweat breaks out, and the heart seems as if it were about to stop. The system, however, gradually becomes habituated to its action, and these symptoms do not reappear. Seeing that this somewhat unpleasant apprenticeship is uncomplainingly served, it is evident that in smoking there must be some powerful attraction. There are many, indeed, who persist in it when it is doing them an inconceivable amount of injury.

It is a fortunate thing that almost all of the nicotine passes off, or is burnt up, or else the effect would be more markedly disastrous. But the pleasurable effects of tobacco are derived in great part from the volatile alkaloids formed during combustion. The alkaloids which develop during the smoking of a pipe are entirely different from those of a cigar. In a pipe, according to Vold and Eulenburg, the tobacco yields a very much larger proportion of volatile bases, especially of the very volatile and stupefying pyridine. On the other hand, a cigar produces but little pyridine, but more of the less active collidine. It is well known that very much stronger tobacco can be smoked as a cigar than as a pipe. As a matter of fact a cigar which could be enjoyed as a cigar, would cause sickness if cut up into small pieces and smoked in a pipe. This pyridine to which reference has just been made has lately been brought forward as a remedy for asthma. Now, the effect of tobacco in cutting short an attack of this latter malady is, at times, very marked. And Professor See, the eminent French physician, believes that the pyridine is the relieving agent.

In the earlier part of this section I have attempted to form a provisional classification of people as far as the effect of tobacco is concerned. Firstly, those upon whom tobacco in any shape or form is an absolute poison; secondly, those who can enjoy a very small amount-daily; and thirdly, those who are able to smoke in moderation. Now, while those who use tobacco with wise discretion appear to be none the worse for it, yet it unfortunately happens that far too frequently there is no limit to this discretion. It is too often the case, therefore, that quite a serious amount of damage to health results from excessive smoking. It requires a good deal of judgment, and even more resolution, to use and not abuse tobacco.

There are certain symptoms which should lead a man either to curtail his allowance, or else give up tobacco altogether. These are marked nervousness, trembling of the whole body, unsteadiness of the hands, and twitching of different muscles. There may be also swimming of the head, severe headache, and a feeling of despondency. In other cases there may be irritability of temper, a want of will determination, and progressive loss of memory. The special senses--sight, hearing, taste, smell, and touch--may all be blunted. The Bight and hearing are often markedly affected. Colour blindness is sometimes a result, and there may be that impairment of vision known tobacco AMBLYOPIA. As regards the hearing, too, there is not unfrequently a drumming in the ears and confusion of sounds.

And more than this, tobacco, when unsuitable or used in excess, has other prejudicial effects. Its action on the heart is well known, and is frequently manifested by violent palpitation and by disturbed action of the heart. There is also a definite disorder known as "the smoker's heart." In this affection the beats, instead of being regular, are very rapid, suddenly becoming very slow. In this way the rhythm of the heart has been aptly compared by Dr. Lauder Brunton to a restive horse, who goes into a gallop for a few yards, next pulls up all at once, and then breaks off into a gallop again. When tobacco has these prejudicial effects upon the heart, it is no good diminishing the allowance. The only way to bring about any good result is to knock it off altogether.

In addition to its direct action on the heart, tobacco smoking may also bring on a sudden fainting, in which there is absolutely no warning. This condition may develop from the tobacco alone, but in many instances nervous excitement or shock are superadded. Professor Fraser, of Edinburgh, has observed that quite a number of his college friends, who smoked to an inordinate extent as students, were obliged to give up tobacco as middle age approached. Several of them had to do so on account of the onset of these sudden fainting fits. Many smokers also suffer from what is termed chronic pharyngitis. In this affection the mucous membrane at the back part of the mouth looks like dirty-red velvet, and there is also a constant hawking of phlegm. And further, indigestion itself is in many eases entirely due to excessive smoking, from which there is no relief except by abandoning the habit altogether.

But even when tobacco does not produce such marked ill effects, it is as well to remember that it has always a definite action from a gastronomic point of view. And it is this, that directly after the first draw of a cigarette, cigar, or pipe, the palate loses its delicacy of perception. As Sir Henry Thompson remarks, after smoke the power to appreciate good wine is lost, and no judicious host cares to open a fresh bottle from his best bin for the smoker. This is perfectly true; under such circumstances valuable wine would simply be thrown away. But, on the other hand, there is an unquestionable sympathy between coffee and tobacco, and a cup of Mocha blends harmoniously with choice Latakia. This is well recognised in the East; and throughout the Continent coffee and temperate habits go hand in hand with the cigar or cigarette. We must also agree with Sir Henry when he declares that smoke and alcoholic drinks are only found associated together in Great Britain and other northern nations, where there are to be found the most insensitive palates in Europe. It is a good thing, therefore, that the habits followed here are unknown to him, or else Australia would certainly have had a rap over the knuckles.

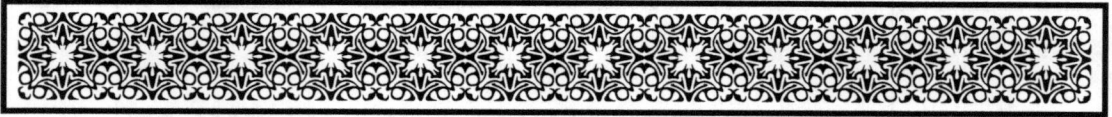

CHAPTER VII.
EXERCISE

This comes last alphabetically of the five essentials concerned in the maintenance of health--namely, ablution: the skin and the bath; bed-room ventilation; clothing; diet; and exercise--but it is none the less important on that account. Exercise may be defined as action of the body, whereby its organs and their functions are kept in a state of health. Each one of us has from the moment of his existence a certain stature allotted, as it were, to which he will attain. In this way some will be tall, others will be short, so that the height of the body is something quite beyond our control, as we know by the interrogation, "Which of you by taking thought can add one cubit to his stature?" But in contradistinction to height, we know that the muscles of the body can be developed and increased in size by use. It is by their action in exercise that the muscles are enlarged, hardened, and brought to their greatest state of perfection. And it is only by exercise, and by exercise alone, that they can be maintained at the acme of physical condition.

Now, in the same way that education develops and increases the power of the brain, so exercise has a similar effect on the body. When the muscles are strengthened, the beneficial effect is also participated in by the heart, lungs, and digestive organs, and thus the removal of worn-out material from the body is assisted. The effect of exercise is thus to remove used up products from the system, and so afford an opportunity for renewed material to take their place. Ceaseless changes are constantly going on throughout the body, and any part which has fulfilled its object is no longer necessary for the requirements of the system, in fact it becomes injurious. Its removal has to take place by one of the various outlets, and it is by exercise that its expulsion is greatly assisted. In this way exercise differs altogether from the part played by food. The latter is the introduction of nourishment into the system for the renewal of its wants, while exercise is the principal agent by which DEBRIS is eliminated.

It was well known amongst the Greeks and Romans that the muscles reached their greatest state of development by means of exercise. Though, therefore, gymnastics formed a great part of their system of education, yet the chief aim in their athletic instruction was the desire to train men to fight their battles, and in those days war was a matter of personal valour and of individual bravery. On that account, therefore, the men who were selected as their soldiers were among the healthiest of the nation. Those who by reason of bodily infirmity or inherent weakness were unfitted for military prowess were left alone. But, as Maclaren has well pointed out, the object of systematic and proper exercise is not for the production of a race of soldiers, though a certain proportion of the population will always be required for military service. With the great majority of men the struggle for existence is keen, and it is simply a question of the survival of the fittest, and of the weakest going to the wall. The requirements of the present time are therefore a capacity for endurance and an ability to withstand the effects of work day after day. We do not require athletes who are capable of performing wonderful feats of strength; but the fight of the nineteenth century is brain against brain, and he will be best equipped for the struggle who has the advantage of good bodily health. In the higher callings, where brain power is everything, the necessity for perfect physical condition is all the more imperative, because the brain is supplied with healthy blood, and the ideas flow with less effort.

The brain is an organ of the body exactly in the same way that the heart, the lungs, and the liver are, and therefore is subject to the same changes which belong to every other part of the frame. It will be at its best when there is circulating through it a full supply of rich red arterial blood, for that means a continual renewal of fresh material to it, and a speedy removal of worn-out products. It is by exercise mainly, whether it be voluntarily undertaken, or whether it pertain to the calling, that the body is kept at the pink of condition, and the brain benefited accordingly. Another great and important result from improving the bodily health is the increased power of what we call the will. The undertaking, say, of a long walk or climb involves the possession of a certain amount of determination, and many people, though perfectly aware of the good to be obtained by a few hours' exercise outside the house, have not the determination to carry it into effect. Once the disinclination to move is overcome, the effort required is less each time, and ultimately the will gains a distinct mastery.

When the muscles are put into action, what is termed their contractility is called into play--that is, the force which was dormant before is roused into activity. This is effected through the nervous system, and it is the will which emanates from the brain and is carried along certain nerves to accomplish definite actions. During the contraction of a muscle its individual fibres change in form, producing an alteration in the shape of the whole muscle; thus it becomes shorter and thicker. At the same time, while it is in action more blood flows through it, hence we see that one of the beneficial effects of exercise is to stimulate the circulation through the muscular system. It has also been ascertained by experiments, that the venous blood which comes from a muscle in action is darker in colour than that from a muscle in repose. When the circulation is quickened by movement, and the blood stream hastened, the vigour of the body is increased, because the used up material is all the quicker taken away, and a freshly created supply of nutrition brought to every part.

The rate of breathing is accelerated whenever the body is engaged in muscular exertion, and with this quickened breathing there is an increased amount of oxygen drawn in, and an increased amount of carbonic acid gas and water exhaled by the breath. The oxygen which is absorbed from the air into the blood is stored in the red corpuscles of the latter, by which it is carried to every part of the body. The venous blood which returns from every portion of the system comes back as a dark crimson, instead of being bright scarlet like the arterial blood. It contains carbonic acid, and returns it to the lungs, where it is exhaled by the breath. The oxygen is necessary to existence, while the carbonic acid is injurious. The effect of exercise, then, in any form, is thus to distribute healthy blood more rapidly through the system, while it removes the injurious matters quite as speedily. The effect of active exercise on the heart, as it is well known, is to make it beat faster; by this the blood is driven through the body at a quicker rate than usual. Sometimes, when the effort is unusually severe, there is a disturbance of the regular balance between the heart and the lungs. There is thus produced an irregular or unequal action of the former, causing what is known as "loss of wind," which is, however, soon restored by resting.

There is an excessive flow of blood to the surface of the body, causing it to redden, and at the same time the perspiration is greatly increased. It is on account of this latter moisture opening up the pores of the skin that the good effects of exercise are chiefly due. The perspiration consists mainly of water containing different salts and organic matters. It is found by experiment that the amount of water passing through the lungs and skin is usually doubled even with moderate exertion.

The result of moderate exercise in benefiting the nervous system is well known, and the effect of a gentle walk in making the ideas flow through the brain is a matter of common observation. At the same time, it must be borne in mind that exercise, when carried to the verge of fatigue, compels inactivity of the brain for a time, since Nature must have repose. But when carried out in moderation with a view of improving the condition of the body, it conduces to the salubrity of the brain as well, for the latter organ shares in the health of the former. The only thing to guard against is irregular and fitful doses; thus it is far better to take a little in moderation daily, than to attempt to make one day's exercise suffice for the rest of the week.

It follows from the foregoing, therefore, that without exercise a perfect state of health is an impossibility. There can be no proper bodily health unless there be daily exercise. It is the same with everybody, no matter what the condition of life may be. Exercise is quite as necessary for the well-to-do man as it is for him who is not so circumstanced. The laws of health cannot be violated, and all the money in the world will not atone for neglect in this respect. Exercise is not a matter that can be carried out by proxy. No; each one must take his own exercise, and he derives all the benefit for himself.

It is a fortunate thing, then, that most people have to earn their own living, for the exertion thereby entailed is actually necessary for health. Yet, while this is the case with those who live by their bodily labour, it hardly applies to those who are more dependent upon mental work. For instance, the latter include literary men and journalists, the members of the professions, and those of the vast commercial world--all, indeed, who have brain strain and clerical occupations. In their case the great fault is that they use their heads too much and their limbs too little. For them walking is one of the very best means of obtaining health, and it should be regularly and systematically practised.

It has been said that no man under sixty, unless he be kept walking while at his work, should walk less than six or eight miles a day, if he wishes to keep well and have healthy children. In the cooler weather in Australia these are certainly suitable distances, but in the hot months half these amounts will be found sufficient, and they had better be carried out in the cool of the evening. Then again, for those over sixty it has been well observed that a daily walk is still the best means of promoting health. But the walk must always be proportionate to the strength, and should be done at nothing more than a moderate pace, if a man wishes to take care of his blood vessels.

There is another matter which calls for notice, and it is that of early morning exercise. Now, I am quite willing to admit that there are many who derive great benefit from their early morning swim, their matutinal walk, or their tennis before breakfast. But it should be distinctly borne in mind that there are others with whom such early morning exercise does not agree. They get as a result a weary, languid feeling which lasts throughout the entire day. Now, they are apt to imagine it is the exercise in itself which produces this effect. But the truth is, it arises from the time of day at which the exercise is taken, and is not due to the exertion at all. It must not be forgotten, therefore, that while many people derive the greatest advantage from early morning exercise, yet there are others for whom it is altogether unsuitable. But, on the other hand, the latter will obtain every possible benefit by taking their allowance of exercise at some other period of the twenty-four hours.

There are other forms of exercise besides walking, and these have their good points. Riding is, of course, invaluable, especially in cases of sluggish liver. As it has been wittily observed, the outside of a horse is the best thing for the inside of a man. In the cool months in Australia riding is a real pleasure, but in the hot season it is hardly so agreeable. Then again, rowing is a magnificent exercise, and has much to recommend it in early adult life. There is no harm whatever in rowing as an exercise, but when it comes to racing that is a different matter. It is the great strain on the heart, together with the excitement which constitute the sources of risk. The other varieties of exercise, namely, gardening, the different games, cricket, football, tennis, &c., need not be particularized as they all subserve the same purposes, and are in consequence very desirable.

In all the preceding I have endeavoured to show that daily exercise is absolutely necessary for the proper maintenance of health. But there is something even more than this. It is that a long life itself is to be ensured by exercise. It is only by exercise, and by exercise alone, that the various organs of the body, the heart, the lungs, the stomach, the liver, &c., are maintained in their normal state of health. Their condition, moreover, is only to be improved by the muscular movements belonging to exercise. The heart itself is intended for action, not for inaction. By action it thrives, and by disuse it becomes weakened. It is so with all the other organs. In conclusion, therefore, it must be said that the whole system can only be kept in perfect health by muscular movements, and that in addition to keeping the body in health exercise actually increases the chances of living to a good old age.

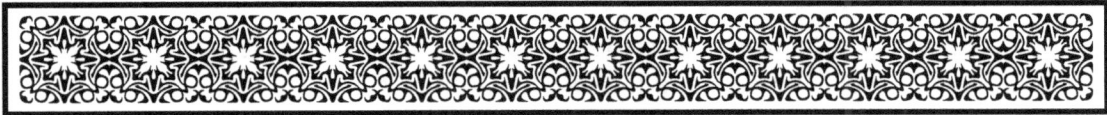

CHAPTER VIII.
ON SCHOOL COOKERY AND ITS INFLUENCE ON THE AUSTRALIAN DAILY LIFE.

"BAD COOKERY DIMINISHES HAPPINESS, AND SHORTENS LIFE."
--WISDOM OF AGES.

In all probability there are but few who have ever had their attention called to certain figures duly set forth within the pages of that mine of information, namely, Mr. T. A. Coghlan's WEALTH AND PROGRESS OF NEW SOUTH WALES. Nevertheless, the facts associated with these statistics so directly concern our Australian daily life that they deserve to be widely known. That portion of the work in which our food supply is considered, therefore, is well worth referring to. It will he found that the consumption of butcher's meat by each inhabitant is greater than in any other country in the world. Thus the amount of meat required for each member of the community every year in New South Wales is 201 lbs.; in Victoria 275 lbs.; whilst in Queensland 370 lbs. are called for. On the other hand, in the United Kingdom only 109 lbs. are similarly needed; in the United States of America 150 lbs. while the figures for the different European countries show an average of no more than 70 lbs.

Another article of commerce which is consumed to excess in all parts is tea. As I have previously stated, it is estimated by Coghlan that the four million people in Australasia use more of this beverage than all the millions who inhabit continental Europe, that is, if Russia be excluded; but he further points out that in Australia itself the use of tea is universal. The tables show that for each inhabitant New South Wales requires annually 7.8 lbs.; Victoria, 7.7 lbs.; South Australia, 6.5 lbs.; and Queensland 8.4 lbs.; and moreover, that West Australia attains a maximum with 10.6 lbs. Now, according to Mulhall, in his DICTIONARY OF STATISTICS, the amount of tea consumed annually for each inhabitant in the United Kingdom is only 5 lbs.; and for the United States of America the proportion is but 1.5 lbs.

A survey of these figures consequently must compel us to admit that Australia is inhabited by a people largely carnivorous and addicted to tea. Surely not one person in a thousand would advocate such a diet under any circumstances. Is it not astonishing, therefore, that innutritious fare of this land is still tolerated in Australia? Facts such as these call for the most serious consideration, since they must irresistibly affect the national life; but though it may seem strange, these matters have never received the notice they stand in need of, if, indeed, they have ever received any notice at all.

There are worlds of interest, however, centred in the notable circumstance that Australia, a new and a semitropical country, is now being peopled by the descendants of those who belonged to an entirely different climate. At the present time the old racial instincts are actively powerful, and exert an influence diametrically opposed to climatic surroundings; and, as a matter of fact, we are witnessing a struggle between our Anglo-Saxon heredities and our Australian environment. But such a conflict against our destiny is one in which the odds are overwhelmingly on one side. For of all forces, that of climate is the most powerful. It is true that man is able almost to remove mountains, and that he can create rivers in an arid land; but to endeavour to resist the dominating influence of climate is to attempt the impossible.

Yet there is something more than all this which should induce us to follow the promptings of nature; this is the fact that Australia will only reach the zenith of her possibilities when her people conform to her climatic requirements. For what would the latter mean? Market gardens innumerable, and a healthy and lucrative life for all concerned; the development of her deep-sea fisheries, and employment, direct as well as indirect, to thousands; the cultivation of the vine, with all the wealth pertaining to smiling vineyards; the growth of the olive and other fruits, and all the other industries which only await their creation; and instead of this, at present, all we possess is the knowledge that we are the greatest meat-eating and tea-drinking race on earth.

PROGRESSIVE CHANGES IN THE THEORIES OF EDUCATION.

We are told that it was Jean Jacques Rousseau who first entirely severed education and learning. In his Emile, published in 1762, he advocated a more natural and less pedantic method of training and developing the physical, mental, and moral faculties of the young. The work produced an astounding effect on its appearance, and has largely influenced the educational methods throughout Europe.

Not so long afterwards, in 1801, Johann Heinrich Pestalozzi, permeated with the atmosphere following the French Revolution, gave to the world his views on education in his work HOW GERTRUDE TEACHES HER CHILDREN.

The essence of his belief being that "sense-impression is the foundation of instruction," he counselled the development of all the faculties in preference to the mere acquisition of words. "Words alone," said he, "cannot give us a knowledge of things; they are only useful for giving expression to what we have in our own minds." Consequently, he believed in imparting instruction by a direct appeal to the senses and the understanding so as to call forth all the powers, selecting the subjects of study so that each step should progressively assist the pupil's advancement. He contended that observation was the method by which knowledge was principally gained, and that the perceptive faculties (intuition) were developed by observation. Even in his own time his ideas were awarded a recognition of their value; in fact, he had the honour of being specially visited by Prince de Talleyrand and Madame de Stael.

In the early part of the present century another reformer, Friedrich Wilhelm August Froebel, arose to influence all future educational methods. As with Rousseau, Froebel held that each age belonged to itself, and that the perfection of the later stage could only be attained through perfection of the earlier. So, too, while Pestalozzi upheld that the faculties were developed by exercise, Froebel went farther, and added that the function of education was to develop the faculties by arousing VOLUNTARY ACTIVITY, in this way becoming, according to Michelet, the greatest of educational reformers. Froebel was convinced that man was primarily a doer, indeed, even a creator, and that he learnt only through "self-activity." In action, moreover, there was not alone the mere physical exercise, but also the actual unfolding and strengthening of the mental powers. To Froebel, indeed, belongs the honour of originating the kindergarten system, which is making such progress at the present time; and more than this, it may be said that while it is employed only in the earlier stages of education, yet his principles are beginning to make themselves felt throughout the entire system of education.

As a matter of fact, what is known in Sweden and in Finland as SLOYD, or manual instruction, may be regarded as a continuation of the Kindergarten system. Through the exertions of Uno Cygnaeus the whole of the national system of education in Finland was reorganized, and manual work was first made a part of the regular instruction in the common schools. In Sweden, likewise, the same principles have been introduced chiefly by Herr Otto Salomon, the director of the great sloyd seminarum at Naas. Sloyd work is used in the schools in a disciplinary way as an integral part of general education; the children, generally boys, are employed for a certain number of hours a week in making articles of common household use. It is maintained that work of this kind is specially invaluable in supplementing the ordinary school education of the three R's. It fulfils the injunction "to put the whole boy to school;" it develops faculties which would otherwise lie dormant, while at the same time it trains the eye and does away with clumsy fingers.

THE PURPOSE OF EDUCATION.

From the foregoing it will be seen that within the last 130 years a striking change has come over the view held respecting education. Prior to that time an artificial and pedantic method prevailed, which received its first check from the pen of Rousseau. The system which he attacked, however, built up as it was upon centuries of mediaeval learning, was not to be disposed of by this one encounter. Such a result was not to be expected in the natural order of things; but as the ideas of Rousseau contained the living truth, they were bound to find advocacy in due course, and though the seed might lie quiescent for a time, yet it was sure to germinate sooner or later. After him the path of educational reform was illumined by the genius of Pestalozzi, and a few years later Froebel appeared to influence for ever the methods of education. Indeed, it was the latter who by his kindergarten system has founded the practical education of our own day.

The vast change, then, along the whole line of education has been from scholastic learning towards that of education in manual training. This is the truest recognition of the fact that the purpose of education is to prepare a child for his journey through life, and not merely to get him ready for an examination; but although the meaning of education has thus become more apparent, there is still too much a tendency in the present day to burden the developing mind with a multiplicity of subjects. We do not wish to produce a living encyclopaedia, but we desire to create a being, well trained in all his senses, and thoroughly competent to take his part in the battle of life. Far be it from imagining that I decry the advantages of learning in the slightest degree, but surely there is the broadest distinction between a scholastic prodigy and a practical well-informed mortal.

This exaggeration of the function of education expressed by the word multiplicity deserves a little consideration, for it would appear that our educationists overlook the fact that the organism with which they have to deal is going through the most critical period of its existence. At the very time that children are rapidly undergoing the process of physical development, there is superadded the acquirement of elaborate mental knowledge, and when bone and muscle and sinew are in the active processes of transformation and growth, then it is that the intellectual faculties are spurred on at a killing pace. The child leaves school in the afternoon with a load of home lessons to be prepared for the following day. The very meaning of the word school has become distorted; instead of being a medium for imparting instruction, it threatens to become merely a building in which the lessons learned at home overnight are heard, and besides this, if the school is thus to become simply a place for hearing lessons, the office of schoolmaster must correspondingly suffer. This I hope will never be, for it would at once take away all personality from the teacher, and transmute him into a mere auditory machine. His individuality would become lost in the official, and teaching as teaching resolve itself into a stereotyped function; and this latter consideration leads me to remark that one man has the gift of imparting knowledge, in which another fails entirely. One instructor has a way of putting things so that they ale retained in the memory of his pupils for ever, while another so fails to express himself that not one clear idea is carried away by his hearers.

The chief purpose of education should be the preparation of the young for their adult life. As Agesilaus the Great observed when one asked him what boys should learn: "That," said he, "which they shall use when men." But the future of the two sexes differs entirely after school life is over. It will follow, therefore, that there should be an essential difference between the education required for the boy and that for the girl. In our present day system of education, however, there is too much a disposition to make no such distinction. The boy in the greater number of cases is the bread-winner, and has to rely on his own exertions, whether they be manual or mental. The girl, on the other hand, looks forward to the destiny of housewife. This aspect of the educational problem certainly deserves to have more attention paid to it than it has yet received. Still a step in the light direction has been made by James Platt, the author of many valuable works on currency, finance, &c., who advocates that business habits and kindred matters should be taught to all youths. Of course it is not intended that the sole object of education should be the principles of money making, but at the same time there is a considerable amount of truth in his contention. But the chief purpose I have in view is to advocate a thorough and systematic teaching of Cookery to girls. In the remaining part of this chapter, therefore, I shall endeavour to bring forward reasons in support of my proposition.

COOKERY INSTRUCTION IN ENGLAND, NEW SOUTH WALES, AND VICTORIA.

Under this heading I propose to describe briefly what is being done in connection with Cookery Instruction in the places mentioned. Now the principal object I have in view is to further the teaching of Cookery to girls during school life. It will, however, somewhat strengthen my advocacy if I refer to the beginning of this movement in England, for it undoubtedly had its origin in causes quite outside of any educational system. There is no question but that the increased facilities for communication, resulting from the advent of steamships and railways, gave to travel an impetus it never before experienced. And as a result thousands of people in the old country acquired a practical knowledge of Continental life, which would otherwise never have been theirs. These travellers saw for themselves the perfection of Cookery in countries like France, and naturally their eyes were opened to the neglect which culinary matters received in their own land; at least, this seems to me a satisfactory explanation of what has occurred, and I put it forward, therefore, purely as a matter of personal opinion, and whether this is the right reason or not, it is quite certain that a desire for improvement in this direction is insensibly coming over our English people.

It would seem that Mr. Buckmaster gave a series of lectures in the Cookery School at the International Exhibition in 1873 and 1874. As a considerable portion of space was devoted to food, it was rightly thought that some practical remark on the subject would prove of distinct advantage. Just about this time, too, in 1874, a good start was made by the establishment of a National Training School for Cookery at South Kensington. From its inception success seemed to smile upon it. Its numbers began to increase, steadily at first, and afterwards by leaps and bounds. It clearly filled a place that had been wanting; and moreover, the objects it had in view were identified with all that was praiseworthy. It was proof positive of the long cherished opinion as to the neglect of Cookery in a girl's education.

Its courses of instruction are for educated persons who desire to qualify themselves to become teachers of Cookery; for students and cooks; and for those who wish to be able to cook in their own homes. Its distinctive feature, however, lies in its artisan kitchen. It is by means of this that families, which spend from seven to twenty shillings weekly in the purchase of food, will be so greatly benefitted. Nothing can exceed this in importance, for any improvement in the Cookery of the whole bulk of the people becomes a matter of national welfare. A conspicuous instance of the success which has attended the establishment of the National Training School for Cookery is the almost annual appearance of a new edition of its hand-book, which is published under its auspices. Therein will be found a most detailed account of the steps necessary for the preparation of innumerable dishes, and the different instructions are given with a minuteness which leaves nothing to be desired.

At this period, also, the Masters of the Cooks' Company, not to be outdone in anything calculated to promote the progress of the culinary art, had several young girls brought from ward schools, and taught in the artisan kitchen already referred to. Indeed, they were instructed entirely at the expense of the Company. This was liberality of the most commendable kind, and it is satisfactory to see a corporate body acting in such a practical fashion. An ounce of practice is worth a pound of theory.

This growing recognition of the importance of Cookery in the old country at last spread to the educational world, although it has not yet obtained that position which it must eventually acquire; but the ball has been set rolling in the right path, and the necessity for instruction in the culinary art is so self-evident, that there can be no doubt as to the ultimate result. It is gratifying in this connection, therefore, to know that the kindred subject of Elementary Laundry Work has now become part of a girl's education. The Education Code of 1890 contains specific reference to the fact that special and appropriate provision has been made for the practical teaching of Laundry Work, and is also accompanied by instructions to the effect that the appliances and methods employed in teaching should be those which are possible in the homes of working people. I have referred to this in passing, as it directly concerns the point at issue.

It would have been a matter of considerable difficulty for a private individual like myself to have collected authentic information relative to the present status of Cookery in English and Australian schools. Under these circumstances, therefore, I deemed it best to apply directly to head-quarters for official statements. Mr. Edwin Johnson, the courteous Under-Secretary for Public Instruction in New South Wales, willingly undertook to place me in possession of all the facts I required as far as England and this colony are concerned. I shall, therefore, give his account of what is being done in the old country; and next condense from his remarks the substance of what has taken place in New South Wales with regard to this vital matter.

In England, the Education Department conditionally wants aid to Cookery Instruction in connection with State Aided Primary Schools under the following stipulations: what provision as to buildings, &c., has been made for Cookery Instruction in accordance with the conditions prescribed. The Department then grants aid at the rate of four shillings per head in day schools, and two shillings per head in evening, or, as they are sometimes called, "continuation" schools, on the number of pupils in the fourth and higher standards presented for examination in Cookery. The classes are taught by ordinary Primary School Teachers who have been trained in Cookery work, and have obtained certificates of qualifications. Under the London School Board, Cookery classes are established in different centres in connection with a large number of the schools; and to a less extent similar classes are organized by the School Boards of some of the larger country towns. Grants from the Education Department are annually obtained for the work by these schools.

In New South Wales, the teaching of Cookery in connection with the Public Schools has long been advocated; and about ten years ago, special lectures on the subject, and demonstrations, were given under authority; these did not, however, then lead to any practical results. Early in 1886, Mrs. Fawcett Story, who had previously taught Cookery successfully in connection with the Sydney Technical College, was appointed, on probation, lecturer and demonstrator in Cookery and Domestic Economy to the students at Hurlstone Training College, the object being to qualify such students as Instructors of Cookery for schools in which they would in the future be employed as teachers. After three months successful work at Hurlstone, Mrs. Story's appointment was confirmed and she has continued to carry on the work. At first appointed "Instructress," she now takes rank as "Directress of Cookery."

In 1889 a Cookery class was established at the Fort Street Public School, and this proving successful, the instruction was extended to other schools. Three classes of work were embodied in the plan arranged to be carried out, namely:--

* 1. An Elementary Cookery Course,
*

* 2. A Plain, or Intermediate Cookery Course,
*

* 3. A Teachers' Course,

*

and at the close of 1890 the numbers receiving instruction had reached 270.

In 1891 the work was extended to the Sydney and Suburban Schools. Classes were also established in connection with those of Bathurst and Goulburn, and arrangements for training a class of Pupil Teachers in this important work were made and carried out. In 1891 the number under Cookery Instruction in connection with the school reached 757, and during the year 1892 arrangements were also made for extending Cookery Instruction among the masses of the people on the basis already described.

It should also be remembered that classes for Cookery Instruction have for some years past been established in connection with the Technical College in Sydney, and more recently in the similar colleges of the larger towns and centres.

As far as Victoria is concerned, I am under considerable obligation to Mr. T. Brodribb, the Secretary of the Education Office, Melbourne, for the following information. It would appear that although the subject has not been systematically taught throughout the schools, instruction in Cookery has been given by experts to the elder female pupils in a number of Metropolitan State Schools for the past two years; two courses of 12 lessons being undertaken in each school between the months of April and November. The instruction has consisted of the preparation of plain wholesome dishes and sickroom Cookery; the proper care and arrangement of the various utensils employed forming an important part of each lesson. Reports obtained from Head Teachers show that, in most cases, the lessons were productive of much benefit to the children, and were thoroughly appreciated. At present, however, the teaching of the subject has been temporarily interrupted; but it is to be hoped that before long a recognition of its vital importance will enable measures to be taken for its permanent continuance.

COOKERY IN ITS RELATION TO HEALTH.

We are drawing nearer and nearer to an appreciation of the power which Cookery wields in the preservation of health, but this awakening as to its value has been too tardy, indeed, it has been from a slumber of centuries. Not that good Cookery has not been practised from time immemorial, but its recognition from a scientific point of view is almost within our own day; and even at the present time, dietetics, or that department of medicine which relates to food and diet, is only gradually assuming a position which is destined ultimately to become second to none. Moreover, there is still ample room for improvement in this direction, and matters will not be rectified till a comprehensive study of food and its preparation, both for the healthy as well as the sick, is embodied in the curriculum of modern medical education.

Not so long ago THE LANCET made reference to the Edinburgh School of Cookery and Domestic Economy, which had been opened by the Princess Louise. It was pointed out that good cookery had more to do with health and comfort, and therefore with domestic happiness, than any other known accomplishment. In the same article, moreover, it was remarked that it would be out of all keeping with the position of Edinburgh as a medical centre, if the importance, in sickness, of good cookery and suitable food were not fully recognised. In conclusion, the same authority expressed the hope that this commendable example would be adopted by many other towns.

All this is satisfactory in showing that the preparation of food for

the table is a subject which can no longer be pooh-poohed, and there
are other signs and tokens which unmistakably point to the same
conclusion. As a proof of this it is only necessary to point to the
fact that eminent physicians have written prefaces to works on cookery,
and more than this, have contributed to the literature of the same.
There is a very excellent handbook by Phillis Browne, to which the late
Sir J. Risdon Bennett, a former President of the Royal College of
Physicians, London, contributed the prefatory note. In it he remarks,
the value of wholesome and properly-cooked food has never been
sufficiently understood or appreciated in the United Kingdom. "In
scarcely any other country," says he, "does so much prejudice and
ignorance prevail on the subject of food and its employment." And in
proceeding to speak of the growing tendency to make instruction in
cookery a part of ordinary education, he adds that this must be a
subject for sincere rejoicing with those who desire both the moral and
physical welfare of the poorer classes. This is not the only evidence
of interest which the same physician took in this matter, for he has
also written an admirable and lengthy article on Food and its Uses in
Health.

But there is another writer to whom the English speaking people are
deeply indebted for a knowledge of all that pertains to food
and cookery; I refer to Sir Henry Thompson, the eminent London surgeon.
His work on FOOD AND Feeding has already run through six editions, and
one can only hope that he will long be enabled to benefit his race by a
succession of issues. He has written other volumes on the same subject,
and further, by his contributions to THE NINETEENTH CENTURY and The
Lancet, he has materially raised the status of the culinary art. And
there are also quite a number of works on diet, and on food, written by
well-known authorities in the medical world, so that the science of
dietetics must eventually attain an unassailable position.

The preceding naturally leads up to the main point, namely, the controlling influence which cookery exercises over health. Now if I were asked to name the one single cause which produces more indigestion than anything else, I should unhesitatingly answer, bad Cookery. Many people Fun away with the idea that good Cookery is necessarily elaborate Cookery, and that in consequence it is quite beyond the ordinary purse. Such is not, by any means, the case, and as a matter of fact good Cookery aims at getting the best possible results at the least possible cost. Herein lies the excellence of French Cookery, and as I have occasion to remark elsewhere, the bulk of the population in that country live infinitely better than does the average Briton.

Indigestion, then, is the great primary result of bad cookery. But, on the other hand, let us hear what Dr. Lauder Brunton has to say on the score of food when properly prepared. "Savoury food," says he, "causes the digestive juices to be freely secreted; well cooked and palatable food is therefore more digestible than unpalatable, and if the food lacks savour, a desire naturally arises to supply it by condiments, not always well selected or wholesome."

But important as good Cookery, in itself, may be in its influence upon health, there is still another essential, which must not be overlooked. And it is that of variety. The oft-quoted phrase of TOUJOURS PERDRIX bears upon this very point. It is a way of saying that even a luscious dish when constantly repeated becomes wearisome, or, in other words, that there is too much of the same thing over and over again. And if a ceaseless repetition of the same dish--however well it may be cooked--palls upon the palate, it is at least certain that it is equally burdensome to the stomach. Dr. Horace Dobell well expresses this fact when he says that it is of the highest importance to avoid unnecessarily limiting the variety of food allowed to all persons, but especially to those of poor appetites and troublesome digestions. Monotonous, uninteresting meals depress the spirits and are subversive of appetite, digestion, and nutrition.

COOKERY AS A PREVENTIVE OF DRUNKENNESS.

Plutarch tells us that Themistocles laughing at his own son, who got his mother, and by his mother's means his father also, to indulge him, said to the boy that he had the most power of anyone in Greece: "For the Athenians command the rest of Greece, I command the Athenians, your mother commands me, and you command your mother." In the same way it is easy to make a defective system of education responsible for much of the existing drunkenness. First of all we have a scheme of education which fails to provide instruction in a girl's domestic duties; then we have the wife who undertakes the task for which she has never been properly trained; next, instead of well-cooked and very much varied meals, we have a conspicuous and a disastrous failure; and finally, we have the bread-winner driven to the public-house--and happiness has left that home for ever. But this is an old story, yet, unfortunately, it is a true one; and it will continue to be true until a clearer perception of what a domestic training should be is more universally recognised. I am sure that I do not exaggerate when I say that millions of our English-speaking race are living this life without the slightest glimmering of what domestic content might be theirs. Surely the word "home" for the artisan should signify something more than a place where he is badly fed. Still, it is a solemn fact that no more concrete definition of the word has ever been forthcoming. Now, such a state of affairs cannot be excused on the score of expense, for the crowning triumph of good Cookery is its very cheapness.

It has already been mentioned that the late Sir J. Risdon Bennett did not think it beneath his dignity to write a prefatory note to a Cookery Book. He has also pointed out that Cookery is a subject which deserves more attention at the hands of those who have the welfare of temperance at heart. He believed that a knowledge of wholesome Cookery would do much to make home happy; to keep the men away from dissipation and intemperance; and to make the children healthy and cheerful. The same idea is expressed by Sylvester, who remarked that Cookery should be most popular, because every individual human being is directly interested in its success. As he says, the real comfort of the majority of men is sought for in their own homes, and every effort should be made to increase domestic happiness by inducing them to remain at home. And long, long ago a quaint old book, Markham's English Housewife, published in 1637, contained the idea in a nutshell, as the following quotation will show: "To speak, then, of the knowledges which belong to our English housewife, I hold the most principal to be a perfect skill in Cookery. She that is utterly ignorant therein, may not, by the laws of strict justice, challenge the freedom of marriage--because, indeed, shee can perform but half her vow--shee may love and obey, but shee cannot cherish and keepe her husband."

Opinions such as these are based on the soundest common sense, indeed no one could honestly oppose them. But it powerfully adds to their weight to find them thoroughly endorsed by the representative medical authority of THE BRITISH MEDICAL JOURNAL and THE LANCET; the
former has from time to time insisted upon the self-same truths, and strenuously urged their practical adoption. These contributions are somewhat too lengthy for complete reproduction, but the views expressed may be briefly referred to. It was maintained that English people have much to learn from the French methods of Cookery; that these are not merely tasteful and appetising, but that they are extremely economical; that materials which the English housewife throws away as useless, her French sister skilfully converts into toothsome and nutritious food; and that it is only an increased knowledge of Cookery which the poor need to render life more agreeable.

THE LANCET also, in an admirable article on "Culinary Civilisation," spoke of the need of women becoming acquainted with the modes of concocting palatable food, if they wished to maintain their domestic power. It was further pointed out that if the husband was to be prevented from neglecting his family, the wife must see that he had well-cooked food at home. And lastly, it was tellingly set forth that when women had fully mastered this lesson a step in civilisation would have been gained, which would show in increased health, increased prosperity, and happier domestic hearths.

But I cannot conclude this portion without a special reference to some remarks by Madame Emilie Lebour-Fawssett. They occur in her most admirable book FRENCH COOKERY FOR LADIES, and are so sensible that they

should never be forgotten. "I like," says Madame, "to place before my husband, who has been hard at work all day long, a nice tempting dinner, very much varied and well cooked; and I cannot, repeat it too often, it is one of the strongest ties of home life, and I am sure many a man in the day, when he is most busy, unconsciously smiles inwardly at the prospect of the nice little dinner awaiting him at home, when his hard day's work is over. Small, dainty, well-made dishes gratify your husband's appetite, help to keep him healthy, prepare him a good digestion for his old age, and save your purse."

In another part of the book, a little farther on, she remarks:---"One of my chief objects also is to teach the great mass of people to make better use of the numberless good things there are to be obtained, and thereby keep their husbands away from the public-house. It stands to reason that if a man who has worked all day comes home and finds nothing warm and appetising prepared for him, he will go away quicker than he came, and spend at the first hotel the money he would otherwise have gladly spent on his family if his wife had tried and knew how to make him comfortable; and, there is no denying it, the greatest comforts a man can have after a day's work, be it manual labour or brain work, are a good meal and a quiet corner in which to smoke his pipe or cigar."

COOKERY IN THE FORMATION OF CHARACTER.

Yet, valuable as it may be in all these foregoing respects, Cookery has something more to recommend it, which gives it precedence before everything else in education; and though this is saying a great deal, I shall endeavour to demonstrate that it is perfectly true. I have already shown that Cookery is of superlative benefit, both in ensuring health and in acting as a preventive against habits of intemperance. But it is as a medium for training that Cookery is at its very best; for it is in reality an art; indeed, it is a master art. At the same time, also, it is a science--the science of applied chemistry. There are no other elements of education which thus blend within themselves these two factors--the practical and the scientific.

To commence with, Cookery requires accuracy. The instructions given with any recipe are sufficient to show this. They tell you to take so much of each thing, to proceed in a certain way, and even what time to take in the cooking. It also calls for attention to detail. Carelessness in Cookery is just one of the rocks on which disaster occurs. An English duke, an ambassador at Paris, was desirous of giving the CORPS DIPLOMATIQUE the treat of a real English plum pudding. The fullest directions were given to his chef--all, indeed, with the exception of mentioning the pudding-cloth. When the eventful time arrived for its appearance, to his dismay several stately cooks appeared, each carrying a tureen of dark-looking fluid. The omission of the pudding-cloth was fatal. Cleanliness is another of the cardinal virtues of Cookery. The very thought of anything else would be repulsive. By the way, that fine old saying, "Cleanliness is next to

Godliness," does not come from the Scriptures, as many suppose, but from one of John Wesley's sermons.

Cookery also exacts punctuality--for have we not Brillat-Savarin's dictum that of all the qualities necessary for a cook the most indispensable is punctuality? If any important matter connected with the process of Cookery be not attended to at the exact moment it is required, nothing can afterwards rectify it. A little delay in attending to this thing, or a little delay in attending to that thing, and whatever is being cooked is irretrievably spoiled. And, moreover, it is not to be forgotten that cookery is of signal benefit in inculcating the advantages of a wise economy. With proper Cookery nothing should be allowed to go to waste, nothing should be thrown away, unless it be absolutely useless. There should be good housewifery; everything, even the veriest scraps, may be turned to the best account. The stock pot will absorb many nutritious and wholesome odds and ends, which would otherwise be consigned to the dirt-box. The loss that actually takes place in many kitchens is without the shadow of an excuse; sometimes the best part of a cold joint is deliberately cast aside.

A NATIONAL PLEA ON BEHALF OF AUSTRALIAN SCHOOL COOKERY.

But there is still something else to be urged on behalf of Cookery, and of School Cookery in particular, which places it immeasurably before even the preceding. I have claimed for Cookery that it develops certain habits which are of the greatest importance in the formation of character; yet, as I have just remarked, there is something more than this, which renders it of priceless value, and of what this consists I shall do my best to explain.

Every one who has the welfare of Australia and of Australians at heart must feel no little concern at that growing indifference to domestic life which is so much the characteristic of our girls. Once a girl has left school, she seems to think that the household is no longer any place for her; she consequently ceases to take any interest whatever in the many matters which constitute the management of a home: her one aim is to get into "business," as it is called. It appears to be immaterial whether she is to be a dressmaker, or milliner, or saleswoman, or employee in a large establishment, as long as she gets away from home.

Now, all this is greatly to be deplored, and has a disastrous influence over the whole of Australian family life, because it must happen that many of these girls eventually marry, and commence their new existence under the most unfavourable conditions. In the first place, they are totally ignorant of everything connected with household management, and what is far worse, they have almost a contempt for it. What the result is, in too many cases, I have already dwelt upon,-- either the husband and the family suffer from the effects of bad Cookery, and unhappiness and ill-health follow, or else the bread-winner flies to alcohol in order to forget his troubles.

It must not be imagined however, that this condition of affairs is altogether beyond remedy, and that our Australian girls are hopeless in this respect. No, on the contrary, those of whom I have just spoken are as attractive and fascinating--as Australian girls always are; but it is a thousand pities that they do not possess a greater appreciation of the importance of home life. Still, after all, may it not be that our educational system is defective in that it does not implant--all through a girl's school life--a love of Cookery, and of domestic management? It is during this impressionable age that all these truths can be so well indoctrinated. Indeed, I am thoroughly convinced that one of the greatest defects in the superlatively scientific education of to-day, as far as the girls are concerned, is the neglect which these matters receive; for it stands to reason that if they are passed by during school life, they are never learnt at all.

And, further, it should not be forgotten that a cook is always able to command high wages. That is a fact which should not be lost sight of, although perhaps it is some what mercenary. A cook need never fear but that she will always be in constant employment. Ah, yes! Max O'Rell got in a home thrust when he declared that "the average woman who finds herself alone in the world could earn her living if she could cook-- but she can't."

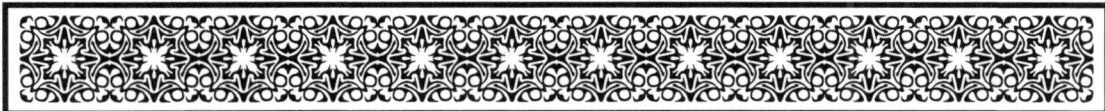

CHAPTER IX.
AUSTRALIAN FOOD HABITS AND THEIR FAULTS.--A PLEA FOR THEIR IMPROVEMENT.

It is somewhat curious that, among the many questions which pertain to the national life of Australia, little, if any, attention has been directed to the influences which the daily food and habitual dietary exercise upon the present, and in what way they will affect the future population. And yet it must be apparent that the life of a nation is moulded in no small degree by its daily fare, by its general food habits, and still more by the fact of its living in conformity with, or in direct opposition to, its climatic requirements. It is evident that the natural dietary of the earth's inhabitants is controlled largely by the particular region in which they dwell. Thus the Hindoos, and contiguous Eastern nations, subsist mainly upon the cereals, in which rice plays so prominent a part. The Greenlander's fare, on the contrary, consists almost entirely of oils and fats; indeed, on this point Sir Anthony Carlisle relates the following anecdote:--"The most Northern races of mankind," says he, "were found to be unacquainted with the taste of sweets, and their infants made wry faces and sputtered out sugar with disgust, but the little urchins grinned with ecstasy at the sight of a bit of whale's blubber." In the same way the Arab is a date-eater and the Kaffir is a milk consumer. These facts being borne in mind, it will be desirable to ascertain whether the usual food habits obtaining in Australia are those which the nature of the climate renders advisable. If, as a result of such an inquiry, it be demonstrated that the dietary customs followed here are not in harmony with the climatic conditions, it would, perhaps, be well to suggest in what direction amendment should take place.

A reference to the isothermal lines in any physical atlas will be of considerable value in assisting us to the elucidation of the subject under consideration. These are certain lines drawn over a chart of the earth's surface, on which are located those cities and regions where the mean annual temperature is the same. Thus the mean annual temperature of Sydney is 62.9 degrees; the corresponding line in the northern world runs through Naples and Lisbon in Europe, and a little below the central portion of the United States and California in America. At Melbourne the average yearly temperature is 57.6 degrees, corresponding in the old world to a temperature met with at Marseilles, Bordeaux, the south of France and Northern Italy, while across the Atlantic a somewhat similar climate obtains about the middle of the United States. The mean annual temperature at Brisbane is 67.74 degrees; this is the same as that of Algiers and the southern shores of the Mediterranean generally, and coincides with that met with in New Orleans and the southern states of North America. At Adelaide the average yearly temperature is 63.1 degrees, and the climate is considered to greatly resemble that of Sicily. Now, no other mode that I am aware of, such as this juxtaposition of localities where the mean annual temperature is the same, will afford such a convenient way of contrasting the mode of living which is practised in Australia with that which is followed by the inhabitants of the regions referred to in Europe. The cardinal difference, and one which stands out in bold relief, is that the Australian food habits are characterised by a preponderancy of meat diet and a corresponding neglect of vegetable products. On the other hand, the dietary of Southern Europe is in rational harmony with its climate, and there is not that insensate insistence of a highly nitrogenous animal fare to the exclusion of all else. The striking features, then, in connection with the Australian dietary are this extraordinary consumption of meat and the faith which is presumably attached to its food value. It is no exaggeration to say that the vast majority of our people believe implicitly in the necessity for meat at their three daily mealy, and not only is this the case in the cooler parts of the year, but it is practised universally during the height of the summer, without being modified in the slightest degree. Thus the student of ethnography is presented with the somewhat curious anomaly of a people living in a summer temperature of 70 degrees or 80 degrees in the shade, eating more meat than do the bulk of the inhabitants of Great Britain and Ireland (with their ice and snow) during their winter months. It is one of the characteristics of the Anglo-Saxon race, however, this inability to appreciate the necessity of conforming to new climatic conditions in which their lot may be cast. It will be the same, too, when the British restaurant-keeper begins business in Equatorial Africa. For an absolute certainty his bill-of-fare for the delectation of the unfortunate colonist will consist of roast beef, Yorkshire pudding, plum pudding, and the old familiar throng. Whether mine host has to consult the taste of his client, or whether the latter has simply to accept what is proffered, is not absolutely decided; probably they are both imbued with a belief in the necessity of solid fare, regarding it as a solemn truth beyond all possibility of cavil.

This abuse of flesh food in a climate like Australia would be serious enough under any circumstances, but it is intensified and aggravated by the direct unoriginality in dealing with meat. Is it not a fact that there is no attempt whatever made to break through the conventional chain of joints, roasted or boiled, and the inevitable grill or fry? In how many houses does the breakfast ever consist of anything but the ubiquitous chops, steaks, or sausages? indeed, one might almost term them "the faith, hope, and charity" of domestic life. I remember reading some little time ago that if a map of the world were made in which lands of utter darkness were coloured black like the coalfields in an atlas of physical geography, certain races would be signalised by their opaqueness. If such a map were ever compiled, Australia would of necessity be characterised by blackness; such a blackness, indeed, that jet itself would be as snowy white beside it. But why should this lamentable state of things be said of Australians, who claim to be progressive in their ideas and advanced in their views, usages, and customs?

In conjunction with this dietetic view of the matter, one of the objects I have in writing is to direct attention to the great neglect there is of vegetables, especially those of the more unknown varieties, as an agreeable, desirable, palatable, and salutary element in the Australian food life. One need not be a vegetarian to properly appreciate the valuable properties of vegetables, and most people will fare better and feel the benefit of a modification of their customary dietary if they decrease the amount of meat they indulge in and proportionately increase their vegetable allowance. Now, there are many vegetables besides those ordinarily in use which might be easily cultivated, and serve to form a pleasing variety at table. Once the demand arises for kinds other than those usually grown, the inducement for market-gardeners to supply them would be no longer wanting. A reference to the catalogues furnished by the seedsmen and plant-merchants of the different Australian metropolitan cities will show that special attention is called to many of these vegetables, and yet I am informed that, although they are continually inserted in the new issues as they appear from time to time, no notice seems to be taken of them whatever. I propose, therefore, briefly to describe some of these comparatively unknown vegetables, and to point out their merits and their claims for recognition.

The globe artichoke might be more frequently grown, as it is really a good vegetable and easily cooked. It constitutes the flower head of the CYNARA SCOLYMUS (one of the thistle family), and is gathered before the flowers expand. The ends of the flower scales attached to the disc, and the central disc itself, are the parts that are eaten, and they constitute a delicately flavoured vegetable. It is extensively cultivated in California, and is there to be met with in nearly all hotels and restaurants. Another thing in its favour is that it is peculiarly one of the vegetables which diabetics may indulge in without fear. It does well in the cooler parts of Australia, and should certainly be more generally grown.

The Jerusalem artichoke is not to be confused with the preceding, as it belongs to a different vegetable genus altogether. It is a species of sunflower, as its name denotes, the prefix Jerusalem being in reality a corruption of the Italian word GIRASOLE, a sunflower. It resembles the potato in that it is a tuberous-rooted vegetable, and grows readily enough--in fact, perhaps it grows too readily, for once it takes possession of the soil it is difficult to eradicate it. The Jerusalem artichoke, however, is comparatively common here, and when cooked properly it is a most delightful vegetable, although it may not be sufficiently appreciated at first. It often happens that these artichokes are of a bad colour, and too crisp when brought to table. This is easily prevented, however, by washing and paring them like potatoes and then placing them in a bowl of clear water, to which a few drops of fresh lemon juice have been added. When boiled with sufficient water to just cover them, and a liberal allowance of salt, for 20 min. to 40 min., they come out a snowy white and quite tender. They are especially delicious when served up with melted butter and egg sauce.

Asparagus.--Although this delicate and luscious vegetable is of the easiest culture, and grows readily along the coast, yet to our shame be it said that it is usually too much of a luxury for ordinary mortal, to afford. Now, it is for the most part such a general favourite that one may well ask why it is not more cultivated. The demand for it in

America is so great, and it yields such a good return, that some growers, make 100 percent; and upwards yearly profit for each acre. Is it not a severe reflection upon our market gardeners, to find that the imported preserved varieties of asparagus are so esculent that the very stalks, are as, luscious as the heads of the vegetable? In its fresh state it should be eaten as soon after cutting as possible, and, like the globe artichoke, is readily allowable to diabetics. It is somewhat curious, too, that the asparagus, and the globe artichoke are the only vegetables which the British race eat as, a single dish.

Brussels sprouts are the most delicate of all the borecoles, and it is a thousand pities that this delightful vegetable is not more often to be met with. These miniature, cabbages, however, require some little care in their rearing, and hence amateurs often fail to reach perfection in their cultivation. They may be boiled like cabbage, in abundance of water and a little salt for 15 minutes, then drained, dried, and finally tossed in butter with a little pepper and nutmeg. They do well enough, as does the borecole or kale itself, in all the cooler parts of Australia.

The cardoon, like the globe artichoke, belongs to the thistle family, yet it is, more hardy and robust than the latter. It is readily grown, particularly in the cooler districts, and, like many other of the more unknown vegetables, is too much neglected. Its leaf-stalks should be at least an inch and a half thick before they are ready for cutting. They are then blanched, and when cooked recall somewhat the flavour of the globe artichoke. These tender leaf-stalks are used in soups and salads, and it may be boiled also in a similar manner to sea-kale, in which latter form it is especially palatable.

The celeriac or turnip-rooted celery is a very choice vegetable, and is much cultivated on the Continent. Its nutty root is not at all unlike the solid root portion of common celery in taste, which by many is considered superior in flavour to the other parts of the latter plant. The celeriac is greatly esteemed, and is known as the CELERI-RAVE BY the French, and as the knoll-selerie by the Germans. The latter, indeed, are so fond of it that they call barely talk of it without moist eyes and watery mouths. It is hardier than celery, and possesses an advantage in that it can be taken up and stored similarly to carrots and beets. The celerific may be boiled as a table vegetable or used for flavouring soups, or it may be sliced for salads. It does well in all the cooler parts, and might be cultivated with benefit, mingled with gratitude.

The egg plant, or aubergine, does so exceedingly well, and can be so highly recommended, that one may well wonder why it is never seen. It is a native of Africa and tropical America, and is very popular both in the East and West Indies. It is cultivated also a great deal in the United States, where it is greatly appreciated for culinary use. In AUBERGINES FARCIES, a favourite dish, they are cut in hakes, the centres chopped and put back into the skins with oil, &c. They are then sprinkled with breadcrumbs, and browned. It is easily grown, and it seems unaccountable why it should be passed over.

The kohl rabi, or turnip-rooted cabbage, is another nutritious vegetable which has inexplicably never been received into public favour. Its delicate flavour should ensure for it a well-established position with those who are fond of good vegetables, as it is more tender and more savoury than either turnip or cabbage, and is not at all unlike cauliflower in taste. For table purposes it should be only about two-thirds grown, for if allowed to go to full size the outside skin becomes tough and hard. It is another of those vegetables which are so highly prized on the Continent, and it is already an acknowledged favourite in America. It does well in all the cooler localities, and gives a larger yield than turnips.

The salsify, or "vegetable oyster," is a typical example of a most unaccountably slighted vegetable with us, and yet it is highly appreciated on the continent and in the United States. The root is long and tapering, becoming fleshy and tender by cultivation, and with a whitish, milky-like juice. It has a rich flavour, not at all unlike that of cooked oysters, whence it derives its value. In preparing salsify for table the darkish outside skin requires to be lightly scraped off, and then it should be steeped for a while in cold water so as to remove any slight bitterness it may possess. Like parsnips, when cooked it requires to be boiled slowly, in the smallest possible quantity of water, until it is almost ready to melt. If boiled fast, in abundance of water, the savour of both parsnips and salsify is to a great extent dispersed and lost beyond recall. One of the most approved methods of cooking salsify roots is to slowly boil them to tenderness in the smallest possible quantity of milk, and then to mash and fry them in butter, with salt and pepper. Cold boiled salsify, with the addition of some chopped herbs, tarragon vinegar, and salad oil, makes an exceedingly good salad. The salsify does well in all the cooler regions, and, moreover, it is easily grown.

Scorzonera.--This Spanish plant is very similar to salsify, and requires the same kind of treatment; but, being a stronger grower, requires more room in its culture. It may be served in soups or treated like salsify. The outside leaves should be removed before the vegetable is cooked. The blanched leaves also are highly esteemed on the Continent, and are used for salad purposes. It grows well in all the cooler parts of Australia, and might certainly be introduced for the public benefit.

Sea kale is one of those vegetables which are brought to perfection in England, so much so that Careme, that mighty CHEF, when he came across them in London went into ecstasies. He described them as resembling branches of celery, which should be served like asparagus, with butter sauce, after 20 minutes' boiling. In some respects this is verily the most delicious of all vegetables, and as it grows well here it should be largely cultivated, yet it is almost unknown. It is fit to rank with, if not precede, asparagus, and as a matter of fact it is far more profitable than the latter, so that market gardeners would have something to gain by its introduction. Like the cabbage, it was originally a maritime plant, and has been brought to its present state of perfection by cultivation. It requires to be thoroughly blanched by exclusion from light, similarly to celery, for when coloured at all it possesses an acrid taste. Of the many ways of sending it to table, one of the best is to boil it and serve it on toast with a little melted butter. It should be largely cultivated, as it does well all along the coastal parts, being, as already mentioned, a maritime plant.

Sweet corn is deservedly a great favourite with those who know of its succulent flavour and nourishing properties. Unfortunately, however, it is with us only in the imported tins from America, and therefore we can only conjecture how delicious it must be when fresh. It is so commonly met with in the fresh form in America that it is found at nearly every dinner table. Large areas where land is not expensive are devoted to its growth, and hundreds of acres are required annually for the New York markets alone. It does splendidly in all parts of Australia, and for growing children it constitutes one of the most nutritious vegetables that can be well imagined. On this latter account alone, therefore, it is really a matter for national regret that it is so improperly passed over. One thing requires to be borne in mind, and it is that the cobs of ordinary Indian corn which are seen in so many country districts must not be confused with this sweet corn, as the latter is entirely different.

These nutritious, although somewhat unknown vegetables, therefore, evidently deserve to be brought into prominent notice, and once public interest is aroused, their cultivation and ready sale will speedily follow. At the same time it must not be forgotten that the tomato itself had a desperate struggle for reception into public favour when first introduced to us. It actually trembled in the balance for no inconsiderable time, and it was some years before its good qualities were universally recognised. To-day, however, it occupies a very different position, and takes rank as a luscious vegetable, appreciated by thousands of people; and besides, it is of undoubted value in many disorders of the liver. But now that the Agricultural Colleges are in full swing in the different colonies, notably in New South Wales, Victoria, and South Australia, it is certain that the greatest possible good to the whole community will result. Their effect, too, in indirectly populating the agricultural areas of Australia will materially aid the great work of decentralisation.

But apart altogether from this matter of the introduction of vegetables which have hitherto been overlooked is another which is hardly less important. I refer to the crude cookery which is bestowed on the ordinary vegetables at present in daily use. That there is sny monotony in an endless recurrence of boiled potatoes, boiled cabbage, boiled this and boiled that, never seems to occur to the vast majority of people in this country, who seem incapable of understanding that these different vegetables are worthy of being served in an infinite number of ways. It will doubtless shock those who cling to this beliefs but the following remarks by Dr. Mitchell, an English physician practising in Paris, directed against his own countrymen be it understood, are forcible enough:--"The plain boiled potato," says he, "whatever else it may be, is clearly a cattle food; so for the matter of that are cabbages, carrots, turnips, beans, peas, and almost every other vegetable when plain boiled. None of them in that condition would be "refused by a cow in fair appetite." Now, there are so many appetising ways of preparing vegetables for table, and at no additional expense, that it is lamentable to find people offering no protest against this feeble exhibition of culinary skill. Why, if there be nothing in the preparation of vegetables for the table beyond plain boiling, it must be acknowledged that Cookery has made mighty little progress since the time it first came into existence.

Having seen, then, what faults exist and what improvements might be made, it may well be asked how these latter are to be brought about, or, rather, how can Australians be induced to life in accordance with climatic requirements? The answer Is by no means easy. It may be said, in truth, that till the great mass of the people recognise their food faults, reform will not be of a national character. As I have already said, the acceptation of that valuable and nutritious vegetable fruit, the tomato, took years to accomplish. In the same way, I fear, a universal recognition that excessive meat indulgence is a climatic error will take many decades before it is an article of national belief. In the schools, Cookery must form an all-important part of a girl's education--not a superficial knowledge of the science, but practical instruction, thorough, complete, real. The dietetic properties of meat, vegetables, of salad vegetables, and of fruit, from an Australian standpoint, should be so thoroughly inculcated that a proper conception of their respective food values should remain for a lifetime. The prizes for proficiency and excellence in culinary matters, too, should be such as to render them worth the winning, and serve as a stimulus for future exertions.

Is it not strange that so far ingenuity, universal approval, or general consensus of opinions call it what you will, has not up till the present given us an Australian national dish? Although tea and damper instinctively arise in the mind when the matter is referred to, yet I take it that we would all repel such an accusation if levelled against us. Does the Australian, moreover, away from his native land perpetuate his patriotism by oft partaking of this pastoral fare? Certainly not. Well, when this national dish is composed and formally approved of by the nation, let us devoutly trust that it will be a MACEDOINE of

vegetables, or a vegetable curry, or some well-concocted salad. It is
true that in one of the cookery books I have seen a dish of peaches,
dubbed PECHES A L'AUSTRALIENNE. It is a sort of compote of peaches, but
to the best of my belief it is simply entitled Australian for the sake
of giving it a name, and for no other reason.

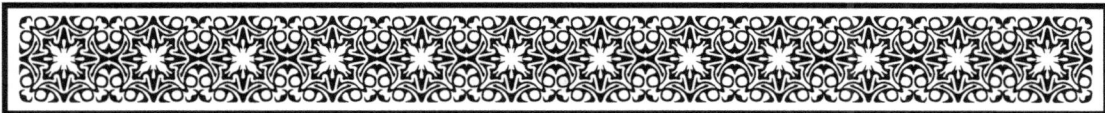

CHAPTER X.
AUSTRALIAN FISH AND OYSTERS--AND THEIR FOOD VALUE.

Anyone looking backwards upon the history of Australia cannot fail to be impressed by one peculiar feature, which is the more distinctive, too, because it is in striking contrast with all else. It is the more noteworthy also, because it affects each individual inhabitant of this island continent, and has a direct bearing on the daily life of every person is the community. Thus, on the one hand, while we are nearing a maximum of progress--or, at any rate, attaining to a high level of success--in political matters, in commercial affairs, and in athletic prowess, yet, on the other, there is unfortunately an apathetic indifference in all that concerns our public and family food habits, which after all constitute the national characteristics of any people. It is true that we have gained the dignity of responsible government, that our wool and frozen meat are entering the markets of the world, and that in the athletic arena our fame is spread both far and wide. Yet it must be confessed that our national food-life has not conformed to climatic requirements in the slightest degree since the memorable day on which Captain Cook set foot on these shores. As those on the Endeavour lived then, so live are now. On the continent of Europe it will be found that the manners and customs, even of contiguous countries, are as widely different as it is possible to imagine. Surely

then, it is, to say the least of it, curious to see the inhabitants of
a semi-tropical country like Australia living in wilful contradiction
to their climatic necessities, and eating the same kind of food as did
their fathers in the old land, with its dampness its coldness, its ice,
and its snow.

Yet, notwithstanding the fact that reflections of this kind are
interesting in the highest degree, I propose to do no more than
consider the matter exclusively from the standpoint of the subject
heading of this chapter. Here, again, we are directly confronted with
an inexplicable anomaly--I refer to the want of enterprise shown in
developing the deep-sea fisheries of Australia. Now, if the dwellers of
this land had sprung from an entirely inland race, this would not,
perhaps, have been so difficult to understand; but arising, as we do,
from a stock the most maritime that the world has ever seen, such a
defect redounds not to our credit as inheritors of the old traditions.
At our present rate of fisheries development it will take centuries
before we will be able to produce anything to even approach the
International Fisheries exhibition of the old country in 1883. At that
memorable exposition His Royal Highness the Duke of Edinburgh, in the
course of his conference paper, gave expression to the following
stirring words:--"From the earliest ages the inhabitants of the coast
of the British Islands have made the sea contribute to their food. This
pursuit has produced a race of men strong, inured to hardship and
exposure, patient and persevering in their calling, brave, prompt, and
fall of resource in the face of danger; intelligent and amenable to
discipline, from the daily habit of subordinating their own wills to
that of anyone whom they know is placed in authority over them for the,
purpose of directing their labours and working with them for the common
benefit; accustomed to co-operate with others for the attainment of a
certain end. These qualities are not only exercised from early youth,
but are inherited and intensified from generation to generation. The
foundations of the great position which this kingdom has attained

amongst the nations of the world must, in some measure, be attributed to our fishermen, for they were our first sea-men; and, from small beginnings, our seamen increased in number and in skill, until the whole nation was leavened with that love of maritime adventure which has resulted in peopling the uttermost parts of the earth with our race, and in establishing that empire upon which the sun never ceases to shine. In earlier times our first maritime commerce must have been conducted by our fishermen, who also manned our fighting navies. The fisheries of the West of England were the nurseries of the sailors who enabled Drake to circumnavigate the world, and, as he said, to 'singe the King of Spain's beard' on more than one memorable occasion."

THE DEFECTIVENESS OF OUR AUSTRALIAN FISH SUPPLY.

That fish should be, comparatively speaking, so scarce in Australia can only be regarded in the light of a national calamity. And not only is the supply deficient, but what little there may be is so outrageously expensive that it is hopelessly beyond the reach of an ordinary purse. It is so excessive in cost that it must almost be bracketed with poultry as a luxury only to be indulged in after lengthened periods. I have been told, when making inquiries on this point, that the reason why fish is so dear is that this is not a fish-eating community, and that consequently there is no demand for it. But, on the other hand, I find that almost everyone I ask is really fond of fish, and that they do not eat it simply because they cannot obtain it at a reasonable price, and this undoubtedly is the true explanation.

But this same scarcity of fish has exercised other people besides myself, for Mr. Alexander Oliver and many others have repeatedly drawn attention to the same deficiency. It has been the primary origin of a Board of Fisheries, it had brought forth Parliamentary Select

Committees, and it has produced endless opinions and suggestions on the part of the public. Now, I am quite willing to admit that there should be proper supervision over the working of the Fisheries Acts, and that existing grievances should be rectified; but, with all due deference, it seems to me that the finger has not been placed on the exact reason why failure occurs in our fish supply. For I say this, that you may do what you will to protect and supervise the shore and inland fisheries, and you may even increase the yield from these sources to an encouraging extent, but that till the deep-sea work is thoroughly taken up and properly developed there will be no cheap fish for Australia. It has been stated that if the deep-sea fisheries of the United Kingdom fell through from any reason, half-a-million of its inhabitants would be brought face to face with starvation. And even these enormous figures include only the fisher-folk themselves, and do not take into account the vast army of buyers, curers, dealers, &c., who are dependent for their very existence upon the fishing industry. Take away the deep-sea fisheries from the old country, and its whole fish supply would practically be at an end. In the same way by the development of our Australian deep-sea fisheries--and by the development of the deep-sea fisheries only--will it be possible, in my humble opinion, to increase the supply and cheapen the price of fish so that it will form part of the dietary in every dwelling.

There was an important select committee appointed by the Victorian Government, a short time ago, to inquire into the unsatisfactory condition of the fishing industry there. It examined a great number of witnesses, and its investigations extended over a large area. Amongst other things, with a view of encouraging trawling operations, it was suggested--

"That a careful survey be made of the sea-bottom in the neighbourhood of our coasts and in Bass' Straits, and the part suitable for trawling properly charted. That a few sets of trawling apparatus of the most modern kind be procured by the Government, and Applications invited from the fishermen at the various ports for permission to use these trawls, free of charge, under certain conditions for a limited period. That the Government fit out a steamer for the purpose of collecting and conveying to Melbourne the fish obtained by the trawlers, the steamer to be provided with cooling chambers, &c."

A number of different matters were also considered, and, in addition, it was thought that, in order to afford the general public greater facilities for obtaining fish, the sale should not be confined to the metropolitan market. It was, therefore, recommended that stalls in the various markets for the sale of fish by auction and otherwise should be opened in the leading suburbs of Melbourne; and that the corporation officer in the metropolitan market, to whom the fish was consigned, should regularly distribute to each of these suburban markets such a quantity of fish as experience would show the particular locality demanded. To a certain extent all this is very satisfactory, but unfortunately select committees have arrived at very similar conclusions over and over again. All their recommendations have never yet been attended by any practical result, and an adequate fish supply for Australia appears to be as far off as ever.

OUR PRIMITIVE METHODS OF FISH CAPTURE.

About the last place one would expect to come across a really fine piece of delicate humour is amongst official correspondence, and yet in a formal letter from Dr. E.P. Ramsay, the Curator of the Australian Museum, to Sir Saul Samuel the following passage occurs. Speaking of the New South Wales exhibits at the International Fisheries Exhibition of London, 1883, the doctor proceeds to remark:--"People here, imagining that we must have already developed extensive fisheries, from the large collection of food fishes which we exhibit, were not less surprised at our very limited materials and methods of capture than at the immense undeveloped wealth of our fisheries and fish fauna." Now, I venture to say that a more unconsciously subtle insinuation at the crude methods of fish capture at present employed in our Australian fisheries was never penned. But what makes it so keenly effective is that it really hits the right nail on the head. In giving evidence, also, before Mr. Frank Farnell's select committee of 1889, Dr. Ramsay, upon being asked whether he thought our fishermen were abreast of the times with regard to appliances, replied:--"They are about 200 years behind the times."

To my mind another most convincing proof of the crude methods of fish capture employed in Australian waters is to be found in the following. In one of the Fisheries Reports it is gravely recorded that "some very valuable gear IN GENERAL USE amongst English, Norwegian, and American fishermen, had been destroyed in the Garden Palace fire, but that the commissioners had been able to replace the otter-trawl and the beam-trawl." The very fact that these appliances, in active use at the present time by those in the foremost front of fishery enterprise, are regarded in the light of curiosities in Australia, proves only too forcibly the correctness-of this opinion as to our primitive fishery appliances.

THE BEAM-TRAWL IN DEEP-SEA FISHING.

It must not be imagined that trawling has never been advocated (indeed, it has even been experimentally practised), for we have only to look through the various Fisheries Reports to find it repeatedly referred to; unfortunately, however, these appeals so far have been without any practical results. It will, therefore, be most instructive to refer briefly to the manner in which trawling and other modes of deep-sea fishing are carried out elsewhere; and more particularly to bring under notice the enormous fish yield effected by them. Trawling, or as it is more properly termed, beam-trawling, may be described as a method of deep-sea fishing, in which a large bag net is towed along the ground so as to scoop, as it were, the fish into its receptacle. There are at least several important stations in England for trawling; some in the English Channel; some on the west, and also on the Welsh coast; and others again (amongst which is Grimsby, the largest fishing port in the world) on the east coast on the North Sea. The trawling grounds of the latter are widely known, and comprise the famous Dogger Bank, which covers many hundreds of acres in area. In its neighbourhood, also, there are numerous grounds such as the Inner and Outer Well Banks, and there are others again nearer the English coast. In addition to these there is the Great Silver Pit, discovered in a severe winter in 1843; and it has been noticed that during the winter months the fish frequent the deeper water, because the temperature is more equable than in shallow places. The depth at which trawling is usually carried on varies from 20 to 30 fathoms; never under any circumstances reaching 50 fathoms--the depth of the Silver Pit being from 35 to 45 fathoms.

It was formerly urged against trawling that it was very destructive to the spawn, at that time supposed to be lying on the sea bottom. But the investigations of the late Professor Sars, for the Swedish Government, into the spawning habits of sea fish, have conclusively revealed the fact that the ova of fish float on the surface of the water during the whole period of their development. Not only have the floating ova of the cod and haddock been reared, but the common plaice, the representative of the flatfish family, including the brill, the sole, and the turbot, is also known to spawn near the surface. The eggs of the mackerel and the garfish have likewise been found floating, and successfully hatched. Now, no fish comes so close to the land as does the mackerel, yet it is certain that it never makes its way into the estuaries and inlets till after spawning is finished--for that it spawns in the open sea is almost without a doubt. These facts consequently do away altogether with the old statements concerning the destructive results of trawling.

The yield from the English trawleries alone is computed to be over 200,000 tons annually, and as the price for trawled fish at the Billingsgate market averages 12 pounds per ton, this represents about two and a half million pounds. And, in addition to these weighty figures, Professor Huxley's words deserve to be well remembered, for, says he, "Were trawl fishing stopped, it would no longer be a case of high prices, but that ninety-nine out of a hundred would hardly be able to afford any at all--herrings and a few other fish caught in the old way excepted." Indeed, it is chiefly by this method of beam trawling that London and the interior are supplied with brill, turbot, and soles; while by it thousands of tons of plaice, haddock, and other fish are brought within the reach even of the poorest.

DRIFT-NET AND OTHER DEEP-SEA FISHING.

Important though the beam-trawl may be, there is another mode of deep-sea fishing which deserves to be well known by us in Australia, and which undoubtedly must come into general use before we can make any pretensions with regard to our fisheries. I refer to that by means of drift-nets. As the trawl is absolutely necessary, on the one hand, for capturing fish which frequent the bottom, so, on the other, the drift-net is essential for those whose resort is the upper portion of the sea. It is by this method alone that fish like the herring, the mackerel, and the pilchard--which may be termed surface fish--are caught in great quantities for food supply.

Now, in Australia, we have vast shoals of migratory fish visiting the coast at different periods of the year. During the winter season enormous numbers of herrings come to these shores, and are permitted to depart without any effort being made to capture them. Attention has been repeatedly called to this strange neglect in our fisheries, for this herring is plentiful and is considered to surpass the famous Scottish herring itself in flavour. The mackerel, too, is to be met with annually, generally about midwinter, in immense shoals, passing near the coast upwards in a northerly direction. The sea mullet also makes its appearance towards the end of the summer months, usually from April to June, at the very time when it is in splendid condition and full of roe. It is always observed to be proceeding towards the north in successive shoals and in great numbers. Many consider its richness and delicacy of flavour to be unequalled. The driftnet system of fishing would be well adapted for it--if the meshes were larger than those for the herring--as when fully grown it is nearly two feet in length. And lastly, it will only be necessary to speak of the "maray," which is practically the English pilchard. As with the fish just mentioned, it is met with about midwinter, passing up north in countless numbers, sometimes covering miles of sea.

As the name implies, drift-nets are not worked from the shore, but they are "shot," as the saying is, in the open sea, and allowed to drift in whatever direction the tide may take them. Each drift-net will measure about 180 feet in length by about 30 feet in depth. They are secured to one another at the ends to form a long single line, perhaps two miles in length. By means of floats the nets hang perpendicularly in the water, thus forming a long wall against which the fish "strike," and get enmeshed by being caught in the gill opening. The nets are kept on the stretch by being "shot" in the face of the wind, and the vessel from which they are paid out, being to leeward of them, drifts more rapidly than they do, and consequently keeps them well extended.

My object, however, is not so much to enter into the details of these different methods of deep-sea fishing as to indicate their value and necessity, if we are to have any fisheries worth speaking of. I shall, therefore, do no more than briefly mention a few other modes of fish capture. Thus, at the mouth of the Thames, thousands of tons of sprats are caught every winter by means of the large bag net, known as the stow net. In shape it is like an enormous funnel, 30 feet high, 20 feet wide, and nearly 180 feet in length. By means of this contrivance the yield of sprats is so great that there is often some little difficulty in disposing of the catch. The renowned whitebait, too, which are believed to be young herrings, are caught by means of a similar, though much smaller, net.

Besides these and various other forms of net fishing, there are the methods in which the long line is employed. For the capture of the cod, both in Newfoundland and in the North Sea, what is called the bultow is used. This is a long line many hundreds of-feet in length, and at every twelfth foot shorter and smaller cords called "snoods" are fastened. These "snoods" are about 6 feet long, and have the hooks attached to their free ends. The bultow is "shot" across the tide to prevent entanglement of the hooks, and is laid in the afternoon. At daybreak, when the lines are hauled in, as many as 400 of the large cod sometimes result from the catch. There are various other appliances used for fish capture in different parts of the world, such as the purse-seine net, the trammel net, the otter-trawl net, &c.; and, as I have already pointed out, the most scathing satire on our fisheries is to find all these necessary means for catching fish regarded as curiosities. When they are no longer considered so, it will be a fortunate time for Australia.

BENEFITS FROM THE DEVELOPMENT OF OUR DEEP-SEA FISHERIES.

What would the proper development of our deep-sea fisheries mean? In the first place, it would lead to a more widely diffused use of fish as an article of diet, within the easy reach of all classes, being thus of incalculable value from a health point of view. Next, it would ensure employment to many hundreds, and eventually to many thousands, both directly and indirectly, and as a natural consequence this would bring about the creation of a sturdy and desirable maritime element in our population. And lastly, it would yield a more than satisfactory return on the outlay invested.

At the present time only the veriest few of our metropolitan population are able to afford the luxury of fish, and people in the country towns hardly see it at all. So, too, we are casting about for this plan and for that plan to lessen a growing difficulty in the Australian metropolitan centres. There are village settlements (which certainly deserve to be successful), and other proposals made to relieve a surplus population, but yet no one has suggested the sea as a means of remedying this congestion. And not only would the fisheries confer upon its followers a healthy calling, but they would raise a vigorous stock of which Australia might well be proud. In addition to all this, a proper development of our deep-sea fisheries would assuredly open up a new avenue for investment. Is it not amazing that men will risk all they have in mines which are not even real, and which exist, only on paper? And besides this, in the most genuine mine that was ever worked there is at least a costly outlay for production, for crushing, or for smelting, before the metal sees the light of day; but in the sea the catch is ready for the market, and only requires the bringing to land.

This matter, therefore, must be taken up earnestly, and there must be a determination to succeed. In the first place, and before all else in the deep-sea fisheries, I maintain that a proper and systematic search for trawling grounds is absolutely essential. Till this is done he cannot for a moment pretend that we have endeavoured to foster them in any way. All the elaboration of your proposed Fisheries Acts, and all the details connected with the working of what may be called shore fishing, sink into nothingness when compared with the results which would follow the working of our deep-sea fisheries. I have already used the argument before, and do so again, and it is this: that if you were to take away from the old country her deep-sea fisheries, she would be practically without any fish supply.

Apparently it is imagined, too, that unless trawling grounds be discovered in the vicinity of Sydney or Melbourne, all efforts will be useless. But it will only be necessary to refer to the deep-sea fisheries elsewhere to at once set this objection aside. Some of the great trawling grounds in the North Sea are at such a distance from port that it would be quite impossible for any vessel to bring its own catch to market for disposal, for the fish would be utterly spoiled before it could be done. But the larger trawling boats go on cruises extending over weeks, and are constantly visited on the grounds by what are called "carriers," i.e. steamers, who run their freights directly into market. The same thing is practised by the Dutch vessels, who fish in the neighbourhood of the Shetland Islands for weeks together. In the same way carrier vessels attend upon their fishing fleets, and carry off the take immediately to Holland. Being in possession of these facts, therefore, we must not be induced to believe that deep-sea fishing is not possible, simply because suitable grounds for trawling, &c., may not be actually within coo-ee of the Australian metropolitan centres.

FISH MARKETS OF SYDNEY AND MELBOURNE.

There are one or two matters in connection with this subject which deserve having attention called to them. In the first place the method adopted in our Woolloomooloo Fish Market of placing the fish in little heaps on the floor itself, when put out for sale, is not satisfactory. In the Redfern Fish Market they are placed in small divisions or receptacles--each lot by itself--and raised above the floor, where they are protected from injury. In the new Melbourne Fish Markets, there are elevated platforms for the fish, and they are thus quite above the cemented floor. Not only are they prevented from being damaged, but it seems to me that the buyers have a better chance of seeing the fish when it is raised a little distance above their feet.

The size of the fish lots for sale in the Sydney and Melbourne Fish Markets varies, and this opens up a somewhat debatable point. with us the lots are comparatively small, both at the Woolloomooloo and at the Redfern Market; while at Melbourne, on the other hand, the lots are much larger. When the lots are small it gives private buyers a chance of purchasing (but how many private buyers are there before breakfast?), and is said in this way to raise the price for the dealers. But with the larger lots the latter are said to be able to buy to more advantage, and thus supply the public with cheaper fish. To say which is the better of the two plans is very much like being asked to solve the query in the story of "The Lady or the Tiger."

But before leaving this matter I should like to refer briefly to the new markets in Flinders Street, Melbourne. They are called the City of Melbourne Meat, Fish, and Farm Produce Markets, and are most extensive in area. The viaduct which connects the two railway systems of Victoria pierces the very centre of these new markets. They are replete with every modern appliance for the storage and disposal of the food supply of a large city. There are numerous chambers for the frozen meat, and by means of what is called a "lock," a whole train can be received into a long covered gallery. The two gates are then closed at either end, and the meat is thus received directly into the freezing chambers, without the slightest loss of any cold air. The fish and game are treated exactly in the same way, except that the receiving and delivery "locks" are not quite so large as in the former case. Still, there is just the same facility for their reception into the freezing chambers set apart for the purpose. The whole arrangements of these new fish markets are very perfect, and leave nothing to be desired.

THE "MIDDLEMAN" CONTROVERSY.

This is one of the topics which is continually cropping up in connection with the fishing industry in Australia. It is noteworthy, too, that the middleman in some shape or form appears to be part of the system of fish selling in every part of the world. At Billingsgate, where they are termed "bummarees," it is stated that they fulfil a useful office in that they act as distributors to the small costermongers, who could hardly get along without them. The "bummarees" watch the market and speculate accordingly, and it must be urged for them that they run great risks from the unexpected arrival of a large amount of fish with a consequent glut in the market. But the "bummarees" pure and simple are comparatively few. Their ranks, however, are swelled in the following way: A salesman, having disposed of his own fish, will "bummaree" for the sake of the possible profit, or a fishmonger, having purchased a double supply for a cheaper price, will "bummaree" half his purchase. In France the procedure is different. First of all there is an agent termed an ECOREUR, deputed by various persons and armed with purchasing power, who is ready to buy the fisherman's catch at once. This simplifies matters wonderfully for the fisherman, who gets ready money and has no further bother. Next, from the ECOREUR the fish is bought by the MOREYEUR, or trader, who despatches it to Paris and the other large cities. Thus, so far, the fish, after leaving the fisherman, has passed through two hands, those of the ecoreur, and those of the MOREYEUR. After this it has to face a most unjust tax--the OCTROI--by which all provisions are specially taxed before entering the "barriers" of any French city or town. Hence the initiated, when travelling in France, often reside on the outskirts of a town, just outside the barrier, where the cost of living is reduced by one-third. On arriving at the markets the fish is publicly disposed of by the FACTEURS A LA CRIEE, or auctioneers, who of course are paid for their trouble. Lastly, it is bought for sale to the public by the POISSARDE, or fishwife. And thus we see from the time of leaving the water till finally it reaches the unfortunate public the fish has passed through no less than six levies, that by the fisherman, the agent, the trader, the OCTROI (I.E. the city toll or town due), the auctioneer, and, finally, that by the fishwife or costermonger.

Having thus explained the system pursued in England and in France respectively, it will be interesting to refer briefly to the different methods with regard to the disposal of fish practised in the Woolloomooloo, the Redfern, and the Melbourne Fish Markets. At the former, the sales are conducted by Mr. Richard Seymour, the inspector and auctioneer of the fish market--with other auctioneers--who act directly from the Sydney Municipal Council; the Redfern markets are conducted by the Messrs. Hudson; while in Melbourne there are licensed auctioneers, who pay for the privilege.

But to return to our middleman, upon whom the whole controversy centres. Indeed, the discussion over him in Melbourne, not so long ago, might be said to have reached to a white-heat phase. But the. premises on which the arguments were based were so hopelessly conflicting that it was impossible to logically settle the point. It was claimed, on the one hand, that the price the fishermen received was cruelly small in comparison with that which the public had to pay. On the other, the contention was that the price paid to the fishermen was fairly satisfactory, and that the public obtained comparatively cheap fish. We have seen, however, what takes place in other parts of the world, and, indeed, every one must admit that there is a remarkable difference between the price which the fisherman gets and that which the public have to pay. Between these two extremes there is an inordinate disparity, and the difficulty is to connect the two together--to bring to light the leakage--and to find out who is living both on the fisherman and the public at one and the same time. On this point a recent Fisheries Report of Victoria says:--"The solution of the very important question of providing a larger and cheaper fish supply for the masses rests mainly in the hands of the public. The present high prices are maintained in virtue of a monopoly which can be only successfully combated by the initiation of a healthy trade competition or a more open fish market. The fishermen, under existing auspices, reap but a small share of the retail produce of their takings, such being further reduced by the high rates for transport they are called upon to pay. In this last-named direction some relief might be afforded by the institution, if necessary by Act of Parliament, of a uniform tariff for the carriage of fish by road and rail throughout the colony."

THE DISTRIBUTION OF FISH TO THE PUBLIC.

This brings me to one of the most difficult matters that has to be dealt with in considering the fish supply of any great city. For you may have the most extensive deep-sea fisheries, you may have the most rapid transit of the fish to town, and you may have the most commodious fish markets; but if you have no proper means of distributing the fish to the public the whole scheme falls to the ground. At present the system both in Sydney and in Melbourne is to have the one principal fish market (there are now two in Sydney, by the way), from which all supplies for the public are derived. Of course it is perfectly competent for the latter to obtain their purchases in the early morning at the time when the sales are conducted; but, on the other hand, the hour is exceedingly inconvenient, and, as a general rule, the lots are too large for the private buyer. Hence the distribution of fish depends almost wholly upon the costermonger or basket-man, who takes his fish round to the public. The basket-man, or costermonger, or dealer--call him what you will--is an indispensable personage, and what is more, he fills a most useful office. It is true that he is given to making strange outcries, and that he is at times boisterous in speech. Yet, notwithstanding these things, he is a valuable member of society, and personally I have a very great respect for him. Indeed, I am certain that he is the food-bearer to many homes, and people would otherwise be put to very great straits in obtaining their supplies. Our friend, however, has usually a long round to travel before he can make a good living, and perhaps he is unable to cope with the requirements of his large district.

It is on account of these difficulties, therefore, that I recognise the value of the French method of distribution, for besides the Halles Centrales, or principal markets, in Paris, there are in all nearly sixty local provision markets where it is possible to obtain, under cover--in all weathers and at any time--whatever is required. It is most desirable that something of this kind should be adopted in Australia. At least it is quite certain that every suburb should possess its own local market. This need not attempt to rival the central depot, but take rank as a local necessity.

FISHMONGERS AND THE SALE OF FISH.

This is naturally in intimate connection with the preceding, and it is very advisable to refer to it in order to direct attention to one or two matters. In the first place, I shall commence by saying that both Sydney and Melbourne are lamentably deficient in fishmongers' shops similar to those which are so common in London. As a matter of fact, the show of fish exposed for sale is in striking contrast to that of meat. For in Sydney and suburbs alone the butchers' establishments run to the number of nearly 600, while in the Melbourne metropolis they even exceed this. One has only to look through the directories of either Sydney or Melbourne, under the heading of "Fishmongers," to see how few their numbers are. In our own city, Chinnery, of Hunter Street, and Matterson, of Pitt Street, make a highly creditable show, and in the southern capital, Jenkins, of Swanston Street, is well known for his excellent display. Otherwise the exhibition of fish for sale in either city is disappointing in the extreme, and is nothing less than an abject confession of our inability to develop our own natural resources.

There was formerly in Melbourne, however, a most admirable firm known as the Mutual Provedoring Company, whose premises were centrally situated near the main suburban railway station. Their show of fish was something to behold, and I do not remember to have seen it surpassed, even in the old country; and, in addition, they hit upon a very excellent device--one so good, in fact, that it is well worthy of imitation. That is to say they gave to every customer a capital fish cookery book, written, indeed, by our own Mrs. H. Wicken. It was a well-compiled production, and contained a goodly number of practical and economical recipes, having special regard to our Australian fish. In this way they did splendid work, as by means of the FISH DAINTIES (the title of the book) they popularised the use of fish. Now, it is greatly to be regretted that this firm no longer exists, because if ever there was a venture which deserved support, it was surely this. But I am no pessimist in these matters, and verily believe that before long this company, or one similar, will be in full swing again, and that the public will thereby benefit in every conceivable way. As far as Sydney is concerned there is a different state of affairs, and it is with genuine pleasure that I refer to the New South Wales Fresh Food and Ice Company, of whose enterprise and praiseworthy efforts I must express my sincere approbation. It is a good thing for the whole community that their endeavours have been crowned with such marked success; and I am very certain that, without any exaggeration whatever, one is justified in saying that this company have been of unmistakable service to their numerous customers, and that by their distribution of fish throughout New South Wales, quite a number of invalids, as well as of healthy people, have every reason to be grateful. Their exhibition of fish in King Street is at all times most satisfactory. Moreover, schnapper and other prime fish are often sold there as low as 4d. per lb., a price at which no one can complain.

THE DEVELOPMENT OF THE OYSTER.

Attention has been thus far entirely directed to the topic of fish, so that it now becomes necessary to turn to that of oysters. It will be found, however, that the actual state of affairs in connection with our oyster fisheries is not at all inspiriting. But before entering upon this matter it will perhaps lead to a better understanding of the whole question if some preliminary remarks are made upon the subject-heading. In doing so it will be most desirable to have recourse to an account given, not so long ago, by Professor Huxley--at that time Inspector of

Fisheries--since he speaks with the weight of authority. Referring to the oysters in the old country, he says that during the summer and autumn months, from about May to September, according to varying circumstances, the oysters pass into a peculiar condition known to the fishermen under the name of "sick." In this state the greater number contain a whitish substance, consisting of numberless granules held together by a sort of slime. The whole is known as "white spat," and the numberless granules are really the oyster eggs. Slowly and slowly the interior of the eggs assumes a darkish hue, tinging the whole mass so much that it is then termed "black spat." Within the space of a fortnight the mass of "black spat" breaks up, and the young oyster is set free.

Mr. Frank Buckland has been fortunate enough to actually see this taking place. The oyster appears to await its opportunity, it stealthily opens its shell, and a lot of spat looking like a dense cloud is ejected. After a minute or two another cloud appears, and this is continually repeated till the performance is concluded. Myriads of young oysters thus liberated from parental control now enter upon the free swimming or locomotive stage of their existence. That is to say they remain near the surface of the sea, although incessantly moving in every direction.

After a variable time, however, they suddenly descend and attach themselves to any suitable substance, on which they at once become distinctly visible in the form of white dots. In their restless stage they are scarcely discernible by the naked eye, but they settle down so rapidly and in such numbers that they appear to fall down through the water. This is known to oyster fishermen as a "fall of spat," and we shall see that this fall of spat is an important occurrence, but that it varies greatly in different seasons.

THE FAILURE IN THE NEW SOUTH WALES AND VICTORIAN OYSTER SUPPLIES.

In both New South Wales and Victoria the condition of affairs in connection with the oyster fisheries and the oyster yield is extremely discouraging. So much so, that unless something is done--and done quickly--we may have to rely mainly on outside resources for our supply. Even at the present time this is the case to a greater extent than most people have any idea of. In support of this statement, as far as New South Wales is concerned, it is only necessary to turn to the last Fisheries Report for the year ending 1890. There it is pointed out that in that year, notwithstanding the enormous length of our oyster-bearing foreshores, we are brought face to face with the fact that we are indebted to other colonies--New Zealand and Queensland--for TWO-THIRDS of our supply. Again, Mr. Lindsay Thompson, the chief inspector of New South Wales fisheries, in his recent official work, THE FISHERIES OF NEW SOUTH WALES, makes the following statements:--In the year 1871 no less than 93,000 bushels of oysters were obtained from the New South Wales beds, which, indeed, helped to supply the Victorian as well as our own needs; in the year 1883 there was a fall to 46,377 bushels; while in 1891 our fisheries yielded only 14,181 bushels. This is a very significant shrinkage, and shows a remarkable falling off in the winnings. It is still maintained by some, however, that there has been a succession of bad spatting years, and that the supply may yet reach to something of its old proportions.

It will be instructive, then, in this connection to refer briefly to the efforts which legislation has made to remedy matters in New South Wales. Under the old Oyster Beds Act of 1868 the areas given to lessees were somewhat large, and consequently what with the prolific natural supply, and a relatively small population, they appeared to be doing too well. It was urged, therefore, that the holdings should be more restricted in size, and that in this way a large number of small occupiers would be afforded a means of living, while at the same time these smaller areas would receive more attention. By the Fisheries Act of 1881 a new era dawned upon the oyster fisheries of this colony, and a system of licensing small holdings was initiated. Under this Act licensed dredging was permitted, but with such disastrous results that within two years a Fisheries Act Amendment Act had to be passed. What happened, in short, was that the beds were actually skinned, so that the total disappearance of the oyster was looming in the distance. But even the passing of this latter Act was powerless to check the evil, and by the Oyster Fisheries Act of 1884 (the present Act) there was a reversal to the old system of long leases and larger holdings. Even at the present time matters are far from perfect, and in the opinion of the Commissioners of Fisheries some radical change is necessary if oyster production is to have a place at all. Now, it is true that the present Act has checked the wholesale extermination of oysters on the part of licensed dredgers. But, unfortunately, in its passage through Parliament, some unhappy amendments totally altered the intention of the Bill. For instance, one clause makes it penal to remove oysters from a reserve or leased area without authority; but omits the protection of oysters on adjoining foreshores which may not be under lease at all; and it has accordingly happened that unprincipled persons have proceeded to rob the adjacent unleased beds of every single oyster they contained.

But while faulty and inoperative legislation may be responsible in part for the failure in our oysteries, it is certain that other causes must be at work to bring about such a disastrous result. And in the different annual reports on the fisheries of the colony this is attributed to various reasons. Thus at some places, between the

Richmond and Port Macquarie, it has been set down to the presence of quantities of decomposing sea-weed on the oyster beds; in the Manning to deposits of mud and sand; and elsewhere again to the ravages of a small worm. Besides these causes, too, it has been ascribed to the long continued absence of floods, with a consequent increased salinity of the water--the latter being considered inimical to oyster life. In the opinion of scientific writers, water containing 3 per cent. of salt is most suitable for oyster development, water above that salinity being too strong, and that below it too weak. It has also been well pointed out by Mr. henry Woodward, in his admirable pamphlet on Oyster Culture in New South Wales, that most of our deep water beds are situated in the rivers, a little way from the sea. Under favourable circumstances there is just that commingling of the fresh water from the river and the salt water from the sea which produces the oyster to perfection. In times of drought, however, the salt water drives out the oysters from the deeper beds by reason of its greater density. On the other hand, the fresh water, being the lighter, floats at the top and enables the oysters to live in the shallower parts, by maintaining the required 3 per cent. of salinity. It is evident from this, that the lessees have acted in direct opposition to this natural law, for they have stripped the oysters from the shallow water, where they would have done well, and laid them down on the deep beds, where the increased percentage of salt water has proved too much for them.

Dr. James C. Cox, of Sydney, the President of the Fisheries Commission, and our best known authority on conchology, has contributed a very valuable paper upon "The Australian Oyster, its Cultivation and Destruction," to the recent official work, THE FISHERIES OF NEW SOUTH WALES, already referred to. A brief summary of his views will, therefore, be full of interest. First of all, then, he separates oysters into three classes, namely, drift oysters, mud oysters, and rock oysters. Now, this classification must be clearly borne in mind, as it will the better enable the reader to understand what follows. He attributes the want of success in our oysteries to several causes, which have not been sufficiently heeded. One of these is that the oyster culturists have expected that the seed oysters which they obtained from between high and low water mark (rock oysters) would produce drift oysters if placed on beds on which drift oysters once throve in abundance. Dr. Cox maintains, however, that these two kinds of oysters, the rock oysters and the drift oysters, are quite different, and, as it will be seen, believes that they require different food. It can be well understood from this, then, that rock oysters will fail to grow on drift-oyster beds.

As to the mud oyster, he thinks very highly of it, and regrets that it has been so ignored by our oyster culturists. He is quite sure that if our mud oyster were cultivated and educated as it is now in Europe, it would be brought to the same perfection as the European and American oyster. It has been said of our mud oyster that it will not keep, and will not carry; but the same was said of its European representative until its cultivators came to discover that by a gradual process of raising it could be educated to keep quite long enough for all commercial purposes.

To come to the real point on which Dr. Cox considers that all oyster culture has failed in Australian waters. It is an established fact that the drift oyster and also the mud oyster require a diatomatic food for their existence. These two varieties of oysters no doubt consume other forms of food, but living diatoms constitute by far the greatest part. On the contrary, the rock oyster does not appear to need the diatomatic nutriment to sny extent, and is fed chiefly by larval forms of marine life. Thus, knowing that the drift and mud oysters require different food from the rock oyster, it is easy to see why our oyster culturists have failed in establishing new beds of oysters in various places. For the whole purport of Dr. Cox's paper may be summarised into expressing his belief that sufficient attention has not been devoted to the replenishment of our natural beds, WITH THEIR OWN KIND.

In former days, when our drift and mud oysters were in their prime, there were many pools of naturally preserved fresh water--in fact, often very extensive lakes--on the banks of many of the estuaries and inlets running up into our rivers and creeks. Now, these reservoirs appear to have been constantly supplied by subaqueous springs of fresh water, and in consequence the supply of diatomatic food was abundant. It was abundant, because, as it is well known, diatomatic life depends for its existence, to a great extent, on the presence of fresh water. These collections of fresh water no longer exist, so that the diatomatic food supply is not forthcoming to maintain the drift and the mud oyster. But there are other additional causes for the disappearance of these latter. The surrounding ground has been cleared for agricultural purposes, and the earth, broken up by ploughing, has been washed into these estuaries, and has suffocated, as it were, the oysters in their natural position. Again, the water which flows over the oysters is continually being disturbed by the different steamers passing up and down. The stirred-up mud they create gets into the gills, and destroys the oysters.

From the preceding it will be seen that Mr. Cox is of opinion that the loss of diatomatic food is one of the principal causes in diminishing the supply of drift and mud oysters, and in addition he believes that this decrease has been also brought about by muddy water. Indeed, fairly clear water is absolutely necessary for their existence. On the contrary, water loaded with any sediment interferes with the functions of the oyster so much as to destroy it. In this way floods are considered to be beneficial, and even almost necessary, to proper oyster development; for they clear out the accumulations of mud, silt, and marine vegetable growth, thus giving the beds every chance. And further, Mr. Thomas Whitelegge, of the Australian Museum, has made some investigations into what is known as the "worm disease," due to the

POLYDORA CILIATA. It was commonly suppose that it was not the worm itself which was fatal, but that by boring through the shell it afforded entrance for the fine mud, which quickly destroyed the oyster. From the result of his researches, however, Mr. Whitelegge believes that the young worm simply swims into the open oyster, and that it immediately begins to construct a tube and collect a large quantity of mud. The worms appear to have the power of collecting a large quantity of mud in a very short time. The mud is covered over at once by the oyster with a thin layer of shelly matter, thus enveloping the worm, together with its mud. After this, one of two things happens: if the oyster be healthy, it envelops the worm and mud so quickly as to dispose of the intruder for good; but, on the other hand, if the oyster be unhealthy, or already infested, the shelly deposition is far slower, as a consequence of which the worm gains the ascendency, and the oyster succumbs.

In Victoria, too, the oyster fisheries are in a most unsatisfactory condition. According to Mr. Saville Kent, the author of THE GREAT BARRIER REEF OF AUSTRALIA and formerly Commissioner of Fisheries in several of the Australian colonies, and who is qualified to speak on these matters, the destruction of the oyster there has been brought about by sedimentary deposits, by parasitic growths, such as sponges, mussels, ascidians, and sea-weed; by the attacks of the dog-whelk and other natural enemies; and by their continual removal by human agency. He points out that there are the remains of magnificent natural beds in different parts, but that they are on the verge of ruin through neglect on the one hand and the invasion of poachers on the other. In short, he very plainly shows that unless active measures be taken for their general resuscitation and development, Victoria will have to look elsewhere for her oyster supply.

THE RE-CREATION OF OUR OYSTER FISHERIES.

If one only looks to the conduct of some of those who have been engaged in our oyster fisheries, the reason for their present defective state will be readily apparent. The Fisheries Commissioners well express it when they state that "If a person takes up ground only for the purpose of collecting and selling whatever oysters he finds upon it, and bestows no care in providing for the continuity of the supply, that ground must cease to be productive." And apart from this it will be found that even when every effort has been made to provide for continuous supply, yet the matter is by no means easy.

The truth is the oyster fisheries have been managed in a happy-go-lucky way. There has been but little care taken in their conservation, and the inevitable result is that the winnings, as the official figures show, are rapidly failing. The same thing is not peculiar to Australia, however, and has happened everywhere else where the same careless policy has been pursued. We have, then, a grain of comfort from the fact that it is not confined to us. In our own case the Fisheries Commissioners have repeatedly called attention to the need for certain legislative reform in connection with our oysteries. They assert, in fact, that "it is absolutely imperative that our oyster beds and deposits must be regulated on quite a different system to that which obtains under the existing law."

Mr. Saville Kent, who has been investigating the cause of failure in connection with the oyster fisheries of Victoria, not so long ago, has made some interesting recommendations. The principle of his system is to establish on selected spots, in the neighbourhood of the formerly most productive natural oyster grounds, small Government reserves, whereon stocks of oysters shall be laid down and carefully cultivated for breeding purposes. He points out that the capacity of oysters for breeding is greatly augmented when they are collected together in a small space, in comparison with that of equal numbers thinly scattered over my extensive area. Each reserve in this way constitutes a prolific breeding centre for stocking the surrounding waters, and by this means alone the process of restoring the natural beds is quickly accelerated.

Indeed, he is particularly careful to draw attention to the fact that in the previously attempted establishment of artificial oyster fisheries a prominent error was in working too large areas. One or two acres intelligently cultivated can be made to produce far more substantial results than a very large area under inefficient management, and at much less expenditure of time and money. A vast amount of money has been expended in different localities on the Victorian coast for the purpose of developing the oyster fisheries. In the great majority of cases, however, the site selected was unsuitable for such a purpose, and the mode of culture adopted impracticable and inefficient. For instance, one place was the recipient of a vast amount of sedimentary deposits. Here he found that they had surrounded the chosen areas with fences of great height and strength, and closely wattled, for the purpose of catching and retaining the young oyster brood. Instead of this, however, they had simply acted as "catch-pits," which had accumulated soft oozy mud to the depth of several feet, and a few dead oyster shells were the only result.

Instead of such an evident failure as this, he recommends oyster-spat collectors of two kinds, one consisting of extra thick split palings 4 ft. long by 8 in. wide, with a brick attached to each end to weigh them down, and at the same time to raise them off the ground. Several of them on being raised for inspection, after three months, were found to have over 1,000 embryo oysters adhering to them. The other form of spat collector he employs consists of cemented slates, arranged ridge-wise on light ti-tree frames, and in some localities these were found to be even more efficacious than the palings.

In the old country the same necessity for oyster culture is well recognised. In an interesting address given not so long ago, Professor Huxley, after referring to the growing scarcity of the bivalve, expressed his belief that the only hope for the oyster consumer was first in oyster culture, and secondly in discovering a means of breeding oysters under such conditions that all the spat was safely deposited. France has done more than any other country in the world in the artificial culture of the oyster. Not many years ago the oyster fisheries there were in danger of absolute extinction--a state of affairs brought about by reckless and unrestricted fishing, without any effort to provide for a re-supply. Mainly through the efforts of M. Coste, the propagation of oysters was scientifically carried out, with a result that has even exceeded the marvellous. According to a recent French official report, the Bay of Arcachon contained in the year 1807, 20 private PARCS, or district oyster beds. In the year 1865 these had increased to the number of 297, with an output of 10,000,000 oysters. In the year 1887, the area under cultivation in the same bay amounted to 15,000 acres, and produced 300,000,000 oysters. In addition to this, a still later report attributes the present flourishing condition of this industry "to the steps primarily initiated by the Government, and to the necessity of upholding this success by continuing the same system of administrative supervision, together with the practical illustration in the Government model PARCS of the most perfected methods of oyster culture, for the benefit of private cultivators."

And lastly, if we require further evidence in support of the necessity for ostreiculture, we have only to turn to America. A falling off in the supply led to an inquiry into the cause by the United States Fish Commission. Professor Goode, in his review of the work accomplished by this body, writes, INTER ALIA:--"The important distinction between the extermination of a species and the destruction of a fishery should be noted. In the case of fixed animals like the sponge, the mussel, and the oyster, the colonies or beds may be practically exterminated, exactly as a forest may be cut down. The preservation of the oyster beds is a matter of vital importance to the United States, for oyster fishing unsupported by oyster culture will, within a short period, destroy the employment of tens of thousands, and the cheap and favourite food of tens of millions." "Something," the professor proceeds to say, "may be effected by laws which allow each oyster bed to rest for a period of years after each season of fishing upon it. It is the general belief, however, that shell-fish beds must be cultivated as carefully as garden beds, and that this can only be done by leasing them to individuals. It is probable that the present unregulated methods will prevail until the dredging of the natural beds ceases to be remunerative, and that the oyster industry will then be transferred from the improvident fisherman to the care-taking oyster-culturists." We are thus led to the inevitable conclusion that if our Australian oyster fisheries are to be re-created, it will be necessary to follow in the same lines. With that object in view, therefore, it will be needful to devise suitable legislative enactments to protect our oyster fisheries and to foster ostreiculture at the same time. We must benefit, in short, by the experience derived from other parts of the world where ostreiculture has been carried to a state of absolute perfection.

THE FOOD VALUE OF THE OYSTER.

In the first place I shall begin by affirming that it would be a difficult matter indeed to say too much in favour of the oyster. It is as highly appreciated at the present day as it was by the Romans hundreds of years ago, and it is certain that in centuries to come it will be found occupying a similar unrivalled position. At the same time, it must not be forgotten that it is not every person who cares for the oyster, showing that there are various forms of affliction; and we find, accordingly, that there is no half-heartedness about the like or dislike for the oyster--it is either held in the loftiest admiration, or looked upon almost with repugnance. It is both food for the sick-room and food for the strong man. It is one of the most valuable forms of nourishment for the growing child, and it gives strength to those of declining years. It is specially appropriate for the brain worker, and yet it is deservedly in great repute with the muscle user--whether athlete or artisan. It is the opening ceremony at our feasts, while it reigns supreme at supper. In short, there is everything to be said for it, while not a single word can be urged against it.

But if it is thus so highly appreciated in health, it is in disease that it is at its best; for here it occupies a place which nothing else can fill. Indeed, after many cases of acute or serious illness, the oyster is one of the first things which the patient looks for. In many chronic disorders, too, it is absolutely without a rival. Thus, in anaemia, where the blood is so poor, it restores the strength; in bronchitis and other chest diseases it helps to relieve the loaded tubes of phlegm; in consumption and similar wasting maladies it conserves the vital powers; in debility it creates new force; in indigestion it is often digestible when all else is indigestible; in nervous disease it renews the nervous energy. The list, in fact, might be multiplied indefinitely, but enough has been instanced to prove the value of the oyster. It should be added, in conclusion, that it is best eaten raw, with its juice, which is its blood mixed with sea-water. A squeeze of lemon is generally employed to bring out its flavour, and, for those who are not invalids, a sensation of cayenne pepper is distinctly an improvement.

THE FOOD VALUE OF FISH.

Along with its great ally, the oyster, fish undoubtedly occupies one of the highest places on the food list. Unfortunately, it is not met with in every home as it should be, its high price and scarcity combining to make it conspicuous by its absence. That such a state of things is actually the case in Australia can only be deeply deplored. Let us suppose, for instance, that we were as well supplied with fish as we are entitled to be, considering that we are of a maritime race and that we live near the sea. If such were the case--and I would it were so-- how would a sudden reversal to the present state of our fish supply be received? Would it not give rise to protestations, to indignation meetings, to questionings in the House, and to the papers being filled with complaints, till matters were put right again? Yes, indeed, all these things would happen! meanwhile, however, we continue placidly in our fishless state of existence, and the finny tribe, outside in the deep sea, have a good time in consequence.

It may seem of little use, therefore, to call attention to the value of fish when we are practically bereft of it. But as some improvement may come about in course of time, the attempt will not be altogether thrown away. First of all, then, it is worthy of note that in the old country that advocate for rational feeding, Sir Henry Thompson, has recently expressed his opinion that a large proportion of the town population would profit by exchanging some of their meat, as an article of daily diet, for fish. He further adds that the digestive system is apt to become overloaded and oppressed by meals consisting chiefly of meat, and that many a constitution suffers from an over-supply in this way, which cannot be remedied without a considerable amount of exercise. That being the case in the old country, with its cold, damp climate, these facts are intensified a thousandfold when they are applied to our semi-tropical existence. Dr. T. K. Chambers, also, another authority on all that pertains to diet, is an advocate for a more general use of fish in our daily life; and, as he sagely observes, every sort is best when it is cheapest, for it is then most plentiful and in fullest season. Then, again, we have Dr. F.W. Pavy, who is well qualified to speak on these matters, observing that fish is an important article of food. For, as he proceeds to point out, the health and vigour of the inhabitants of the fishing towns, where fish may form the only kind of animal food consumed, show that it is capable of contributing, in an effective manner, to the maintenance of the body under active conditions of life. Dr. Horace Dobell, too, tells us how nearly fish represents in food value as equal weight of meat, and how important it is to other forms of animal food as a mixed diet. Indeed, it would be possible to adduce similar statements to an indefinite extent, but my main object in making these references is to call attention to the value of fish as ordinary diet. And although it hae an every-day value of this kind, there are in addition certain qualities ascribed to fish which render it particularly appropriate for a large and important section of our population.

I refer to the brain workers. I say large and important, because in their ranks are to be found literary men and journalists, members of the professions, active-minded, busy men of the commercial world, and the vast array of those having mental work and clerical occupations. In one of the latest books on the subject of food and diet by Dr. Burney Yeo, he remarks that it is the custom to speak of fish as an "intellectual" or "brain" food, on account of the phosphorus contained in it. But he adds that much of its reputation in this respect may be due to its being readily digested by persons of sedentary and studious habits. He proceeds to quote Louis Agassiz, the famous naturalist, who bestows upon fish the following:--"Refreshing to the organism, especially for intellectual labour; not that its use can turn an idiot into a wise or witty man, but a fish diet cannot be otherwise than favourable to brain development."

But if fish is thus a necessary and desirable element in the dietary of our active daily life, it is not to be forgotten that it is at least equally valuable for the invalid. It is often tolerated by the stomach when the digestive powers are weakened from any cause. When the system is recruiting after any exhausting illness, it is usually amongst the earliest forms of nourishment allowed. In many chronic disorders, likewise, it is just one of those things whose place it would be impossible to fill. And, lastly, it should be ever remembered that many men whose lives are passed in a state of perfect thraldom by reason of their extravagant use of butcher's meat would find themselves better in health, better in spirits, and better in temper, were they to curtail their allowance, substituting fish in its place.

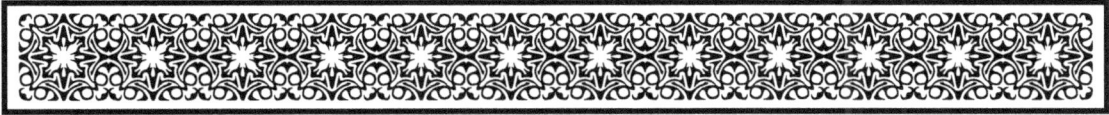

CHAPTER XI.
ON SALADS; SALAD PLANTS AND HERBS; AND SALAD MAKING.

"A SALAD IS A DELICACY WHICH THE POOREST OF US OUGHT ALWAYS TO COMMAND."

Although for some years past any information pertaining to salads and salad-making has been eagerly welcomed by the writer, yet it must be admitted that great difficulties in obtaining such know-ledge in Australia do exist, because the use and value of salads are not widespread and understood, and thus it is that their health-conferring properties are passed by seemingly without regret. And if the topic, therefore, is one possessing an attractive personal interest, for that very reason it is felt that the present chapter falls far short of what might be achieved; yet it may be permissible to plead in extenuation thereof that its composition has not proved the easiest of tasks, and its shortcomings must consequently be condoned by an indulgent public. I shall begin, then, by saying that if ever there was a form of food which was intended for our semi-tropical climate it is undoubtedly the salad, and as thus constituting an article of diet so well adapted for Australia it should certainly be seen daily in every household. It is so appropriately suitable for use amongst us that it deserves to be intituled "the sea-breeze of the table," for in addition to its invigorating qualities, it cleanses, while at the same time it enriches, the blood. The late gifted George Dallas did not go too far when he asserted that a salad was not merely food, but that it had also an exhilarating effect and a distinct action upon the nervous system, which was immensely agreeable and acted like a spell.

It seems more suitable, however, instead of abruptly plunging into the matter of salad concoction, to say a few words from a culinary point of view on the art of making life enjoyable, and thus to draw attention to the curious neglect which is shown to a form of food within the reach of all classes, and whose use would be of the greatest advantage to the health and pleasing to the palate. At the same time, although an ardent believer in the distinct benefit which would be derived by the entire community from the adoption of a mode of living more in harmony with their climatic surroundings, yet I must disclaim any desire to pose as a "faddist." In truth, there are too many worthy people who would submit all the world to their theories in a Procrustean fashion, and who see in their particular hobby a panacea for the whole of human frailties and human sufferings. Instead, therefore, of dilating on the undeniable consequences attached to the reasonless use of animal food at present followed throughout Australia, I shall content myself with a few remarks on the art of living. By far the greater number of people pay too little attention to the present, and imperil their happiness with the hope that at some future period, when they will have put a little together, they will be enabled to thoroughly lay themselves out for enjoyment. But in the vast majority of cases these halcyon days never arrive, or, if they do, it is more than probable the health is undermined by the neglect of those very matters which should form part and parcel of one's daily existence. It is the exact parallel to a man hurrying through many fields and parks and gardens for the purpose of enjoying, from some high eminence, the scene through which he has passed. In his desperate haste to attain his object he disregards all that is beautiful and interesting, only to find that his travelling is nearly over, and that his steps cannot be retraced. On the other hand, a far more philosophic frame of mind belongs to him who, as he proceeds onwards through life's journey, gets a rational enjoyment out of his existence, so that his days pass pleasantly and his health receives the consideration it deserves. It will appear somewhat mundane in this connection to assert that the latter and, therefore, happiness are to a great extent dependent upon the mode of living, but nevertheless it is absolutely true, and thus it is that I come back to the quotation at the beginning of this chapter-- "A salad is a delicacy which the poorest of us ought always to command."

You will remember that the Duc de la Rochefoucauld, in those marvellous essays and maxims of his, says that notwithstanding the disparity of men's fortunes happiness is equally distributed. He was doubtless right, more especially as he looked at the matter from a Frenchman's point of view, for it must be remembered that to the great body of people in that country life is more pleasant than to the rest of humanity. Indeed, on this point Mr. Sept. Berdmore declares that in France dishes are cooked by the humblest which would be appreciated if they appeared on the menu of the best club in London, and he avows, moreover, it possesses the greatest national school of cookery that has ever existed. But, on the contrary, as far as Australia is concerned, the state of affairs in the culinary art with the bulk of the people is simply deplorable, and it seems. well nigh hopeless for any improvement to be brought about. There is, however, one little ray of light at the end of this dark tunnel we are in, and it is the knowledge that the cookery classes in the public schools will by-and-by bring about important changes, resulting in the amelioration of the whole of the culinary habits at present, curiously, supposed to exist. And it is gratifying to know that the admirable cookery classes at the Technical College, under the able guidance of Mrs. Wicken, are making the most excellent progress and producing brilliant results.

These altruistic reflections, however, have somewhat drifted us
away from the matter under consideration, so that it becomes necessary
to revert again to the main subject. Now, even at the risk of being
regarded as wearisome, I propose to consider somewhat fully the
different steps to be followed in the preparation of a simple salad,
for it will be noticed that in all the cookery books the directions
given for the concoction of a salad are most meagre and wanting in
detail. In addition to this want of information, too, it is quite
evident that the instructions have never been actually followed by the
compilers of these works themselves, or they would signally fail if
they attempted to follow their own advice. Furthermore, even those who
pride themselves on the knowledge of the preparation of food for the
table are often surprisingly misinformed on the subject of salad-making.
It will be as well at this stage, consequently, to refer to the
plan usually followed by English people, so as the better to contrast
the two methods--the faulty or English with the correct or French.
Well then, English people almost invariably cut their lettuce first
into halves, and next into quarters. These latter are then placed in
water to soak for some time, and are afterwards laid on a plate to
drain. In this way the leaves are supposed to be thoroughly cleansed,
but as a matter of fact deep down between the leaves are the minute
insects, which are left undisturbed. The next proceeding is to cut the
leaves into very fine shreds, to add a few slices of hard-boiled egg,
and finally to pour over the whole a mysterious mixture known as
salad-dressing. Thus is produced the orthodox English salad, which
everyone, probably from patriotic motives, pronounces to be extremely
nice. In the French preparation of a salad, however, each single leaf is
detached and carefully cleansed, some needing simply wiping, while
others require absolute washing. Every leaf, be it borne in mind,
before going into the salad bowl must be perfectly dry, or else
the first great principle of salad making will be infringed, for oil
and water refuse to mingle. In preparing a French salad, too, the
stalks or coarse ribs are removed from the middle part of each leaf,

and the larger leaves also are carefully divided into halves. The whole leaf is not chopped up into shreds, as in the English salad. After this the drying of the leaves is best accomplished by placing them within a clean towel. Instead of the towel a wire basket, panier a salade, is more convenient and is generally used in France; it should be easily obtainable for a shilling or two. In using the towel the four corners are held together in the right hand, and the whole is repeatedly brought sharply round with a swing of the arm, stopping with a sudden jerk, till all the water is driven off 011 the floor. Herein consists the excellence of the French method, for the leaves are thoroughly cleansed, the acrid parts are removed, and the leaves are perfectly dry. On a small plate, near by, are usually three or four heaps of finely-chopped herbs (FINES HERBES), namely, burnet, chervil, chives, tarragon, mustard and cress, or even parsley; these constitute what is known as "the fourniture" of the salad. The lettuce leaves, on being taken out of the towel, are then placed within the bowl, and over them is daintily spread whatever is required from each of the little heaps of herbs already referred to. A little salt is next to be quietly tapped over the salad, and the spoon salad-server is then filled once or twice with the best salad-oil, and this is now sprinkled on the salad, carefully turning the leaves over the while so as to obtain the thinnest possible film of oil equally distributed over the whole surface of each leaf. The salad spoon is next half-filled with the best vinegar, and the latter liquid is now most carefully added, only a drop or so at a time, so as to diffuse it uniformly throughout the whole. The thorough incorporation of the oil, but more particularly of the vinegar, with the salad requires to be done with a light hand to avoid bruising the leaves, and consists in stirring it and dexterously bringing up the under leaves.

This comparison, however, between the methods of preparing salads according to the English and the French fashion is not quite complete, and consequently it will be advisable to refer to one or two other matters, of which it is necessary to be apprised in order to produce a perfect salad. In the first place, the form of the salad bowl itself is very important, for it will readily be apparent that it must be of such a shape as to facilitate the complete blending of the oil and vinegar with the materials used. That which is nearest to half a perfect sphere is by far the best; and another essential is that it should be of sufficient size to afford room for free manipulation. On looking in the windows orle is fairly astonished at the diversity of shapes that are exposed for sale. In most of them the floor of the bowl is flat, with a sort of recess all round its margin. This, of course, is most ill-adapted for the purpose for which it is intended. Nearly all of them, again, are by far too small; it is impossible to mix a salad properly in a vessel very little larger than a soup plate. So that in the selection of a salad bowl see that it is the nearest approach to half a perfect sphere in shape, and take care that it is roomy enough for freely working the salad. Lastly, do not waste money on the meretricious ornamental world which besets so many of the bowls exposed for sale. A very good substitute can be made in the ordinary large earthenware basin used in the kitchen, the deeper the better, which will be found to answer every purpose, and its cost brings it within the reach of every purse. Next, with regard to the servers, these are usually supplied with the bowl, but wooden servers are considered by many to be the best, and price is certainly no drawback. The oil, too, must be the purest you can buy, and Crosse and Blackwell's is as good as any; at least, I do not know of a better oil at present, as it is sweet and without the slightest suspicion of rankness. So, too, with regard to vinegar: pay a little more for a good article, and you will have no cause to regret it. The best French, or Crosse and Blackwell's white wine vinegar, is good enough for anybody. You will find that the oil and the vinegar will last a long time, and that the cost of making a salad is actually the veriest trifle. In making a plain lettuce salad such as has been described, you will, of course, have to do without the chopped herbs, because, unfortunately, we in

Australia have not risen to the necessity for their cultivation, but you can make shift with small pieces of celery, which taste admirably in the salad, or little bits of radish, or thin slices of cucumber-- whatever, in fact, happens to be in season.

There is a remarkable condition of affairs obtaining in Sydney, and the same applies to the other metropolitan centres of Australia. On turning up our directory for the current year it will be found on reference that the number of butchers for the city and suburbs is nearly 600. On the other hand, the number of those whose calling is given as that of greengrocer does not reach 300. Now, it is not to be denied that a goodly proportion of vegetables are sold by dealers whose address is not to be found under the latter heading. Nevertheless, it is still a significant fact that while many of the butchers' establishments possess quite an attractive and inviting appearance, on the contrary those devoted to the sale of greengrocery are represented by dingy-looking places, and by a collection of faded vegetables which seem always to be apologising for being on view at all. The show of meat which is to be found in our Australian capitals is certainly worthy city in the world, and if the display of vegetables were only equal to it, as it assuredly should be, there would be at least something on which we might congratulate ourselves.

Another fact which is equally to be deplored with this small display of vegetables seen throughout the city is the few varieties which are cultivated. In a former chapter attention was drawn to the nutritious properties and exquisite flavour of many vegetables which are easily grown, but which are most unaccountably passed over, and it will be remembered that the tomato was instanced in particular as having a desperate struggle for existence, and that it was years and years before it was finally received into favour. Similarly in the case of salad plants there is the same matter for complaint, and beyond the ordinary cabbage lettuce, celery, cucumbers, and radishes, there is nothing grown. And yet there ought to be inducement enough for many of our young men to devote themselves to such a healthy occupation as market gardening, with profit to themselves and with benefit to the community. The market gardens around Paris, although small, are cultivated to perfection. The French market gardeners, moreover, are, as a rule, a very prosperous class; they keep to themselves, and marry among themselves. On making inquiries from the leading seedsmen throughout Australia, and asking what varieties of salad plants are mostly in vogue, you find that the cabbage lettuce is almost the sole representative. And thus it is that in the very climate where the system calls for salads, so to speak, there is absolutely no attempt made to supply a crying want. A brief reference to a few of these salad plants will better illustrate the importance of their culture. Here, as with the different vegetables, I applied to headquarters for information, namely, to Mr. F. Turnen, of the Department of Agriculture, Sydney, who once more came to my assistance and courteously indicated the localities in which they are likely to do well. And it only seems fitting and appropriate here to remark that Australia's road to prosperity lies through her agriculture; the hydro-cephalic growth visible in every colony is unnatural and needs rectification.

Lettuce.----Of this there are two varieties, the ordinary cabbage lettuce and the cos, so named from the Island of Cos in the Aegean Sea, which is also known as the upright, or smooth-leaved lettuce. Although this latter is to be obtained, yet in nine cases out of ten only the cabbage lettuce is procurable. But, as a matter of fact, the upright or smooth-leaved cos lettuce is of a more delicate flavour, and when grown properly by having the leaves loosely tied together at the top about ten days before cutting, it is more crisp and juicy, and better adapted for saladings. In the old country, too, the cos variety, with its long leaves, is common enough, and is there preferred to the cabbage lettuce. It is to be regretted, therefore, that we see so little of it.

Endive.--Now, here is a noble salad plant of which even the very name is hardly known by the greater number of our people. There are practically two classes of endive, the broad-leaved or Batavian variety, and the curly-leaved endive. Both sorts, however, must be well blanched if perfection is required. It is true that the curly-leaved endive is at times to be obtained here, but it is extensively cultivated in England, as it is very crisp and tender, while it also possesses a piquancy which is greatly appreciated. Nevertheless, the plain or Batavian kind (the ESCAROLE of the French) has also its admirers, particularly for salad purposes. Now, it is to be carefully noted that the accompaniments, or "fourniture," of these two varieties of endive are vastly different. With the Batavian it usually is formed of chervil, tarragon, and that delicate alliaceous salad herb, chives. On the other hand, a chapon is used with the curly endive; it consists of a crust of bread over which a clove of garlic has been rubbed. This is thrown into the bowl and tossed about during the process of mixing the salad, and gives to it a delightful effect. In addition to its use as a salad, the curly-leaved endive makes a particularly good garnish for grills, such as chops, steaks, &c.; and, by the way, Sir Henry Thompson, the eminent surgeon, remarks that the sauce PAR EXCELLENCE for grills is mushroom ketchup. But before leaving the endive it is as well to refer to a blood relation, namely, the wild endive or chicory. When its large, fleshy roots are dried in a kiln, roasted and ground, they become familiarly known by their admixture with coffee. This plant, the succory of former days, is greatly esteemed by the French, by whom it is known as barbe de capucin. To meet the great demand for it large quantities are sold in the neighbourhood of Paris in order to produce this salading. Its young leaves are used for this purpose, but they must be thoroughly blanched so as to take away every particle of bitterness.

Corn Salad.--This hardy annual salad plant is believed to derive its name from the fact that it grows spontaneously in the grain-fields. It is also known as lamb's lettuce, and in America as fetticus. Here is an example of a once well-known plant dropping out of use, for one of the earliest-known salads was this same corn salad, on which was laid a red herring. But now-a-days it is called MACHE in Covent Garden Market, where it has been sent over from France. This lamb's lettuce is greatly appreciated on the Continent, and makes one of the best of salads, especially when mixed with celery. As it can be easily grown in all the coastal districts and in the cooler parts of Australia, it is certainly a matter for regret that we are not favoured with it.

In addition to the preceding, namely, the cos lettuce, the two varieties of endive, the chicory, and the corn salad, or lamb's lettuce, there are one or two other salad plants which require a brief notice. Now, as far as celery and radishes are concerned, we may be said to be fairly well off; but the same is not the case with mustard, with garden cress, or even with watercress. The latter is to be obtained from John Chinaman, it is true; but it is curious that in Australia we see none of the watercress vendors so familiar in the streets of the old country.. Yet there is really a good living to be made out of it, and its use would prove of benefit to hundreds of families, as with a little salt it makes an exquisite sandwich between two thin pieces of bread-and-butter. A wise physician, Dr. T.K. Chambers, uttered a great truth when he remarked that the pale faces and bad teeth which characterised many of the inhabitants of cities were due to their inability to obtain a proper supply of fresh green vegetables, and that thus the watercress-seller was one of the saviours of her country. So great is the demand for watercress in New York when it first comes in that the prices range from 2s. to 4s. for a basket holding only three quarts. At this rate an acre of watercress under cultivation would represent almost a fortune. Of course all watercress should be thoroughly washed and then dried in a towel, like the lettuce for the salad, before it is eaten. Lastly, it must never be used from a source where any sewage contamination is suspected.

Now, although these different forms of salad plants are not cultivated to any considerable extent, yet when we come to inquire into the salad herbs, we find that they are not grown at all, and indeed they are practically unknown. They constitute, however, the crowning grace of a proper salad, and confer upon it a delicacy which is unrivalled, and thus it is that any traveller will tell you that a salad in France tastes so infinitely better than one elsewhere. Now, these salad herbs are readily grown, and do not require any care in their cultivation, so that there is no opportunity for excuse on that score. In order, however, to prevent this paper becoming too diffuse, I must confine my remarks to those salad herbs which it is almost impossible to do without--that is, if we wish to have any salads worth speaking of. It will be convenient, for this purpose, to refer to the word "ravigote"; and by this term is meant a collection of four herbs, namely--burnet, chervil, chives, and tarragon. As has been already mentioned, each of these herbs, chopped up very finely, is usually placed in a little heap by itself on the one plate, and from these four heaps is selected whatever is required for the salad. This invariably forms the garniture of any lettuce salad, whether cabbage or cos, and also of the Batavian endive, though, as we have already seen, the curly endive is best suited with the chapon--i.e., the crust of bread rubbed over with a garlic clove. The very derivation of the word "ravigote," from the French verb RAVIGOTER, to cheer or strengthen, shows that certain exhilarating virtues are ascribed to these herbs.

Burnet.--This is also known as salad burnet, and is a hardy herb, which will continue green during the greater part of the year. The young and tender leaves possess a smell and taste almost identical with cucumber, and greatly enhance the flavour of the salad. These leaves, when blanched, are sprinkled over the latter; but in addition burnet enters into the composition of ravigote butter, and helps to form green mayonnaise. It hardly requires any culture whatever, and will do well in the coastal districts and in all the cooler localities. With all these advantages, therefore, we can only marvel why it is denied us.

Chervil.--Of the two varieties which are cultivated elsewhere than in Australia--namely, the common chervil and the curled variety--the latter is generally considered the better. It grows about twenty inches high, and has deeply divided leaves, which are aromatic, and which are thus absolutely a necessary component of any well-ordered salad. The plant will grow everywhere, and, as it is never seen, it is only one instance out of the many which might be adduced, that much is neglected in Australian cultivation which would be of advantage to the whole community.

Chives.--This is the most delicate of all the onion family; it occupies the one end of the scale, while garlic presides at the other; and midway between these we find the spring onion, the shallot, and the onion itself. It is a delightful salad herb which is too much neglected, and it is worthily entitled to cultivation in Australia. It gives to the salad a piquancy and an agreeable pungent flavour, which, while it faintly recalls that of the onion, is yet free from the accentuated properties of the latter. In addition to lending such an enhancement to salads, chives may be used for soups. The plant itself is a hardy bulb, growing to a height of about eight inches, and it is the tender tops which are used for saladings. It can be easily propagated, and will grow readily in all the cooler districts.

Tarragon.--This used popularly to be known in the old country as "herb dragon," whereas it is now vested with the newer title. It is frequently to be found there is the country gardens, where it is in repute for the preparation of tarragon vinegar. It, however, occupies a position second to none as a salad accessory. It is one of the most odoriferous of the pot herbs, and gives to a salad a delightful aromatic warmth. At present all that one can do in the concoction of a salad is to make use of the tarragon vinegar, which is so admirably put up by Messrs. Crosse and Blackwell. Those who are fortunate enough to possess the plant itself should keep the leaves, as when dried they retain their flavour for some time. It is recommended, however, that the young plants should be propagated each year by division of the roots, as the plants of the first and second years are more delicate than those of older growth. It can easily be grown over the greater part of Australia, but I am not going to say more than that we are needlessly bereft of what we might enjoy.

In drawing attention to any matter connected with the subject of this chapter, a brief reference to mayonnaise sauce must necessarily find a place. This may be used with all endless variety of salads, but it is particularly concerned in the preparation of chicken, and also of crayfish salad. On looking through the cookery-books one gets perfectly bewildered with the different directions laid down by the various authors. This mayonnaise sauce, however, is so very important that it becomes an absolute necessity to know the successive steps in its preparation, for, though easily made, yet there is a right and a wrong way of going about it. Through the kindly offices of that accomplished aristologist, Dr. A. Burne, I was enabled to have some practical instruction in making mayonnaise sauce at the hands of the CHEF of the Cosmopolitan Club, and I will endeavour, therefore, to give an account of how he went to work.

The bowl he employed to mix it was about 9 in. across at the top, and its floor was rounded in shape, just as a salad bowl should be, to facilitate the thorough incorporation of the ingredients. Then, taking a couple of eggs, he broke each one by knocking its side midway between the two ends against the rim of the bowl. The greater part of the white of the egg was allowed to escape into a small vessel next the bowl, as it is not required for the mayonnaise, but comes in handy for other culinary purposes. He now, with the yolk in one half of the shell, poured away all the white remaining in the other half. Next he dexterously turned the yolk into this latter emptied shell and then got rid of the white left in the half previously occupied by the yolk. One egg was thus served in this way, and then the other, and the two yolks were slipped into the bowl and broken up with a few stirs of the egg-whisk. This latter is readily purchased from any ironmonger for the modest sum of one shilling. The next proceeding was a wrinkle which is worth knowing, and it consisted of placing, within the bowl about a salt-spoonful of the ordinary dry mustard. This was well beaten up in a second or two. About a tablespoonful of good vinegar was next added, the whisk going vigorously to work, and thus blending well together egg yolk, dry mustard, and vinegar. At this stage occurred a sort of halt or breathing time in the manipulation, as the chief peculiarity of the mayonnaise now began. The CHEF, with his left hand, managed to tilt up the salad bowl and to hold a bottle of salad oil at the same time. The latter being inverted, he kept it over the contents of the bowl in such a way as to allow only a drop or so of the oil to escape at a time. Drip, drip, drip, went the oil, and as his right hand kept unceasingly plying the mixture with the whisk I could not help noticing what a fine wristy action he had. Almost directly as the oil touched it the mayonnaise began to thicken, to swell, and to change in colour. The remorseless whisk almost seemed to lash it into foam, and now the oil came faster and faster till the amber-looking sauce was ready, and all this within the space of at most two or three minutes. I suppose he must have used quite a teacupful of olive oil. Only one thing more: after stirring in a sufficient quantity of pepper and salt, the CHEF desired me to taste the result, and as I did so I read the triumph in his eye--it was superb.

It has been my aim, indeed my only aim, all through this chapter, to bring into prominence the important fact that the salad is a dish which is at once within the reach of every family, and moreover that it is one which is fairly a necessity in our semi-tropical climate. For these very reasons, consequently, I have endeavoured to give the fullest directions for the mixing of a simple salad. But it may be that after becoming thoroughly expert at making this latter, and being flushed with success, the aspirant for saladic honours will be desirous of a more ambitious essay. Some instructions for the famous herring salad have therefore been added, and it can be reserved for high days and holidays, or as a lordly dish wherewith to entertain a much-esteemed guest. It is slightly altered from a valuable recipe given to me by my very good friend Mr. Ludwig Bruck, and is made as follows:-- Two salt Dutch herrings are to be obtained. These are imported in casks, and when purchased have a somewhat pronounced odour, which is removed by the soaking. If milt herrings are used, the milt should be moistened with a little vinegar and rubbed up into a paste, and this should be kept to pour over the salad just before the dressing is added. If roe herrings are bought, the roe should be soaked in vinegar for a few minutes, the eggs then separated and kept for sprinkling over the salad similarly to the preceding. The herring heads and tails are to be removed and discarded; the bodies should be gutted, skinned, and washed, and then they must be soaked in water or milk for three hours-- the latter enhancing the flavour greatly. After the soaking the bones should be removed and the flesh cut into small dice-like cubical pieces, and the latter are then set aside in a basin. The next thing is to peel and core two sourish apples, and then to cut them up into small cubes like the herrings. To the apples should DOW be added two pickled gherkins, and, if you like, some boiled beetroot and a few capers, and these--excepting, of course, the capers--should be divided into the same small pieces. If you wish to have the real herring salad, a quarter of a pound of cold roast veal, also in small pieces, will likewise be required. Whatever you may choose to use of these is now to be well mixed together while the next direction is attended to. It is only fair to note here that Mr. Lang, formerly of the German Club, who prepares the best herring salads in Sydney, always adds a little cold roast beef, cold ham, and boiled ox tongue. While all this is being prepared two potatoes should be boiled with their jackets on.

They should then be immediately peeled and cut up into small pieces like the other ingredients. While now hot the potato is added to the preceding, and everything is thoroughly mixed together; it is necessary to use the potato warm, for if cold it would set hard. The methods of using the milt or the roe of the herring have already been respectively indicated, and after this matter has been attended to, all that is now needful to complete the herring salad is to pour over it some mayonnaise sauce, the preparation of which has been previously described.

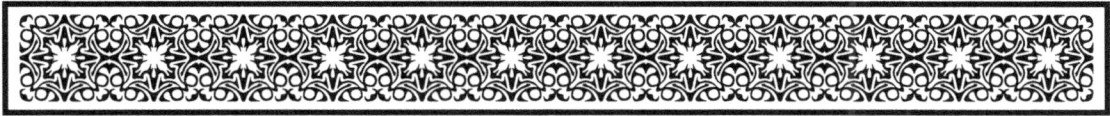

CHAPTER XII.
ON AUSTRALIAN WINE, AND ITS PLACE IN THE AUSTRALIAN DAILY DIETARY.

"WITH TIME AND CARE AUSTRALIA OUGHT TO BE THE VINEYARD OF THE WORLD."--
GREATER BRITAIN.

Were I asked to name the one industry on which the prosperity of Australia must sooner or later rest, I should unhesitatingly answer, "On the cultivation of the vine." And this must be so; for while there is every reason to know that it will be called for from abroad, it is absolutely certain that it will be required in our own territories. The chief purpose of this chapter, indeed, is to insist upon the value of our own wines as the most healthful and the most wholesome drink for Australian use. It is a strange anomaly this, that at the present period of our existence a declaration of this kind should be necessary. Yet it is only in keeping with the rest of our food habits, with their perpetual challenge to our semi-tropical environment; and hence we are confronted with the astounding fact that although we are practically Southern Europe, yet we follow a mode of living suitable only for a rigorous climate and a land of ice and snow.

Moreover, as I shall attempt to show, the Australian climate and soil are beyond all question naturally intended for the cultivation of the grape, so that there is no occasion to overcome the forces of nature; on the contrary, they are unceasingly giving us the greatest encouragement. Then, again, think what widespread prosperity the use of our own wine would bring about. Apart from its beneficial influence on the national health, it would cover the land with smiling vineyards, and give to enormous numbers a healthy livelihood; it would absorb thousands from the fever and fret of city wear and tear into the more natural life of the country; and lastly, it would relieve the abnormal congestion of our crowded centres, and do more to bring about widely distributed employment than any other industry.

The history of the introduction of the grape to Australian soil deserves more than bare reference to that event It will be remembered that Captain Cook discovered this territory in 1770; in November 1791, barely more than twenty years afterwards, the first vine was planted at Parramatta, near Sydney. Nothing can demonstrate the suitability of the climate and the soil for its cultivation more than this one fact, namely, that at the very beginning of Australian settlement it was plain enough that the land was meant for the grape; and there is an interesting historical association, well worthy of note, attached to this circumstance. By order of the Emperor Napoleon, the Great Napoleon, a voyage of discovery to the Southern Hemisphere was performed by a fully equipped expedition during the years 1801, 1802, 1803, and 1804. One of the naturalists, M.F. Peron, has given us an excellent account of his New South Wales experience, and after referring to the Parramatta vineyards as likely to be followed by the most excellent results, he goes on to say:--"By one of those chances which are inconceivable, Great Britain is the only one of the great maritime powers which does not cultivate the vine either in her own territories or her colonies, notwithstanding the consumption of wine on board her fleets and throughout her vast regions is immense." This is another illustration of the old adage that lookers-on see most of the game, for this observant Frenchman has recorded an opinion the very truth of which comes well home to us. His remarks, moreover, open up a vista of what a great trade might be done with India in connection with our wines; indeed, it is this interchange of products which keeps the circulation going in the blood-vessels of commercial life.

Yet, although the vine was thus early started in Australia, it has since made but little progress, relatively speaking, in comparison with the great industry of wool-growing, and it will be appropriate to make this reference to the grape and the fleece conjointly, for the same name--that of John Macarthur--is intimately associated with both. In a small way sheep-breeding had been initiated soon after the settlement of Australia. But it was John Macarthur, by his introduction of the merino sheep in 1797, who gave the first impetus which led to the subsequent creation of the Australian wool trade. It was John Macarthur, too, who formed the first vineyard in Australia at Camden Park in 1815; though, as I have already said, the growth of the vine industry has not advanced with anything like the same rapidity as that of wool; if it had, Australia would now occupy a position second to none in the world.

It seems most fitting and opportune also to mention the fact that at the very time I am writing there is a proposal in the SYDNEY MORNING HERALD to do something to perpetuate our gratitude to John Macarthur. It is not often that one man has the opportunity of establishing two such great industries as wine-making and wool-growing. The benefits to Australia which have followed from the latter are altogether beyond calculation; for which alone the name of John Macarthur deserves to hold a place in the memory of Australians for ever, and if the wine industry had only been developed in like proportion, Australia's prosperity would have marvellously increased. Knowing, therefore, what John Macarthur has done for Australia, it is to be hoped that before these lines see the light of day what is now proposed will be an accomplished fact.

The next most notable occurrence in the history of Australian
viticulture is undoubtedly the action of James Busby who in 1828, says
Mr. T.A. Coghlan in his WEALTH AND PROGRESS OF NEW SOUTH
WALES,
returned from Europe "with a large collection of cuttings from the most
celebrated vineyards of France, Spain, the Rhine valley, and other
parts of the continent of Europe, and started, on his estate at
Kirkton, in the Hunter River district, a vineyard which has been the
nursery of the principal vineyards of the Colony." This was a more
important event than would be imagined from a bare recital of the fact,
for Busby has conferred upon Australian vines a high quality for all
time to come in this way. His collection of cuttings from the best of
the vineyards in Europe consisted of the choicest varieties or
"cepages," and this has been a matter for congratulation ever since.
Fuller reference, however, will be made to this important subject a
little farther on. what is certainly interesting also is that Busby was
so impressed with the future of the Australian wine industry that in
1830 he published his MANUAL OF PLAIN DIRECTIONS FOR PLANTING
AND
CULTIVATING VINEYARDS, AND FOR MAKING WINE, IN NEW SOUTH
WALES; and, as
I have just said, the high qualities of our wines are due to him alone,
so that the name of James Busby must always be gratefully remembered by
all Australians.

It makes one think that these sturdy pioneers of former times had a
greater belief in Australia and her possibilities, and more energy and
foresight, than are apparently possessed nowadays. But while I am on
the subject of the literature of Australian viticulture I must not
forget to mention an excellent little pamphlet by James King in 1807,
entitled, AUSTRALIA MAY BE AN EXTENSIVE WINE-GROWING COUN-

TRY.

Indeed, James King was another of those far-seeing men who were convinced that there was a great future for the Australian wine industry; moreover, he did a good deal in the way of developing it by cultivating the grape and by making wine.

Now, there are certain figures connected with vine-growing and the consumption of wine which possess a great value in relation to Australian viticulture, inasmuch as they enable us to see more clearly its relative progress, and, what is more, they indicate its future possibilities. It is only by methods of this kind that we are enabled to form an accurate estimate of the condition of any industry. And besides this, too, they act as a--stimulus to increased exertion. But it will be still more interesting and instructive to make a comparison between the little which has been done in wine production and the almost incredible proportions of our wool industry. And when it is remembered that there was nothing to prevent the wine trade from attaining a magnitude very like to that of wool, it will be seen what magnificent opportunities have thus far been practically thrown away.

At present the whole of Australia annually produces only a little more than three million gallons of wine, while the yearly yield of France is 795; of Italy, 798; of Spain, 608; of Hungary, 180; and of Portugal, 132 million gallons. And another thing is that the whole of the five colonies of Australia and Tasmania have altogether no more than 48,099 acres under vine cultivation. The total amount of wine made in the six foregoing colonies for the year ending March 31st, 1892, was only 3,604,262 gallons. The city of Paris itself requires nearly 300,000 gallons of wine daily, so that this single city would consume in 12 DAYS all the wine which the whole of Australia takes 12 MONTHS to make. So far back as 1875 the production was 1,814,400,602 gallons. And lastly, there is just one more fact worth remembering which is that the approximate value of the 1890 vintage to France was nearly

40,000,000 l. sterling.

Let us see, on the other hand, the gigantic strides on the part of wool. In 1805 the amount of wool exported from Spain was 6,895,525 lbs., and from Australia NIL. In 1811, however, Australia exported the modest quantity of 167 lbs. In 1861 the exportation from Spain had fallen to 1,268,617 lbs., while from Australia it had increased to 68,428,000 lbs. In 1891 New South Wales alone produced 357,096,954 lbs., representing a value of 11,036,018 l. And lastly, the wool exportation of Australia and Tasmania (not reckoning New Zealand) for the same year reached the enormous figures of 593,830,153 lbs., with a value of 20,569,093 l.

The disproportion between the attention which has been given to viticulture and that which has been bestowed upon wool-growing is well brought out in the following table:--

TABLE showing the value of the total amount of WINE produced in the FIVE COLONIES OF AUSTRALIA (including both that for local use and that for export) for the year ending March 31st, 1892; and the value of WOOL (only that exported, and therefore irrespective of that locally required) for the FIVE AUSTRALIAN COLONIES and TASMANIA alone, and not including that exported from NEW ZEALAND, for the year 1891:--

Pounds (value).

Total value of Australian wine (local use as well as export) produced for the year ending March 31st, 1892, only about..........800,000

Value of wool exported from Australia and Tasmania alone in 1891 (and therefore irrespective of the additional value of that locally required), not less than...............................20,569,093

From the foregoing, therefore, it will be apparent that the
whole subject of Australian viticulture is one of tremendous
importance; and I am strongly of opinion that practical results will
only be brought about by awakening in the mind of the Australian public
an active interest in everything connected with this, though yet
undeveloped, great wine industry. With that object in view, therefore,
it will be my endeavour to bring forward those main points of
viticulture which it is most desirable should be widely known. But such
an attempt, to be successful, must largely depend upon the arrangement
which is adopted, for it is impossible to do more than take up the
principal matters concerned with the space which is at my disposal. The
scheme which has been devised will, it is hoped, help to a clear
understanding of the subject.

THE CLIMATE.

If there is one reason more than any other why the wine industry should
sorely reach to colossal dimensions, it is that the climate is
naturally adapted for the cultivation of the vine. Although human
effort and human skill can overcome what looked to be almost
insuperable difficulties, they cannot, as we know, fight against
climate. Hence, having a climate created, as it were, for the growth of
the grape, there can be no possible excuse offered for its neglect.
Indeed, as I have already shown, the suitableness of the climate for
this purpose directly attracted the attention of the first arrivals,
and as a consequence the vine was actually planted a few years after
the discovery of Australia.

There are three constituents, namely, heat, light, and moisture, which in varying proportions make up what is known as climate. The first two, heat and light, are derived from the same source--the sun--and may, therefore, be conveniently considered together. The more heat and light a vine receives the more vigorously it grows. What is more important, however, is that the wine from it becomes stronger. It gains in strength because the percentage of glucose increases in the must: the must being the juice pressed from the grape, but in which fermentation has not commenced. Accordingly we find that the wines of the warmer regions in new South Wales, Victoria, and South Australia are much stronger than those from the cooler parts.

It is important to remember that the unripe berries of the grape contain several acids, notably tartaric, citric, and malic acids. As the fruit begins to ripen, these acids act upon the various substances, namely, starch, gum, dextrine, lignine, cellulose, &c., also contained within it, and grape sugar or glucose is formed in consequence with the advent of ripening, therefore, the fruit becomes richer in sugar and poorer in acids; part of the acids, in addition, is neutralised by the mineral salts which are absorbed by the roots. These acids, however, are not so thoroughly neutralised in a cooler climate, and as a result the wine has often a sour, crude taste. The warmer the climate the more alcohol the wine will contain; indeed, it may become too strong. On the contrary, the cooler the climate the more of acid there will be, and it may possess in consequence a crude, sharp taste. But these are matters which can be rectified by choosing the right varieties of grape for the different localities, and by their proper cultivation.

The third element concerned in the climate, namely, moisture, has now to be considered, and it is important from the fact that in a moister climate the percentages both of glucose and of acids in the grape are diminished. It is also important for another reason, namely, that while heat and light are unalterable, moisture may be produced by irrigation.

This constitutes one of the vexed questions connected with viticulture, and the most diverse opinions have been expressed about it. Some believe that irrigation is of great value, while others cannot say enough against it. But it would seem that when judiciously employed it is of unquestionable advantage. It renders the cultivation of the grape possible in places where it would otherwise be impossible; it largely increases the yield; and, what certainly must not be forgotten, it enables a lighter wine to be produced in the warmer regions. And another argument in favour of irrigation is this, that there is far more fertilizing matter in river water than in rain water. Hence it is that irrigation greatly enriches the land and increases the yield. It is thus a powerful aid, and because its advantages have been abused, that is no reason why it should not be made use of in a rational and scientific manner.

There is still another matter connected with this question of climate, namely, the aspect of the vineyard, which should be referred to because many different views are held upon it. But, as in all similar cases where there are such decidedly antagonistic opinions, it will be found that the arguments are not maintained from the same standpoint. So in this case the importance or non-importance of the aspect depends altogether upon the climate, and upon the locality--whether it be level or hilly. On level ground the aspect is not nearly so important. On hilly land it makes a considerable difference, from this circumstance, that in Australia the northern side of a hill is always hotter than that facing the south. In the hot regions, therefore, a hill slope facing towards the south is preferable; while in the cooler districts, since more warmth is required, a situation with a northern aspect is necessary. It is often said that hilly ground is better for the cultivation of the vine than level land. This is certainly true as far as cold localities are concerned, because a warmer aspect can then be chosen, and there will also be more shelter and better drainage.

THE SOIL.

People as a rule run away with the idea that the soil for the grape must necessarily be of a rich character. Even the farmer, thinking of wheat growing, and the market-gardener, thinking of his turnips, are apt to entertain a similar belief. But the truth is that the vine is a hardy plant and will grow in almost any place that is not water-logged or otherwise unsuitable. In America the definition of a soil adapted for the grape is expressed in the following phrase:--"Land that is suitable for vine-glowing is land that is not suitable for anything else." This is of course an extravagant way of stating the matter, still it is worth recalling. We may say this much, however, that almost any soil will do for the vine, provided that it does not bake and crack in the summer, nor get wet and boggy in the winter. A simple test is said to be adopted by the vine-growers of the Rhine. A specimen of the soil is put into an earthenware vessel into which boiling water is poured to cover it, after which it is undisturbed for three days. If the water on being tasted gives a mouldy or salty taste, the soil is believed to be unsuitable.

In considering the soil we must pay heed to its physical and its chemical characters. By its physical characters we mean its looseness or stiffness, its depth, and its colour. This looseness is a matter of much importance. It fulfils the great indication required in a soil for grape-growing; that is, a soil which will not remain damp after having been well wet. There is a marked difference between a stiff clayey soil which dries up and cracks in summer, and a loose soil which is always moist a little below the surface.

The depth of the soil is a matter that varies in accordance with the climate. In warm districts the vine requires more room for development, and goes deeper. In the cooler regions it has a sufficiency of moisture, and can content itself with a shallower soil. The colour of the soil, like its depth, is a matter of consequence according to the climate. A dark soil absorbs heat, becoming hotter consequently, while it reflects but little on the plant above. On the other hand, a light-coloured soil absorbs very little heat, but reflects almost the whole of the rays upwards upon the vine. From this it follows that a dark soil is better in a cooler climate, because there is generally an excess of moisture; while a light colour is more suitable in the warm regions, for the moisture is then retained.

The chemical constituents of the soil play no inconsiderable part in assisting the development of the vine. Of these, however, there are only five--namely, nitrogen, phosphorus, potash, calcium, and iron-- to which it is necessary to draw attention. For the successful cultivation of wheat and other cereals a richly nitrogenous soil is invaluable; for turnips and maize one rich in phosphorus is of great advantage; but for the vine potash is of considerable importance. It is true that nitrogen and phosphorus are necessary for the production of the vine wood, but it is for the fruit itself that the potash is so much required. As it is well known, the deposit known as winestone or "cream of tartar," on the inside of the cask by the fermentation of wine, is really tartrate of potash. In a similar way the potato is a plant which requires a supply of potash, and without it there is a manifest diminution in the crop. But in the case of the vine, unless there is a sufficiency of potash, the leaves do not attain to their full development; the stem is stunted to one-fourth of its natural size; and there is little or no fruit at all. Calcium or lime has a marked effect in increasing the strength of the wine. For this reason, therefore, this element is more necessary in the cooler than in the warm regions. And finally, there is that other chemical constituent of the soil, which deserves a brief notice, and it is iron. Now, the presence of iron therein has a distinct effect in deepening the colour of a wine. This is without doubt the reason why our Australian wines, as a general rule, are so rich in colour.

"CEPAGE," OR VARIETY.

Many words connected with viticulture are of French origin, as might be expected considering that it is a land where the wine industry is such a source of wealth. The term "cepage" (pronounced say-pazh) is one of these, and it possesses quite a distinctive and particular significance, so that a little explanation is necessary. The vine family is divided into several species, of which the ordinary grape vine, VITIS VINIFERA, is the most important. Of the VITIS VINIFERA there are many, more or less distinct, sorts of "cepages"; and the value of the word lies in the fact that it serves as a means of distinguishing all these different varieties. Originally a native of Asia Minor, there are now over a thousand sorts of European vines. Of these quite a number are already cultivated in Australia, and a brief reference to a few will help to a better understanding of the term "cepage."

Of the red grapes the following may be instanced:--The Carbenet (pronounced Car'-ben-ay); of which-there are two varieties, the GROS or large, and the SAUVIGNON or smaller kind. The latter is perhaps the choicest of all the red wine grapes, and has a characteristic flavour, with delicious bouquet and perfume. It forms the basis of all the best vineyards of Bordeaux, and is largely cultivated in Australia, for it does well in the cooler parts. And it will be just as well to take this opportunity of referring to the word "Carbenet," as in Australia it is much too often erroneously spelt "Cabernet." The best authorities, however, are all in favour of "Carbenet" as the proper mode of spelling. In the same way an unfortunate orthography in the case of

Riesling, which was given as "Reisling" in the London
exhibition of 1886, gave a writer in the SATURDAY REVIEW the
opportunity of a tirade against Australian wine-makers.

The Pinot (pronounced Peen'-o) Noir or Noirier will serve excellently
to demonstrate the significance of the word "cepage." This is the
dominating grape of the best vineyards of Burgundy, and enters into the
composition of many famous wines, such as Romanee-Conti Chambertin,
Corton, &c.; just as the Carbenet Sauvignon belongs to the renowned
clarets of Bordeaux, Chateau Margaux, Chateau Lafitte, and Chateau
Latour. This black Burgundy does well in our cooler regions, and is
usually pruned short, although it gives far better results with long
pruning.

Shiraz (pronounced Shir-az') is another red variety which is
extensively cultivated in Australia. It is the grape from which the
celebrated Hermitage red wine of France is made, and was first planted
by a monk, who brought the cuttings from Shiraz, in Persia. It is one
of our most reliable red varieties, and prospers best in a moderate
temperature. But the white varieties will perhaps afford us a better
idea of the expression "cepage," for three different varieties may be
adduced, whose characteristics are well known. First of all there is
Riesling (pronounced Rees'-ling, but too often, as I have just
mentioned, erroneously spelt Reisling), whose prototype is that
delicate Riesling of the Rhine, from which those famous wines of the
Rheingau, namely Steinberg, Marcobrunner, Johannisberg, as well as
Hock, are made. It is probably the best of our white wines, and does
well in the cooler districts. But it should be borne in mind that long
pruning is indispensable for it, as it gives very poor crops when
pruned short.

Then we have Tokay (pronounced Tok'-ay), so nearly corresponding to the
Furmint, which is the chief grape grown in the well-known Tokay

vineyards of Hungary. It yields a most excellent wine, and does well in the same regions as the preceding. And lastly, Verdeilho (pronounced Ver-dell'-o) deserves to be referred to amongst the white wines. It is the principal white variety grown in Madeira, and Madeira is a wine that is especially held in repute. It is better suited for the warm districts, and requires to be completely ripe before vintage.

It was a most fortunate thing for Australia, therefore, that her pioneers in viticulture were men like James Busby, who obtained their plants from the finest "cepages" in Europe. And this is a magnificent legacy which must inevitably exercise a powerful influence for ever on the Australian vine. Mr. Hubert de Castella drew special attention to this very fact in his paper read before the Royal Colonial Institute, London, in 1888: so that a beginning was made under the most auspicious conditions.

There are some interesting facts in connection with the different "cepages" which are certainly worth noticing. If the climate and the soil in one place be similar to the climate and soil in another, each variety--LE CEPAGE--of the grape will always produce the same wine. Thus some vineyards on the Yarra, Victoria, having a similar climate and similar soil to one of the great Bordeaux districts of France, produced a wine hardly to be distinguished from that of the latter. Then, again, one vine may produce a choice wine in one locality, but only an indifferent growth in another; and, conversely, a different "cepage" which does well in the latter region is almost a failure in the former. For instance, in France, the Gamay in the Beaujolais district, in which the soil is granitic, gives a superior wine to the Pinot; but, on the other hand, the Pinot in the Burgundy country, where there is a limestone formation, gives forth a world-famous wine, whilst the Gamay is nowhere in comparison.

Next, it is necessary to remember that the effect of a warmer climate is to increase the alcoholic strength of a wine. At the same time, however, it must not be forgotten that this effect is greater in some varieties than in others. One "cepage," giving in a cool region a wine of 18 per cent. of alcohol, when transported to a warmer locality may show an increase to 26 per cent. of alcohol. Another "cepage," showing 20 per cent. in the lower temperature, may only develop 23 per cent. in the hotter districts.

It will be evident from the preceding that the greatest discrimination is necessary in the selection of the variety for any particular region; and from the knowledge at present at the vine-grower's command he can do no more than form an approximate opinion of the "cepage" likely to suit his locality best. It is recommended, therefore, that new planters, before starting their vineyards, should carefully observe what varieties are giving the best results at any neighbouring vineyards; if some appear to be doing better than others, they should stick to the successful kinds. And again, it is advisable that they should be chary of what plants other wine-growers extol, when perhaps the latter are in another part of the country altogether and under totally different conditions of climate and soil. Instead of committing themselves to a large purchase, therefore, they should plant a selection of several varieties, and find out those which are the most suitable.

THE GROWING OF THE GRAPE--THE PREPARATION OF THE SOIL.

It is not my purpose to enter fully into the entire subject of grape-growing, for that is too extensive to be dealt with here; nevertheless, there are many points about it of Australian concern, over which there has been considerable discussion. This shows that our vignerons, instead of placidly following out old lines, are determined to find out for themselves the methods which will give the best results. That such a spirit is in active existence is unquestionably a source of satisfaction to those who have the welfare of Australian viticulture at heart, for it is only by a determination to find out the best course to be pursued in the many points connected with grape-growing, and more especially with wine-making, that we can hope to reach perfection.

And although we have the climate, and the soil, and everything in our favour, yet it must be recollected that there are vignerons of the very highest excellence in the old wine-making countries, and that it will only be by surpassing them that we can hope to secure the markets of the world. As I have already said, my own belief is that the best way of infusing vigour into our wine-making industry is to arouse public interest in the subject; and with that object in view, therefore, I shall endeavour to bring forward those matters which are of Australian viticultural importance.

Even at the outset we come against a disputed point, about which there has been, and is still, considerable diversity of opinion. It is to what depth the ground should be cultivated. On the one hand, there are some who affirm that a shallow depth of 8 or 9 inches, or even of 6 inches, is quite a sufficient penetration of the soil for most land; but, on the other, there are many who, while conceding the fact that a superficial cultivation like this may be successful for a few years, are strongly opinioned that a deeper working is eventually necessary. More than this, they contend that, even admitting good results were obtained by simple ploughing, yet they would have been still better with a deeper working. It would seem, however, that climate has a good deal to do with the matter. In the hot districts the vine attains a far greater development than in the cooler parts, and the roots require a deep soil. And besides this, in the warm regions the wine is naturally too strong, and the deeper the soil is worked the lighter the wine will be.

But there is one thing in particular which should not be overlooked, and it is that the land should be in a state of fine sub-division. One American writer insists that the ground before planting should be "as fine as bolted flour." This expression serves very well to show the importance of a thorough pulverisation of the soil; and the best results are certainly obtained .where this is energetically carried out.

THE GROWING OF THE GRAPE--LAYING OUT THE VINEYARD.

The next thing in order is that of laying out the vineyard, in which it will be desirable to consider what distance apart the vines are to be planted. This matter of spacing the vines is one about which there is still considerable disagreement; and the question as to whether they should be planted near to one another, or far apart, is yet unsettled. But the truth is no inflexible rule can be laid down, as the climate, the soil, and the "cepage" all exercise a controlling influence. It seems to be generally admitted that in the warm districts the vines should be planted farther apart than in the cooler regions.

In a hot climate the vigour of the plant is increased by the great amount of light and heat which it receives. The must will be too strong, therefore, and it is only by planting the vines at a greater distance apart than usual, and also by pruning very long, that the resulting wine will be rendered sufficiently light in strength. In a cooler region, on the other hand, where the vigour of the plant is less, the crop on each vine must be reduced by short pruning, so as to increase the percentage of glucose in the must and ensure a good wine. And where the size of the plant is lessened by this method of pruning, the vines must be placed closer together in order to make use of all the available soil. This latter itself has also to be thought of in this matter of spacing the vines. In a rich soil, where the vigour of the plant is increased, the vines should be placed farther apart; in a poor soil, on the contrary, they should be planted closer together.

Mr. Francois de Castella, formerly Expert to the Board of Viticulture, the author of THE HANDBOOK ON VITICULTURE FOR VICTORIA, and who is now the proprietor of the Tongala vineyard, in an instructive article on viticulture in Victoria lays down the following rules with regard to the spacing of vines:--"THERE IS FOR EACH LOCALITY, WITH THE SAME CONDITIONS OF SOIL AND CLIMATE, A CERTAIN DISTANCE, WE MAY CALL THE OPTIMUM, AT WHICH VINES WILL THRIVE BEST; IF THIS DISTANCE BE INCREASED THEY WILL NOT IMPROVE, AND MAY EVEN DETERIORATE. Unless this be a distance which cannot conveniently be worked by horse labour, it would evidently be a waste of land to plant any wider, and would entail the use of unnecessary labour for its cultivation. It would be just as foolish to plant vines any closer than this, as it would give unnecessary pruning, disbudding, tying up, &c.--that is, if the climate be such that grapes will ripen satisfactorily.

"I have come to the conclusion that in our district (Lilydale, a cool region) the optimum distance is 4 1/2 by 4 1/2 feet, practically 2,000 vines per acre, at least in the poorer soils; and, after careful observation, I am of opinion that vines planted any wider will not bear more fruit. This is, however, rather too close to be conveniently worked by horse labour. I should, therefore, recommend 5 by 5 feet. But on the Murray (a warm region) this distance would not suit at all, and I believe that the vine-growers are right to plant 8 by 8, and even 10 by 10 feet, in that district.

"In conclusion, I would advise every vine-grower starting in a new district to determine by experiment what is his optimum distance. He can make a pretty good guess from observations of soil and climate, and for the rest let him, instead of planting all his vineyard on one scale, plant different blocks at different distances apart, so that if he wishes to extend his vineyard later on he may know what is the most suitable way to do so. By a careful consideration of these and other points which regulate the growth and development of the vine, and a practical application of the deductions drawn from them, it is possible for the intelligent vigneron to obtain from his land a maximum of return with a minimum of labour, and also to regulate the strength of his wine so as to suit the requirements of trade, thus making viticulture one of the most remunerative as well as most attractive branches of agriculture."

In France, especially in the northern districts, the vines are placed much closer together than ever they are in Australia, and this means that only hand labour can be employed. But it has to be remembered that the scarcity of manual labour with us makes it necessary to arrange the vineyard with enough width between the plants for a horse. rt is desirable, however, not to go to the other extreme and space the vines at too great a distance from each other; indeed, in favour of a closer planting, the following influencing circumstances should be borne in mind. In the elevated regions, where the rainfall is ample, the vines may be planted closer together than on the plains or on the lower slopes; firstly, because there is no fear as to a sufficiency of water; and secondly, for the reason that the vines, by being nearer together, protect one another from the inclement weather. Spring frosts also are very liable to occur in certain localities; and here again the vines, by being brought closer together, afford shelter to each other from the direct rays of the sun, which are particularly injurious when coming on top of a severe frost.

Then again, although some believe that in dry districts it is better to give each vine plenty of space, yet there are others who are of opinion that a closer formation is rather an advantage. And on this account: that since the roots come in contact with one another, they are compelled to strike deeper in search of water--just in the very place it is desirable they should go. In addition to the foregoing, it must not be forgotten that a dark-coloured soil absorbs more of the sun's heat than one of lighter colour; just as a dark coat is hotter to wear than a light-coloured one. For this reason, therefore, it is better for the plants to be closer together in a dark soil, since the shadow of the vines will then be over the root-producing areas.

In the SOUTH AUSTRALIA VINEGROWERS' MANUAL, which has been prepared by
Mr. George Sutherland, under instructions from the Government of South Australia, the author expresses this conviction: That a very large proportion of the new vineyards of South Australia will be planted wide, especially in the warmer districts and on the lower rises of the foothills; but that after all 6 feet may be found the most suitable on more elevated localities, where we shall have to look for some of the best wines of the claret and hock type. One leading Californian authority, according, to Mr. Sutherland, was a great advocate for wide planting. After an exhaustive inquiry into the matter, however, throughout the wine-producing countries of Europe, he became quite converted, and believed in closer planting. Mr. Francois de Castella also records the fact that in a block of vines at St. Hubert's (Lilydale, Victoria), every second vine was rooted out on one-half of the block. After ten years it was found that on the whole the closer

wines had done better than those from which every alternate vine was rooted out.

THE GROWING OF THE GRAPE--WHETHER TO PLANT CUTTINGS OR ROOTED VINES.

There is another somewhat disputed matter connected with viticulture, which deserves a little notice; and it is the relative merits of planting cuttings or rooted vines in the vineyard. The majority of the witnesses examined by the Royal Commission on Vegetable Products in Victoria, 1889, admitted that cuttings ultimately produced a better vine. But, as in some of the preceding points at issue, may it not be that climate and soil have a great deal to do with the results? Signor Romeo Bragato, the Expert to the Board of Viticulture in Victoria, in his HINTS TO INTENDING VINE-GROWERS, recommended cuttings, not only for cheapness, but because if planted in the vineyard at the first they did not require removal.

In the course of his advice he proceeded to remark:--"The ways used here and elsewhere by the vine-grower are two--namely, by cuttings, and rooted vines--but they do not always agree which of the two is the better. There are many who say that, for the new plantation, rooted vines must be preferred; others maintain that it is better to plant by cuttings, because they grow more nourishing and give the vine a longer life. Both these methods are good and to be recommended; but, in a general way, I would advise you to stick to the cuttings, and that not only because by planting them you will have a sensible economy, but also because if you plant the cuttings in the vineyard you will never have to more them. If you use rooted vines, it is impossible, notwithstanding all your care and attention, for you to carry them from the nursery to the vineyard without hurting their roots, which are very delicate.

" But if the ground which you intend to plant with vines were loose and arid, then I would never hesitate to advise you to always use in that case rooted vines, because the cuttings without roots would not absorb the rainy water which in such kind of soil runs away in the same time it takes to fall. This is the reason why, in such a soil, the cuttings seldom strike.

"On the selection of the cuttings depends the future of the vineyard, but of this the vine-growers are not sufficiently persuaded, because they do not pay all the attention required for this delicate operation. In fact, when in the vineyards in order to cut the cuttings, they take the thin and thicks--those growths on the new wood and on the old--without making any distinction, and without knowing if the old vine gives fruit or not. Many also, without other care, leave their cuttings in the vineyard for months exposed to the air, sun, and rain; not thinking that the very porous wood gets dry very quickly, and becomes weak near the buds. Others, again, buy their cuttings without knowing to what variety of vine they belong, and how they were preserved. It is not surprising, therefore, that these negligent vine-growers, after having incurred great expense in preparing the soil and planting the vineyard, besides having their vineyard planted with so many varieties, are compelled to pull up a great number of cuttings that have not struck, or, having struck, do not carry fruit."

THE GROWING OF THE GRAPE--THE HEIGHT OF THE VINE ABOVE THE GROUND.

The young vine takes about four years to reach its fruit-bearing stage. During this time the plant requires to be properly trained so as to obtain the best results from the growing grape. Now, although there are many different systems of rearing vines, yet in the main they consist of an upright stem or trunk, and an upper part or crown--the latter varying considerably in shape. Thus we have the "gooseberry-bush" style, which is employed for those vines requiring short pruning. Then there is the "trellising" style, for the long-pruned varieties, in which the vine is trained to a great distance along a wire. Indeed, these two methods may be taken to represent the two main styles of training the vine; although the different modifications used in various countries are almost endless.

There is, however, one important point which requires attention, no matter what system is adopted, and it is the height of the vine above the ground. The nearer a vine is to the ground, the more radiated light and heat it receives, and as a consequence its resulting nine is stronger. In vines so near the ground, also, the alkaline dust arising from the soil neutralises the natural acid of the fruit, and prejudicially affects the fermentation of the wine.

As a matter of fact the earthy taste--GOUT DE TERROIR--which is sometimes present in wine, is believed to be caused by a certain amount of soil being present on the grapes during fermentation. This must be looked to, especially in the warmer districts, where by giving the wine a greater distance above the ground, a lighter, more delicate, and better wine, quite free from the foregoing demerit, is produced.

The testimony of experts throughout Australia is unanimously in favour of raising the vine sufficiently above the ground, so as to keep the grapes well off the soil, and also to provide for the free circulation of air beneath. It is true that in some parts of the Continent the practice for ages has been to keep the vines well down against the earth. But this is done to secure the advantages of the radiated heat, and enable the grapes to ripen. In Australia, however, even in the elevated districts, the sun is usually warm enough to ripen the grapes without this being necessary.

THE GROWING OF THE GRAPE--ON PRUNING.

Before leaving these references to the growing of the grape I purpose making a few remarks upon pruning, a subject which is as interesting as it is important. The objects of pruning are manifold. By it the cultivation of the wine is facilitated; the best results are obtained from each variety of grape; the yield is increased; the product is more uniform in character; and the quality of the wine is vastly improved. But a great deal of the work of pruning is so entirely technical that it would utterly fail to possess any attraction for the general reader. Consequently I shall attempt no more than to briefly refer to those particular matters which are of Australian concern.

Now, it is laid down as a rule for pruning that some vines should be pruned short, while others require long pruning; that is to say, one variety of wine requires to be repressed, as it were, and in another the branches have to be kept long to produce a superior quality of wine. The explanation is that while the sap is on its way through the roots, the stem, the branches, and the shoots of the vine, for the production of fruit, it is distilled out, so to speak, during its passage from the earth to the fruit. As Mr. George Sutherland prettily puts it, the grape is, in fact, the crowning product of the whole plant. In this way, the farther the sap has to travel through the whole vine on its way to the growing fruit, the better will the resulting wine be.

To a certain extent this is true of all vines, but more especially so in the case of Shiraz and some of the Pinots. In various districts of France, in order to bring the grape to perfection, the vine-growers will train out their main branches along trellises to a length of 50 and even 60 feet, so as to give the sap the longest possible distance to travel; and, further, for the purpose of concentrating into the fruit the whole result of the wine, all the buds and little shoots, which would distract therefrom, are carefully taken away. This gives to the vine a very curious look, but it serves well to illustrate how greatly wines differ as to whether they require short or long pruning. It also helps to a better understanding of the two main styles of training the vine already mentioned, namely, the "gooseberry bush" and the "trellising."

The fact that this elaboration of the sap in long-pruned vines requires a long distance to intervene between the roots and the fruit itself, is one of considerable importance. It is necessary to remember, however, that cultivation of this kind requires additional labour. Moreover, one of the principal reasons why the short-pruned vine has become such a favourite in Australia is that it is a labour-saving vine, and therefore its adoption is almost a necessity. But, as Mr. Sutherland remarks, "there is no doubt that Australia can never hope to produce in any quantity the finest qualities of wine until the vignerons attend more to those practices which depend essentially upon the fundamental fact that the sap flows with different habits through different varieties of vines; and, therefore, that some vines require short pruning, while it is even more important to remember that others will only yield satisfactorily under a system of long pruning."

In a paper on viticulture, at Mildura, which was drawn up for the Royal Commission on Vegetable Products in 1890, Mr. Francois de Castella, a former expert to the Board of Viticulture, Victoria, has condensed so much knowledge within a small compass that I have quoted the following:--

"Most of the settlers I met told me that they intended to prune their vines short. Now, in my opinion, they could not make a greater mistake --for wine-growing, at least; as for raisin-growing I have never taken any interest in the subject, and, having no experience, do not wish to express an opinion on it. I must say that all the settlers I had occasion to speak to were raisin-growers, but I should warn any future wine-grower at Mildura, who may chance to read these few notes, to beware of short pruning.

"Most of our vineyard labourers come from the cold parts of Europe, such as Switzerland, where grapes ripen with difficulty under ordinary circumstances, and where the vine does not take any considerable development. There, short pruning has to be resorted to in order to make a drinkable wine. When these men arrive in Australia they bring all their old habits and prejudices with them, and tell the inexperienced vineyard proprietor that long pruning weakens the vine. The proprietor, thinking that they know more about the subject than he does, allows them to do as they like, and they set to work to cut the vine down to such an extent that, unable to take advantage of the genial climate to which it has been transplanted, it gives only one-eighth or one-tenth of the quantity of grapes it could be made to bear with intelligent pruning, besides being much weakened; whereas long-pruning strengthens a vine if the climate be favourable to its development.

"Another disadvantage of short pruning in warm climates is the well-known fact that the less grapes you have on the vine, the more glucose the must will contain; therefore, instead of making much more per acre of a drinkable wine, which they easily could do, they content themselves with a much smaller quantity per acre of a wine which ferments so badly that alcohol has to be added to prevent the production of lactic acid, resulting from the excessive temperature reached during fermentation favouring the development of this particular germ.

"The resulting wine, a curious mixture of alcohol, sugar, lactic acid, and water, is most unpalatable, sour, uninviting, and unwholesome. besides ruining the name of Australian wine when sold as such.

"I may here warn vine-growers against the advice given to them by some would-be authorities, who tell them they can make a light wine by picking grapes before they are ripe. This is absurd. The unripe grape contains a certain percentage of vegetable acids, such as tartaric, malic, &c., &c. some of which are themselves converted into glucose during the process of ripening, whilst others are eliminated after helping to transform the starch of the vegetable tissues into glucose. It stands to reason that if the fruit be picked before complete maturity, these acids, which are not capable of fermenting, will be found unchanged in the wine produced, thereby rendering it acid and undrinkable. It is, of course, necessary, in warm climates, to pick the grapes before they get over-ripe or shrivel up; but it would be just as foolish to rush to the other extreme, and pick the fruit too soon.

"If, instead of blindly following the mode of culture which has been adopted in a cold climate, the vine-grower would listen to the dictates of reason, and were to try a few inexpensive experiments, he would soon find out his mistake, and confer a boon on himself as well as on his neighbour, not to speak of the consumers of his wine.

"Even in the cooler districts of Victoria, such as the Yarra Valley, I do not know of any variety of vine which is weakened by long pruning, even in a series of years; while certain varieties are so influenced by short pruning as to bear no fruit at all. If this be the case on the Yarra, how much more must it be so on the Murray?"

Mr. de Castella then referred to some other matters connected with the practices followed at Mildura, and concluded with these encouraging words:--

"I contend that no other culture will give such magnificent returns, do so much good to a country, or have greater attractions for the happy proprietor of the vineyard, as there is no branch of agriculture which presents such a vast field for experimental research, or which is so extensively benefited by the practical application of scientific laws and principles, as viticulture."

THE MAKING OF THE WINE--THE CELLAR.

Up till this time our whole attention has been taken up with everything that has to do with the production of the grape. But with the gathering of the crop a complete change has taken place, for nature no longer exercises such a controlling influence. At this stage the art of winemaking really begins, and the climate, the soil, and all the other factors that have so much to do with the growth of the grape assist us no longer. From the moment that the grapes are gathered till the wine is ready for bottling is a most eventful period; for, during this important time, under proper treatment, wine may be made to reach perfection.

Indeed, it is only by paying the most minute attention to all the details connected with the making of wine that Australian vignerons will succeed in placing our wines before all others; because it is very important to remember that the must produced in Australia is equal, if not superior, to any in the world. Now, all that follows this portion relates to wine-making alone; and it should for that very reason, therefore, possess a special interest for us. Moreover, it will be a good thing for the wine industry, for Australia, and for her people, when such an interest becomes part of our daily life.

Naturally the first thing to suggest itself, therefore, in the making of the wine, is the place in which it is made. There is no doubt that in Australia the importance of a proper cellar has never been sufficiently appreciated. But the French have a proverb, "the cellar makes the wine," showing that it plays no inconsiderable part in the production of good wine. As Mr. Walter W. Pownall, the representative of the Australian Wine Company, explained before the Vegetable Products Commission in Victoria, a knowledge of cellar routine and cellar work would aroid the spoiling of much good wine. A man thinks when he has grown the wine that is all that is necessary. But the fact is, a wine-grower has never done with his wine till it has passed out of his hands.

There was a valuable pamphlet on Australian wines written by the late Doctor Bleasdale, of Melbourne, in 1876. It is now out of print, and regrettedly so, for the worthy Doctor was one of the best connoisseurs of wine Australia ever had. Mr. L. Bruck, the well-known medical publisher of Sydney, however, has placed me under considerable obligation by giving me his own copy, and in the preface therein I note that the author, in speaking of this very question, remarks:--"I would here reiterate what I have often stated, namely, that if the cellar management in the three colonies were equal to the magnificent produce of the vines, no "country on the earth could surpass, in quality and variety "of kinds, Victoria, South Australia, and New South Wales."

Then again, Mr. James Smith, of Melbourne, in the course of his admirable prize essay on Australian wine, which appeared in GREVILLE'S YEAR BOOK OF AUSTRALIA for 1886, has these observations on this subject:--"It is, however, in the management of the cellar that one must look for the most efficient means of securing that uniformity of quality which I regard as such an important desideratum. If it be not a science, it is certainly an art requiring special knowledge, training, and experience, combined, perhaps, with natural aptitude. And it is precisely in this respect, I fear, that our deficiency in Australia is greatest.

"In the wine-making countries of Europe the cellarmaster is an expert who inherits the skill, traditions, methods, and usages of many generations of men who have adopted and followed the same calling. His organs of smell and taste have been educated to practise the nicest discrimination of flavour and odour, and if the vintage of a particular year differs in quality from that of its predecessor, he knows how, by a judicious blending of the old with the new, of the highly-coloured with the pallid, to arrive at that uniformity which is so indispensable."

The cellar must neither be too damp nor too dry. Any excess of dampness would rot the casks and give a musty taste to the wine; while, on the contrary, in too dry a cellar the staves of the casks would shrink and cause leakage. The cellar is usually kept somewhat dark. The openings for the admission of air and light should be provided with shutters, so that the atmosphere and temperature may be under control. The floor of the cellar should be paved or cemented, be well levelled, and cleanliness throughout should be strictly and strenuously maintained.

But the following remarks of Signor Bragato as to what a cellar ought not to be will perhaps be more instructive, and besides they contain a

vast amount of information on the subject. In referring to some
of the cellars he came across during his tour of inspection through one
of the Victorian districts, he writes:--

"The majority of the buildings used as cellars are nothing less than
wooden sheds, with galvanized iron roofs. Here the air has a free
circulation day and night, and the cellerman is thus rendered powerless
to control the temperature, which very often, from 100 degrees in day
time, goes down to 54 degrees or less during the night. The appliances
required for winemaking are all round badly preserved, and are covered
with mouldiness and dust. The floor of the buildings is not paved or
cemented, and it consists of earth, so that it has the power of
absorbing the wine that gets spilt and becomes the source of pernicious
germs, which will spread all over the cellar and in the air, to be
finally deposited in the must and in the wine, causing irreparable loss
in the quality of the wine. There are a few good cellars, but these,
also, are badly kept and badly used.

"The casks are neglected, and the coat of tartar is scrupulously left
in the cask, with the erroneous idea that it tends to preserve the
wine. All the empty casks I have smelt in the cellars inspected are
impregnated with bad odours, which are not detected by the majority of
the owners, in consequence of having accustomed their olfactory organs
to the predominant odour of mouldiness in their cellars, and so they
are unable to detect if the odour of their casks is healthy or not.

"With the bad cellars which the vignerons have at their disposal,
combined with the neglect of the casks and other appliances, and the
little care in the preservation of the wine, it is only natural that a
large quantity of the wine produced is spoiled, and condemned to the
still to be converted into inferior brandy of bad taste and colour,
which is often used to fortify the wines, with the result of rendering
them unfit for consumption. "Amongst the wines I have tested, I found

some really very good ones, presenting all the characteristics required in a fine wine. But if there are good wines, there are also very bad ones, and these, I am sorry to say, represent the bulk in every cellar I visited. Some of the wines are cloudy, sweetish, with a good deal of asperity. Others present tartaric, lactic, and acetic fermentations."

After some further comments on various other matters, the same gentleman concludes his report with the following:--

"Finally, I may say that by what I have seen I cannot help expressing the opinion that Australia is capable of producing really fine wines, to be highly appreciated in the world's markets. But to produce an appreciable wine, it is necessary that the vignerons should improve in their system of wine-making, and substitute for their sheds cellars constructed on a rational principle; and by devoting more attention to the cleanliness of the casks and other cellar appliances. A modification in the system of cultivation and pruning of the vines will also be factors in improving the quality of the wine.

"There is in this country good soil, and a climate which cannot be equalled for the successful cultivation of the vine. Capital is plentiful, and the people very enterprising; so there remains only the want of Technical Instruction, by the institution of practical schools of Viticulture, without which it is doubtful if ever its vignerons will succeed in making wines likely to be appreciated in the foreign markets."

In the same way Mr. J.A. Despeissis, of the New South Wales Department of Agriculture, also insists upon cellar cleanliness. And it would seem, indeed, that there is ample justification for his deprecatory remarks. It appears that on several occasions he has noticed fowls and pigeons roosting in the wine cellars. Now, as he pungently observes, the wine cellar was never intended for this sort of thing. Another way of putting the matter would be to point out what a mad thing it would be to use a fowl house as a cellar. Moreover, he gives minute directions for disinfecting the cellar, in order to destroy any germs or minute organisms which may be lurking in crevices or in odd corners. This is best accomplished by burning some sulphur in earthenware pots, distributed over various parts of the cellar; previously seeing that all the windows and gaps are rendered air-tight by means of bagging. The fumes should be left in the cellar--for a day or two, after which the doors are opened, and a free current of air allowed to sweeten the whole place.

Moreover, a model cellar is necessarily a very elaborate affair, considering it is the laboratory, so to speak, in which the wine is created. A model cellar would consist of the following six compartments:--

* 1. The section for the first treatment of the grape.
*
* 2. The fermentation department.
*
* 3. The section for the preparation and storing, of the new wine.
*
* 4. The underground cellar for the storage of the matured wine.
*
* 5. The bottle department.
*
* 6. The distillation department and for the utilization of the refuse of wine.
*

The cellar of Mr. Henley, near the Ovens River, in Victoria, is very complete. It is provided with a steam lift, a steam crushing machine, and a steam pump, while there is perfect ventilation and a uniform temperature. His cellar is divided into three compartments: the fermenting house in the middle, the cellar for the new wine, and the cellar for the old wine. The building is 83 feet by 80 feet, built of brick, with double walls 9 inches thick outside and 4 inches inside, and between the walls there is 4 1/2 inches of space. The temperature on the hottest days in the summer never surpasses 80 degrees Fahrenheit; and, lastly, the floors, both of the cellars and the fermenting house, are cemented for the purpose of absolute cleanliness.

THE MAKING OF THE WINE--THE GATHERING OF THE GRAPE.

At the very beginning one of the chief matters to be looked to is the selection of the time at which the grapes should be picked. The proper period is that when the interior of the grape contains its principal components, the sugar and the acids, in the right proportions. In the warmer districts the grapes are sometimes allowed to become too ripe. In such a case there would be an excess of sugar and a deficiency of acid, and a regular fermentation would be impossible. On the other hand, it will be remembered in the course of the remarks upon pruning that I quoted Mr. Francois de Castella to show what a mistaken idea it is to pick the grapes before they are thoroughly ripe in order to produce, as it is erroneously supposed, a lighter wine. It is of the greatest consequence, therefore, to choose that particular time for gathering the grapes when they contain the respective elements in their strictly proper proportions.

On the eventful day for the picking of the grapes the weather should be fine and bright, and in the warm districts they should be picked early in the morning and late in the afternoon, so that they are not too warm. The grapes should never be taken to the fermenting house when too heated; indeed, it would be better not to crush the grapes at all than to have them in such a state. As Signor Bragato observes, if they are too warm the fermentation will start with too high a temperature in the must, and very likely the result will be the formation of lactic and acetic germs. In Algiers and other warm regions the grapes picked in the day are left outside during the night; by this means the temperature of the must is lowered.

In the picking of the grapes the greatest care should be taken to discard the mouldy, dry, and dirty grapes, and leaf insect worms should likewise be got rid of. Once the gathering of the grapes is commenced it should be concluded as quickly as possible, and therefore a sufficient number of hands must be engaged for the purpose. For instance, with the Riesling, if the grapes are left on the vines on a hot day twenty-four hours after they arrive at perfection, the wine will not be nearly so good.

THE MAKING OF THE WINE--VARYING ADDITIONS TO THE MUST.

On the arrival of the grapes at the press-house, the first thing to be determined upon is whether the stalks are to be used or not. In the case of white wines it is not customary to separate them from the grapes. A good deal, however, will depend upon different circumstances. Thus, when grapes are grown in flat, damp places, or during wet seasons, it is often advantageous to ferment the berries with part of their stems; but, on the contrary, those grapes which contain a sufficiency of tannin will not require the latter. For example, in the production of white wines at Mr. Hans Irvine's ("Great Western") vineyard in Victoria, the grapes are first crushed with the mill, the mill consisting of two grooved wooden rollers working against each other. After this the skins, together with the stalks, are placed in the wine-press. In the case of red wine, however, the grapes are separated from the stalks by means of an iron griddle, so that only the skins are employed in the formation of the wine.

The methods pursued with regard to the elimination or retention of the grape stalks vary in different parts of the Continent. The most careful vignerons remove the stalks in the case of the finest growths of Burgundy; but in the making of champagne, and also in the Rheingau, from which part come the famous Hock wines, the stalks are allowed to remain. In the Medoc districts, which produce the finest clarets, the stalks are likewise put into the fermentation vat; but this is considered to be a great mistake, since a long time elapses before the astringent taste of the wine subsides. With the far-famed Red Hermitage wine of France, too, the stalks are permitted to pass into the vat, and in the case of sherry and port, as well, the stalks all take part in the fermentation, though it is believed that better results would be obtained by their removal. But in all these old wine-producing countries of Europe the same customs have been followed from time immemorial, and they are not likely to be altered at present.

THE MAKING OF THE WINE--THE MUST ITSELF.

The must--that is, the juice expressed from the grape, but in which (juice) fermentation has not yet taken place--is a fluid of very complex composition. It is made up of a variety of ingredients, with which it is necessary to become familiar in order to follow, during the process of fermentation, its change into wine. We find, therefore, that a large part of the must consists of water; this serves to dissolve the other constituents, and to dilute them to the required extent. For instance, the sugar in the must needs to be considerably diluted for the purposes of fermentation. In too concentrated a form it actually prevents it, as we see when fruits are preserved in syrup.

Next to water, sugar is the material which exists in the largest proportions in the must; it is, however, that peculiar kind of sugar termed "glucose," which may be described as uncrystallisable sugar, and as consisting of half grape sugar and half fruit sugar. It possesses the property of being able to ferment, which cane or crystallisable sugar cannot do, unless, indeed, it first be changed into glucose. Now, it is a curious fact that although cane sugar can be transformed into glucose, yet the latter form of sugar has never, so far, been changed into cane or crystallisable sugar. As Mr. J.A. Despeissis points out, the invention of a process that would achieve this would be worth more than all the mines of New South Wales put together.

In the process of fermentation the glucose is broken up into a number of substances, which differ entirely from it; and as these different bodies are very important they deserve much attention. Under the influence of fermentation glucose undergoes a great change, of which the principal products are alcohol and carbonic acid gas. The alcohol is, of course, the one predominant feature in wine; and according to the amount of alcohol which wine contains, so it varies in strength.

In addition to these two main products of glucose by fermentation, namely, alcohol and carbonic acid gas, there are glycerine and succinic acid, as well as a lesser proportion of other derivatives, very much akin to alcohol. Of all these glycerine is by no means unimportant, as it confers a blandness or mellowness upon the wine. The succinic acid, also, is distinctive for this reason, that it is the source of that characteristic flavour in wine known as "vinosity."

Besides the water and the glucose, the must likewise contains quite an appreciable amount of those important bodies, the various acids. These consist of tartaric acid, so frequently met with all through the vegetable world; of malic acid, which is the acid almost distinctive of apples; of tannic acid or "tannin," and of other acids. These different acids play an important part in the production of wine; without them, in truth, it would be a mere admixture of spirits and water--a colourless, flavourless, and insipid product. By their assistance, however, wine is endowed with the brilliancy it possesses. And more than this, the action of the alcohol on these acids develops those exquisitely delicate ethers--the oenanthic and other ethers--which constitute, in fact, the bouquet of the wine. At the same time, it has also to be remembered that while these many acids constitute the life and soul, so to speak, of the wine, their very presence is absolutely necessary for the process of vinous fermentation. That is to say, the active agents of vinous fermentation are only enabled to work perfectly in a liquid which is somewhat acid.

There is an astringent principle, named tannin, which calls for attention in any reference to wine-making. It is almost the same body-- not quite--as the tannin obtained from galls, and so largely employed in tanning. This vine-tannin, if it may be so termed, does not exist in the juice of the grape, but in the stalk and the skin. The white wines, in which the juice is almost always freed from the skins and stalks, contain but little tannin; while, on the contrary, most red wines, in which juice, skins, and stalks are all included together in the fermenting-vat, contain a good deal. Some white wines derive their tannin from the oaken casks which hold the wine; and their colour, in consequence, subsequently deepens. Other red wines, strange to say, gradually lose their dark colour from a certain action of the tannin. So that tannin is the cause of some white wines deepening in colour, while it renders other red wines of a lighter colour. Now, tannin has the effect of preserving albuminous substances, and in this way it may be beneficial in rendering red wines more durable. But although this may be advisable in wines which are liable to turn, it is certain that excess of tannin is most undesirable. In fact, the practice of placing the stalks in the fermenting-vat is in many cases, as I have previously stated, an unnecessary proceeding.

The mineral kingdom is not unrepresented in must, and certain saline substances are found in it. Of these, the salts of potash are uniformly present, and the most important is, without doubt, the acid tartrate of potash. This is the salt so well known in commerce under the name of cream of tartar. The lees of wine contain it in considerable quantity, and it is also found as a crystalline deposit in the inside of the casks. As the alcohol begins to develop in the must this salt is precipitated, and the more so the lower the temperature. Thus it is that a light wine of low alcoholic strength, if it be markedly acid, will lose the acidity in a cool, underground cellar. And, as a matter of fact, the proper maturation of a wine is impossible without a due amount of tartar; besides this, it develops in the wine a well-defined vigour and tonicity, which improves its taste, while it also increases its alimentary qualities.

There are a few other ingredients in must, namely, the colouring matters and essential oils, and the albuminoids, or nitrogenous substances. The colouring matters and oils appear to be contained in the cells of the inner side of the skin. Of these, the purpose of the colouring matter is obvious; while the essential oils are believed to contribute to the "aroma" of the wine. The albuminoids or nitrogenous substances are of the nature of white of egg; and, when in small proportion, are necessary for the due performance of the fermentative process. But, in excess, they are a source of considerable anxiety to the vigneron, in that they are the cause of much of the wine going wrong.

THE MAKING OF WINE--FERMENTATION.

The must, as we have already seen, is the juice of the grape, which has been squeezed out by the grape-mill or from the wine-press. The murk, or pomace as it is called in America, on the contrary, is the mass of grape skins, stalks, &c., left behind in the press. A clear apprehension of these two terms is required in order that no confusion may arise. The fermenting-vat is the cask in which what is called the strong, stormy, or tumultuous fermentation takes place. The "cuvage" is the length of time the contents are left in the fermenting-vat.

The whole phenomena of fermentation are too complicated and profoundly scientific to be dealt with here. I shall do no more, therefore, than briefly refer to the behaviour of the must in the fermenting-vat. Fermentation sets in soon after the must is placed within the latter. The germs of vinous fermentation are contained in abundance in the air of the wine cellar, as well as being on the grapes themselves. M. Pasteur, who has contributed so much to a proper understanding of fermentation, has proved that the yeast fungi come from the external surface of the grapes, and are not derived from the interior. Hence it follows that the skins are to be well crushed before fermentation begins, to ensure proper action in the must.

The temperature of the must soon begins to rise, and the fermentative agencies break up its glucose into alcohol and carbonic acid gas. There is a bubbling and seething in the liquid during this action, which gradually subsides. The increase of temperature in the fermented fluid begins to abate; the skins and husks subside to the bottom of the vat; the liquid itself becomes slightly less turbid--and the first stage of wine-making is at an end.

A clearer insight into this important part of the process will perhaps be gained by noting some of the practices followed on the Continent, as regards the duration of the vattage. The length of time the various contents--whether they be the grape juice alone, or the grape juice together with the skins and stalks--remain within the fermenting-vat, varies greatly in different parts. In the Champagne country, the must is allowed to stand for twelve or eighteen hours, during which time a froth arises to the top and a sediment descends to the bottom. Without disturbing either of these, the precious liquid is carefully withdrawn into small barrels, and the fermentation is then allowed to proceed. This purification is one of the most important matters connected with the making of champagne.

The Medoc districts, in the Bordeaux territory, produce the finest of the clarets. The grapes are detached from the stalks, and subjected to pressure. The must is put into the fermenting-vat, to which is added the murk resulting from the pressing, and the stalks which were previously separated from the berries. The time necessary for vinification varies; in good years it is no longer than four or five days, and the future wine will then be at its best with regard to taste, delicacy, and softness.

In one case, that of the Red Hermitage wine of France, the grapes are unstalked and crushed before being placed in the vat. The contents of the latter are then stirred twice a day, and ultimately once a day. This is continued for about a month, and in one of the best vineyards for forty days. This long "cuvage" appears necessary from the fact that the large amount of sugar in the must is but slowly transformed into alcohol.

There is a curious incident which occurs in connection with the world-renowned wines of Burgundy, which is worth recording. As the fermentation proceeds, the murk, as in all similar fermentations, rises to the surface of the vat, and forms what is called the "hat," or CHAPEAU. The fermentation proceeds till all is ready for the wine to be drawn. At this time the "hat" is so dense that it will bear the weight of two or three men. Each of them now begins working with one foot till he gets it through the crust, and the whole CHAPEAU is eventually broken up and mixed with the wine.

But to return to our subject. As soon as the stormy or seething fermentation is over, the young wine is drawn off from the fermenting-vat into the maturing-cask, at which time it may be quite warm and turbid. In a cool cellar and with perfect quiet it gradually becomes clearer; it deposits on the bottom of the cask many of the substances it contains, and the fermentation becomes no longer visible. The time which this "slow fermentation" takes to occur will vary with the type of wine, with the nature of the must, and with the influence of the season. Speaking generally, it may be said to be from two to eight weeks after its entrance into the maturing-cask. The wine is considered to be ready for its first racking when it has become clear and transparent, and when its lees have subsided to the bottom of the cask.

In racking there is a withdrawal of the wine from the sediment which it casts down, and which is known as the lees. It is an important operation because irremediable damage is caused to wine by allowing it to remain in contact with the dregs. A knowledge of their composition is of great value, since it serves to explain their injurious influence. The lees deposited from vinous fermentation consist of mineral salts, tartaric acid, and organic matters. Of these the 'organic substances are the most to be dreaded, and for this reason, that they are very prone to rapid decomposition. They consist of yeast-cells, cells of other micro-organisms, of DEBRIS and minute particles of grape stalks and skins, and of other bodies, all readily liable to decompose. All these various materials, therefore, are continually a source of peril, for the slightest thing may start action in them, which spreads throughout the wine and simply ruins it. By removing it from such undesirable company all these risks are avoided, and the best possible qualities of the wine are afforded the opportunity to develop. In the performance of racking definite changes take place in the vine, which are assuredly important. For it must be remembered that the nearly fermented young wines contain an excess of carbonic acid gas; and this is rightly regarded as possessing great preservative properties, in that it prevents the dangerously spreading growth of the little micro-organisms and germs present in all new wine.

In the course of racking, however, a certain amount of the carbonic acid gas must be lost, and fresh oxygen is absorbed from the atmosphere. The oxygen is invaluable from the fact that it exerts a powerful chemical influence upon the wine; as a consequence fermentation is slightly renewed if there be any grape sugar remaining. At the same time the colour of the wine is also modified, and any rawness or harshness in its taste quality is enormously increased by the development of those delicate and subtle ethers which have so much to do with the flavour and bouquet of all wines.

The operation of racking, consequently, is one of great importance, as it requires to be repeated from time to time. A copious deposit of lees generally takes place after the first racking, and a second one should speedily follow. During the first year young wines are often racked off as many as three times, but with the older wines once a year, at the beginning of spring, may be sufficient. But it is precisely in matters of this kind that judgment and experience are so much needed.

Now, it has been pointed out over and over again that it is solely by a correct treatment of Australian wines in the cellar that we can hope to attain to excellence; in fact, the whole secret lies in this direction. And it is very much to be regretted, therefore, that cellar management and wine treatment have not yet been conceded their proper position, that of being the principal factors in the success of Australian wine. Amongst others, this very truth was pointed out by Mr. Pownall, to whom I have previously referred. In giving evidence before the Vegetable Products Commission of Victoria in August 1889, he observed:--"In some of the cellars I have been horrified with the amount of wine which I should describe as 'perished' and as 'perishing.' It is astounding, I can hardly express the quantity. And very often the vine-grower is so ignorant of his business that he shows one wine which is 'tart' and 'sour,' and even praises it. I find those wines are generally exceeding three years old, and I attribute it to the lack of cellar knowledge and treatment, because in the same cellar where I find large quantities of bad wine I find this year's and last year's wine good, and promising well; but if longer kept, and so treated, after a few years it will be utterly useless."

It will only be by paying attention to all the details connected with the cellarage of Australian wines that the victory will be ours. I have said so before, and now say it again, that our Australian must is quite equal to, if not superior to, any in the world. But it is from that very time that the critical stage in the making of our wines begins. It behoves our vignerons, therefore, to concentrate their energies mainly upon that vastly important period which follows onwards from the very beginning of vinification.

THE TASTING AND JUDGING OF WINES.

Of the five senses, namely, seeing, hearing, feeling, smelling, and tasting, the last is by no means the least important. It is a wise provision, this sense of taste, in that it enables us to relish our food, and also to select that which is suitable at the same time. If we took no pleasure in eating we should probably cease to eat at all, and die of starvation. And if we had no taste we might eat that which was unsuitable. In illness, almost the first things that the sufferer will complain about are that he has lost all desire for his food, and that everything tastes alike to him. The true taste impressions are limited to the following, namely, bitter, sweet, sour, and salt. The best substances to mark these four varieties of taste are quinine for the bitter, honey for the sweet, vinegar for the sour, and table salt for the last. The sense of taste is closely associated with that of smell; indeed, the sense of smell has nearly all to do with the perception of flavour. There is an inseparable connection between the two senses of smell and taste, for when anosmia or loss of the sense of smell occurs, all taste, except for bitterness, sweetness, sourness, and saltness, is completely lost, so far as ideas of flavour, &c., are concerned.

Brillat-Savarin, the high-priest of gastronomy, quaintly puts it that smell and taste form only one sense, having the mouth as laboratory, with the nose for the fire-place or chimney; the one serving to taste solids, the other gases. George Dallas, too, the gifted author of THE BOOK OF THE TABLE, also expresses the association of taste and smell in an apt way. He makes reference to the fact that the other senses are not dependent on each other, but that the hearing becomes more acute in a blind man. On the contrary, taste is made for marriage, and smell is its better half. Taste loses, as he says, all its delicacy when it cannot mate with a fine olfactory nerve. The late Dr. Druitt has likewise noted that the union of smell with taste is essential for the enjoyment of wine.

From the foregoing it will be seen that when we speak of taste we refer to a complicated and extremely delicate process. There is this also to be remembered, that it is a sense which can be cultivated to a high degree; and in the wine-taster it is brought to the very pitch of excellence. Yet, notwithstanding all this, it must be a matter of every-day experience, that people will profess to an ability to judge wine when they know absolutely nothing of the various points, so to speak, to be looked for. What I mean is this, that there are many different things to be observed when a wine is tasted, and that each one requires to have proper judgment bestowed upon it. What these are I shall endeavour to speak of in due course.

Wine tasting is a fine art as seen with the COURTIERS or experts who are employed by the large houses in Bordeaux. There are exceptional qualifications required for this office, for its holders must possess a delicate and highly trained palate, and an exquisite and perfect sense of smell, while at the same time a lengthened experience and unerring discrimination in the value of the wine submitted to them are also called for. Mr. James Smith, in his prize essay, already referred to, quotes with approval the following passage from a French authority:-"The COURTAGE of wines is, then, a true science, which is acquired by long observations, by numerous tastings, extensive practice, and a correct judgment; a science which has rendered, and is daily rendering, true and important services to our vinicole department (that of the Gironde); for, by this means, intelligent classifications have given to our GRANDS CRUS a universal reputation, and have made our best wines known and appreciated throughout the civilised world. In the judging of wines, therefore, at least four essentials are necessary: two of the senses--the taste and the smell must be perfect--while great experience and special knowledge must be equally present."

Now, there is an old saying, DE GUSTIBUS NON EST DISPUTANDUM, and consequently every person has a perfect right to like what pleases him; so that in this way anyone may prefer to drink whisky, or any other form of spirits, and he is quite entitled to believe there is nothing so good for him; but, on the other hand, an habitual spirit-drinker must not claim to possess a correct judgment in estimating the qualities of a good wine; for, as a matter of fact, the daily influence of whisky on the palate is absolutely fatal to its delicacy of perception. There are none of the graceful flavours, none of the delicate ethers, none of the perfumed bouquets in whisky that belong to a wholesome wine. No, there is only the coarse spirit which benumbs the palatal nerves, and renders them incapable of picking out these vinous attributes. Moreover, it would almost seem that a person's very thoughts are controlled by his customary beverage. It is evident, indeed, that Richard Bentley, one of the greatest scholars of modern times, believed in this doctrine; for did he not make this memorable remark to one of his pupils: "Sir, if you drink ale, you will think ale"?

Is it not true, also, that with many people champagne is regarded as the highest type of wine? This is more likely to be the case with those who are beginning to realize the pleasures of life. Indeed, as it has been acutely remarked, a youngster from college, when invited to dinner, thinks himself badly treated if he does not get it. Now, it is not to be denied that champagne is, in its way, an imperial drink, and that it has a specially exhilarating effect. But, at the same time, it must be remembered that it is on the other side of the champagne stage of life that the appreciation of really great wines begins.

Take, for instance, a comparison of the wines of Bordeaux and of Burgundy. These are two distinct classes of wine, and, according to Mr. Sept. Berdmore, should be imbibed different days. That they are entirely distinct wines might only be expected, seeing that the geographical positions of the two districts are so far apart. The Bordeaux wines come from the south-western or Bay of Biscay side of France, while those of Burgundy belong to her eastern portion. It is almost universally a matter of belief that the red wines of Bordeaux should be warmed gradually--taking some hours--before they are drunk. The temperature of these wines should be as nearly as possible the temperature of the dining-room itself. The finest clarets are often utterly spoiled from the fact that this has been disregarded, and they have been brought to table without ally preparation. In the case of Burgundy, however, an opposite treatment is required, and by many connoisseurs it is considered to be best when brought up from a cool cellar shortly before use. All these are matters of considerable importance, and show that the judging of wines requires something more than a mere off-hand opinion. There are certain descriptions of the different varieties of wines, given by Thudicum and Dupre, Vizetelly and others, which are of great assistance in helping to a knowledge of the various desiderata to be looked for. Moreover, much will be gained by collecting them together, as their principal characteristics will be better remembered when they are thus contrasted with each other. It is not my wish to laud the wines of other countries to the disparagement of Australian growths, but it is my object to show clearly those desirable properties which all good wines should possess. A knowledge of these lofty standards will do more to better the quality of our Australian wines than anything I know of.

The wines of the Medoc, that district of the Gironde which produces the finest clarets, namely, Chateau Margaux, Chateau Lafitte, Chateau Latour, &c., possess distinguishing features peculiar to themselves. They have a certain slight distinctive roughness; are fine, juicy, marrowy in the mouth, and after having been in bottle some years they acquire a very beautiful bouquet. They have, moreover, this remarkable hygienic quality, that they can be drunk in large quantity without, as the French say, "fatiguing" either head or stomach. But there is another portion of the Bordeaux country, namely the GRAVES, which produces both red and white wines. The latter include those magnificent Sauternes, Chateau d'Yquem and La Tour Blanche, which take such high rank; Chateau d'Yquem, indeed, has been likened to liquid gold--liquid gold in a crystal glass--and is one of those most luscious and delicately aromatic of wines, with an exquisite bouquet and rich, delicious flavour.

As it has already been stated, Bordeaux and Burgundy are entirely different wines, and this fact must be well remembered. The wines of the latter comprise some of the most famous growths of France, and are distinguished by the suavity of their taste, their finesse, and spirituous aroma The red wines have a fine colour, a good deal of bouquet, and a delicious taste. They give tone to the stomach, and facilitate digestion. Of these red wines of Burgundy the Romanee-Conti is among the first growths, and it is renowned for its fine colour, its aroma, its delicacy, and the superb quality of its delicious taste. Clos de Vougeot is another great growth, which is slightly more alcoholic than the preceding. Chambertin, also, possesses a good deal of seve, delicacy, perfect taste, and pleasant bouquet; moreover, it has a softness which made it an especial favourite with the great Napoleon. Corton, likewise, is of high colour, corse, and, as it gets older, acquires a great deal of seve and bouquet.

The white wines of Burgundy however, must not be forgotten, for amongst them is the renowned Chablis. This, with the oysters, the squeeze of lemon juice, and the brown bread and butter, usually heralds in any large dinner. Although slightly alcoholic, it is not heady, and possesses body, delicacy, and an agreeable perfume, with that distinguishing PIERRE A FUSIL taste--that flinty flavour--which is its recognised characteristic.

Leaving the Bordeaux wines and the wines of Burgundy, it is next desirable to speak of one which belongs to the South of France. It is well known, at least by name, to most Australians, and any description of its properties, therefore, will be the more appreciated. This is the Muscat of Rivesaltes, in the department of the Oriental Pyrenees. By some it is esteemed the best liqueur wine in the world. A good sample of it possesses great finesse, a good deal of vinosity, and that wonderful muscadine bouquet which gives to it its celebrated characters.

There is another wine, coming from the valley of the Rhone, in the south-eastern portion of France, whose name is equally familiar to most Australians; this is the Red Hermitage, or, as it is perhaps more commonly known amongst us, Shiraz, wine. A genuine wine is distinguished by great richness, a lively purple colour, and a special bouquet; and it becomes, by these united qualities, the best wine of this region.

Turning to the German wines, those of the Rheingau must claim our attention. This district borders on the Rhine, and it is said that the river acts as a mirror, in reflecting the rays of the sun towards the vineyards. The Rheingau must not be confused with the district of Hochheim, which is situated on the Maine. Yet it is curious that the first syllable of the latter district (Hochheim) has furnished the monosyllabic English word Hock, under which are confused ALL the Rhine wines. Amongst the wines of the Rheingau may be enumerated Steinberg, Marcobrunner, and Johannisberg. With regard to the wines of the Rheingau, Mr. Henry Vizetelly observes: "Although the flavour and bouquet of the grand wines of the Rheingau are equally pronounced, it is exceedingly difficult to characterise them with precision. After gratifying the sense of smell with the fragrant odour which they evolve --and which is no mere evanescent essence vanishing as soon as recognised, but often a rich odour which almost scents the surrounding atmosphere--you proceed to taste the vine, and seem to sip the aroma exhaled by it. Now and then you are conscious of a refilled pungent flavour, and at other times of a slight racy sharpness, while the after-taste generally suggests more of an almond flavour than any other you can call to mind. No wines vary so much in their finer qualities as the grand growths of the Rheingau. The produce of a particular vineyard, although from the same species of grape, cultivated under precisely similar conditions, will differ materially in flavour and bouquet, not merely in bad and good years, but in vintages of equal excellence. Moreover, these wines need the most skilful cellar treatment during the long years they are maturing. All great wines, it should be remembered, ripen slowly, and cannot be 'pasturised' into perfection--that is to say, cannot be rapidly matured by heating them to a certain temperature, as ordinary wines may be."

The Hochheim vineyards are situated, as I have previously indicated, on the banks of the Maine, several miles above its confluence with the Rhine. There is one exceptionally fine Hochheim growth which comes from the vineyard of the "Dechanei," or deanery. True Hochheinner is a remarkably aromatic wine, and possesses both body and fire. Indeed, it contains as large a percentage of alcohol as the so-called noble Steinberger--the most spirituous of the Rhenish growths--with more sweetness. It consequently lacks that subdued acidulous freshness of flavour which is such a marked characteristic of the wines of the Rheingau.

Some reference to sherry and port is necessary, because they are both types of wines that are widely known, and consequently ally remarks concerning, them are of value by comparison. It would appear that with most sherry, and certainly with all port, there is an addition of alcohol to the wine. Even the wines which are sold in England under the name of "natural sherry" contain from 13.2 to 15.5 per cent. of alcohol. Beyond all question, therefore, from 1 1/2 to 3 1/2 per cent. of alcohol must have been added, for no "natural sherry" should ever contain more than 12 per cent. of alcohol. Some sherries, however, have been introduced with an alcoholicity of from 12 to 13.6 per cent., with the following, characters: The taste is freely vinous, rich, pure, mellow, and quite free from heat or the taste of added spirit. But fashion has much to do with the type of sherry in request; thus the colour has varied from time to time. In the same way, too, a taste for dry sherries arose with the Manzanilla epoch, only to be carried to excess. As with all other wines, a certain age in sherry is desirable; the ethers become developed during this period, and impart a rich flavour to it. In the course of time, however, sherry falls off so much that it is only fit for giving flavour to young wine.

In the matter of port, also, it may confidently be asserted that not a single drop is sold that does not contain a certain amount of added brandy. That is to say, all port wine, without exception, is brandied. The effect of the brandy is to keep the wine quiet; it prevents it from undergoing any fermentation; and, what is more, it keeps it from changing, no matter whether the climate be hot or cold. Messrs. Thudicum and Dupre state that a perfectly natural port has 9 per cent. of alcohol as the lowest, and 13.8 per cent. as the highest limit.

A sample of Alto Douro wine submitted to these gentlemen, although it was slightly alcoholised, yet possessed the following desirable qualities: it was fine, because it was derived from the finest and ripest Alto Douro grapes, the Verdeilho and Bastardo; it was full, owing to its great vinosity and high amount of natural alcohol, yet free from adventitious syrup; and it was pure, because free from all those faults which depreciate so many southern wines, such as the fousel flavour, or the burning taste of distilled spirit. Besides all these great qualities, it characteristically possessed the very essence of an ideal port wine flavour--without the saccharine and spirituous taste commonly found in port wine--and it had a natural smooth astringency such as pleases the palate and imparts keeping qualities.

Moreover, it was very unlike the artificial sweet and burning products commonly called port wine. It was thoroughly fermented, and contained such a minute quantity of grape sugar that the latter could not be possibly detected by the taste. It was perfectly dry, and thereby differed entirely from ordinary port wines, which contain from 2 to 6 per cent. of sugar. Its alcoholicity was certainly below all the port wines usually sold. With all these desirable qualities, therefore, it possessed high dietetic and hygienic virtues, and refreshed the system like Burgundy or Medoc wine.

It will be convenient to make reference here to two terms about which there is a great deal of confusion. It is the difference between the "aroma" and the "bouquet" of wine. Now, the Settimana Vinicola has recently well observed that although these two are usually supposed to be the same, yet they are entirely different. The aroma of a wine is altogether distinct from those agreeable and delicate odours known by the name of "bouquet." For instance, some American grapes have what is called a "foxy" smell, and the wine prepared from them has this aroma, which is perceptibly disagreeable. Aroma pre-exists in certain grapes, and during vinification will pass into the resulting wine. On the other hand, perfume, the bouquet of the French, as it has been pointed out by Professor G. Grazzi-Soncini, is the complex sensation produced simultaneously on the palate and nose, owing to the intimate connection between these two organs, and which has already been referred to. This bouquet is due to the action of the ethers, which are formed during the life of the wine. The CORRIERE DEL VILLAGIO remarks, in addition to the preceding, that there is a chemical difference between the "aroma" and the "bouquet" of wine. The former is produced chiefly by one or more carburets of hydrogen, and their oxidation derivatives. The bouquet, however, results from the admixture of aldehydes with one or more essential oils and various ethers, produced by combination of fatty and other acids with ethylic and other alcohols, and from these changes result the different ethers which constitute the bouquet of wine.

One of the most valuable books published on vine-growing and wine-making is that by the justly celebrated Dr. Jules Guyot. The greater part of one particularly important chapter is wholly taken up with the most graphic and lucid description of wine-tasting with which we are acquainted. Besides this, it contains such an amount of information on the subject, that no remarks in this connection would be complete without reference to it. For the following vivid rendering of a good deal of this very chapter I am very much indebted to my friend Dr. John Steel, of Sydney:--

"Wine put upon its trial is subjected to two jurisdictions; the one altogether belonging to the senses, the other wholly physiological. The appreciation of wine by the senses is referred to three of our organs of sense--the eye; the nasal chambers, in front and behind; and the mouth, equally at its anterior and posterior part.

"WINE JUDGED BY THE SIGHT.--Wine pleases the eye by its clearness and colour: and be it ruby, rose, amber, or white, it ought always to have perfect clearness and freshness of colour. Neither of these latter tones will be out of harmony in a really good wine, even in extreme old age. If you will not take upon yourself to decide whether a wine is good when it is attractive to the sight, you can always say that it is not good or at least that it is not in the best condition, when its transparency and shades of colour are questionable. Freshness of colour and clearness are good signs. Though they are not to be regarded as qualities, yet any appearance to the contrary betokens real defects in the wine.

"WINE JUDGED BY THE SENSE OF SMELL; THE TWO ODOURS OF WINE.--Wine reveals itself by two sorts of odours (the aroma and the bouquet) to the outer organ of smell--that is to say, when that sense is exercised by inhaling (or sniffing) the wine. The first, or aroma, is the general and common odour peculiar to most wines. It is always strongest when the wine is newest, but it always characterises good wine, however old it may be. This first odour seems to be due to the volatilization of the spirit, which holds in solution an essential oil, more or less volatile, more or less powerful, and more or less characteristic of each kind of wine. This aroma is a sign of real quality in the wine, and is generally very strong and very noticeable during the first years; it becomes concentrated, refined, and attenuated as the wine ages. The second kind of odour the bouquet, on the contrary, is developed with age, and would appear to be owing to the reaction of vinous acids on the spirit, which gives rise to certain ethereal combinations.

"WINES ARE NOT MADE CHIEFLY TO PLEASE THE SENSES OF SIGHT AND SMELL--
Aroma, like colour, is a favourable or unfavourable sign, agreeable or disagreeable. Yet before everything wine is a nourishing beverage. It is a very good thing that sight and smell should be gratified in this way, but it would be puerile and ridiculous to exalt beyond measure the importance of these organs of sense; and to pretend that the superiority of wine rests almost exclusively on the pleasurable impressions which are derived therefrom. I have seen many hosts bother their guests with vexatious insistence to look at, hold up to the light, sniff their wine, even the empty glasses, almost throughout the whole duration of a banquet--at the risk of making them well nigh die of thirst. The true amateur, the wine-taster, knows perfectly well how to look at and how to smell his wine; but he knows full well also that these two preliminaries ought to be immediately followed by the taking of the fluid into the front part of the mouth. Colour and smell are merely two notes introductory to a gastronomic theme; if they are only by themselves they lose their relative value, and the theme is not properly understood.

"WINE JUDGED BY TASTE; THAT IS, BY THE MOUTH AT ITS ANTERIOR AND
POSTERIOR PART.--Before speaking of the impression wine gives to the sense of taste, I ought to say that this sense is the only one in the animal organization which possesses a double apparatus for perception-- one at the tip and edges of the tongue, the other at its root and at

the soft palate. The first perceives acid or electro-positive tastes through the two lingual nerves; the second detects alkaline tastes by the two glosso-pharyngeal nerves. Tastes perceived by the front part of the mouth, in the case of liquids as well as solids, are not the same as those discriminated by the back part of the mouth. An alkaline salt, for instance, gives to the front part an acid, styptic, salt, or sweet taste, but communicates to the posterior part a basic, bitter, or saponaceous taste.

"WINE-TASTING PROPERLY SO CALLED.--Wine taken into the front part of
the mouth gives rise to acid, sweet, and styptic tastes at the outer edges and tip of the tongue. All shades, in harmony, ought to give a pleasing sensation to the organ, when neither acidity, sweetness, nor astringency predominates. Next we pass the wine to the posterior part of the mouth, and delay it there by a kind of gargling. It is now that we get the smack of the soil, the taste of cask or wood, the insipidity of salts, or any bitterness. If the whole effect is pleasing to the back part of the mouth, with the absence of all disagreeable impressions, we must, to put the finishing touch on the wine-tasting, not spit it out, but swallow it. As soon as the wine has passed over the root of the tongue and the soft palate and its pillars, a most pronounced odour ascends from the pharynx into the nasal cavities, and gives forth newer and more powerful revelations, AS to the qualities or defects of the bouquet of wine, than can ever be obtained by the outward sense of smell. Moreover, the last contact of wine with the mucous membrane of the pharynx and of the base of the tongue leaves a lasting impression of taste, and when this sensation is disagreeable it is designated under the collective name of 'after-taste.'

"GOOD AND BAD WINE JUDGED BY THE SENSES.--If, then, a wine pos-sesses
perfect clearness and freshness of colour, if it has an agreeable

odour, if the combined effect of the acid, sweet, and astringent tastes
is gratifying to the anterior part of the mouth by a fusion, seeming to
form a unique taste like many notes in a complete harmony; if to this
harmonious impression the back part of the mouth adds a feeling of glow
and vinous richness, without alcohol being noticed; and if, at last,
the act of swallowing crowns the whole with a natural bouquet, not
followed by any 'after-taste,' we may pronounce the wine to be good as
judged by the senses. But, on the other hand, the wine is
unsatisfactory if it fail in any of these points. It will be inferior
in proportion as the acids, sugar, and the salts become individually
perceived by the tip of the tongue. Again, it is imperfect when the
chilliness, flatness, the essential oils, the taste of earth and of
cask, and above all, an excess of froe spirit, are manifestly noticed
at the base of that organ. And lastly, it is defective just as the
'ARRIERE BOUQUET' is less pleasant, and the 'after-taste' more
disagreeably prolonged.

"THE DIFFICULTY OF JUDGING BY TASTES.--In this unfolding of the
process of wine-tasting I have endeavoured to be clear, and yet I feel
I have not been sufficiently so. It will be impossible to judge by
tastes until science has laid down signs or words representative of
their quality, of their stamp, or of their harmonious relations. The
science of tastes has yet to be founded. Till then, chefs de cuisine
and the clever caterers for banquets will remain isolated geniuses or
empirics; while, as regards wine-tasters and gastronomists, they
approve or they criticise, but they do not establish any rules. It
would be a curious collection that would comprise all the expressions
used by wine-tasters, wine-merchants, commercial travellers, amateurs
(by far, indeed, the most numerous class), to express the feelings they
experience in tasting wines. I know an English traveller who only liked
a wine when it caused a 'peacock's tail in the mouth'; and
everybody knows the expression of the Auvergnian drinking a glass of
generous old wine--'It's a yard of velvet going down the throat.'

"THE PHYSIOLOGICAL EFFECT OF WINES.--The inhabitants of a beer-drinking
or spirit-drinking country will never possess the vivacity of
wit and the light-heartedness of those who live in a wine-producing
land. It is not by any means the alcohol in itself which constitutes
the worth and goodness of wine, for beer may contain as much, and
spirits certainly contain more. To be more or less spirituous does not
constitute good wine. All natural wine is good, whether it be strong or
weak in spirit, if it keeps its organic life. It is good, too, if it
reveals itself by a fresh odour, by a union of all its elements in a
taste harmonious to the palate, by being easily digested, and by
causing greater activity of body and mind, and a sensible augmentation
of muscular force. Be the taste of the wine fresh, sharp, or delicate;
be it soft, unctuous, or rich; be it acid or strong, the wine is good
if it supports and increases the forces of body and mind, without
wearing out the digestive Organs.

"WINE IS GOOD RELATIVELY AND NOT ABSOLUTELY. WE OUGHT TO HAVE BEFORE
EVERYTHING GOOD COMMON WINES.--A wine is good according to the use to
which we put it. Even an excellent liqueur or dessert vine is
undesirable and out of place for ordinary drinking purposes or for
nourishment. We must distinguish between wines for ordinary use, those
for side dishes (ENTREMETS), and those for dessert. And these again
should be differentiated into wines for small, medium, or large
glasses, relatively, proportional to the quantity which we can or ought
to drink. A good cake is always good if we only eat a little at a time,
and seldom take it; but bread is infinitely better and preferred by
everybody to eating cake always. It is vastly more important to have
good ordinary wines than to have good VINS D'ENTREMETS or good liqueur
wines. And, indeed, this very matter affects the total consumption
within and out of France, and the interests of producer and consumer,

as well as the interests of public hygiene. Good ordinary wine, alimentary wine--for wine is a real and excellent food--by no means a wine strong in spirit, nor is it a wine of great age; but it is a wine of fine CEPAGE, not going beyond 10 per cent. of spirit, or even 6 per cent."

UNIFORMITY IN AUSTRALIAN WINES.

This is a subject the importance of which cannot be over estimated. And it is one markedly calling for consideration, as there have been, and still are, grounds for complaint in this direction. It will be advisable, therefore, to look well into the question, because it will amply repay the trouble bestowed upon it. First of all, then, let us refer to the remarks of Mr. Francois de Castella, the author of the Handbook on Viticulture for Victoria. He points out that in each district there will be one class of wine which will surpass all others in excellence, and that this is the type which the grower should produce. All the vine-growers in any one district should endeavour to make their wines of the type specially adapted for that particular district; and of course the type will vary in different districts. In this way, and only in this way, will it be possible for the public to obtain an unvarying article.

At the present time there are in each district a number of wines possessing various names, such as Hermitage, Shiraz, Carbenet, Burgundy, Chasselas, Riesling, Tokay, &c., but these names actually mean nothing. Each district should produce a different type of wine. A Riesling from the Yarra and a Riesling from the Murray are as distinct as Hock and Sherry. Mr. de Castella further advises that each vine-grower should join the Vine-Growers' Association in his locality. In this way the members of each district can agree amongst themselves to produce one class of wine, or at most two--say one white and one red. Instead of the same names being applied to entirely different wines, the nine will come to be known by the name of the district in which it is produced. One will then be able to have some idea of the contents of a bottle, from the label upon it. At present the name on the bottle is no indication whatever of the wine within; indeed, the same name is on the outside of many totally distinct wines. This change must assuredly come, and the sooner it does the better for Australian wines.

Mr. Pownall, in the course of his evidence before the Royal Commission on Vegetable Products in Victoria, also drew attention to this same want of uniformity. He believed that each vineyard ought to aim at making a standard quality of wine, so that wine-merchants might know what to expect from that vineyard. The wines throughout Australia should likewise, as far as possible, bear uniform names. He stated that he had met wines in various vineyards grown from the same grape, and called by different names; and though this might seem a trivial matter, yet it led to endless confusion. Moreover, it should not be permitted to continue, especially as it could be so easily rectified.

It must be said, however, that at the Great Western district, in Victoria, a start has been made in the right direction. A report on the vineyards of that locality referred to the gratifying fact that a marked tendency existed towards the adoption of a rational nomenclature of wines. Many of the leading growers were confining themselves to one red and one white wine. Some of them called their wine by the name of the vineyard, adding the words Hock, Chablis, Claret, &c. after them. This is unquestionably so far an improvement, and it is to be hoped that before long the wine will be known by the name of the vineyard or district, and by nothing else.

Mr. James Smith has also strongly insisted upon the supreme importance of this uniformity, especially as regards the quality of the wine. And this is perfectly true. The quality of any particular wine is solely dependent upon the season, but the produce of any given vineyard should surely possess, as he remarks, a distinctive CACHET, by which the palate is enabled to recognise it. For instance, an expert would not fail to distinguish between a Chateau Margaux and a Chateau Lafitte, nor between a Chateau Latour and a Haut Brion. Notwithstanding the different vintages, there is always a uniformity and continuity of flavour maintained through all these great growths. But in the case of our Australian wines there is a lamentable difference. Wines of the same denomination and from the same grower DIFFER SO MATERIALLY one year from those bearing a similar name, and coming from the same cellar, in another, that it is difficult to believe they are the same. As Mr. Smith justly observes, this is an unpardonable defect in the estimation of connoisseurs; more especially such as attach themselves to a particular kind of wine, and naturally drink it by preference. Constancy of type should be unremittingly aimed at by the vigneron. And this can only be possible by continuous attention to each individual factor concerned in vine-growing and wine-making.

THE FUTURE SUCCESS OF THE AUSTRALIAN WINE INDUSTRY--AND UPON WHAT IT DEPENDS.

Figures help us considerably more than words in enforcing a proper idea of the magnitude to which the Australian wine industry should develop. It will be appropriate, therefore, to preface this portion by bringing forward a few speculative data. In an earlier part of this chapter it was stated that the city of Paris alone requires nearly 300,000 gallons of wine daily, and that this single city would consume in 12 days all the wine which the whole of Australia takes 12 MONTHS to make. The population of Paris is nearly two and a half millions, while that of Australia is three millions odd. By considering these together it will be seen that the wine which it takes over three million people all the year to make, lasts another two and a half million people only 12 days.

Now, the total annual wine yield of Australia, including both that used here and that which is exported, is only worth about 800,000 L. It follows from the foregoing, then, that Paris will in 12 days consume about 800,000 L. worth of wine, and for the whole year the Parisian figures for wine consumption will reach to something like 20,000,000 L. Let us suppose that Australia were only a wine-drinking community, as her climate unceasingly calls for. It would be fair to assume that her yearly wine bill would be in accordance with the following rule of proportion. If Paris with her two and a half millions annually consumes wine to the amount of 20,000,000 L., then Australia with her three millions odd would surely require for her own use at least 20,000,000 l. worth year by year. And when it is remembered in addition that the export trade should be enormously in excess of any local requirements, it will readily be see what a magnificent future only awaits its calling into being.

We cannot hope that our Australian wines will take a high place amongst those of the world as long as they are not in general use by our own people. There can be no keener reproach than to have it said: "Why, even the Australians themselves do not drink their own wines." And this is regrettedly the fact. It is necessary, therefore, that first of all our people should take a very deep interest in all the details connected with vine-growing and wine-making, and thus give some encouragement to those who are doing their best to establish what will ultimately become Australia's brightest glory. And it will be a good thing for this land when a knowledge of every point in the growing of the grape, and every step in the making of the wine, becomes part and parcel of our daily life. The very hoardings of our streets are covered with advertisements of countless brands of whisky, and of numberless varieties of ale. But those setting forth the virtues of our wines are conspicuous by their absence. It would seem that Australia, where our own wine should be the national beverage, is almost the last country in which to find it.

It may be asked, what are the reasons which lead to this disregard of the virtues possessed by our own wines? The reply to this question is not an easy matter, but I shall endeavour to answer it to the best of my ability. The probability is, if a dozen people were asked, at random, why Australian wine is so little used in Australia, that at least that number of different explanations would be forthcoming. The truth, however, is more likely to be found in a combination of reasons, rather than from any one single cause. These are obviously worth considering, from the very fact that the knowing of what they consist is of the first importance in rectifying them.

I shall begin, then, by saving that the label on the bottle has much to answer for, in that it is misleading. It does not give any idea of what is to be found inside. Thus the word Riesling, on one bottle, may be attached to a wine grown on the Hunter, in New South Wales, and on another to a wine from the Yarra, in Victoria. It is true that the wine from these two places may be grown from the same "cepage." But while the river Yarra wine will contain perhaps 11 per cent. of alcohol, that from the Hunter River will have quite 20 per cent.--so much does an increase in the warmth of the climate increase the alcoholic strength of the wine.

And while we are on the subject of labels, I must certainly take exception to the unattractive character of those employed on the bottles of our Australian wines. There is no reason whatever why a little consideration should not be paid to the artistic sense in this respect. Our wine merchants, it would appear, fail to understand the selling power which belongs to the "get-up" of the label on a wine bottle. I feel sure this attractiveness has a great deal to do with the success of many products, notably in the case of the American preserved fruits. Some of these are labelled in a manner which is creditable in the highest degree--and what is more, from a practical point, it is no unimportant factor in their huge sale.

Then again, there is that want of uniformity which Mr. James Smith has so ably descanted upon, and to which I have already referred. It is bad enough to have a wine labelled Riesling, or whatever it may be, from one place differing entirely from a wine of the same name which comes from some other locality. But it is a far more serious defect when the wine of any particular place one year differs entirely from the same wine coming from the same locality at another. For the same variety of wine, of the same vineyard, thus to vary, year by year, is simply unpardonable. This must not be allowed to continue, for while it exists Australian nines will always be subject to reproach--a reproach, indeed, which cannot be explained away.

And while dealing with these shortcomings I propose to speak of another matter, which is by no means unimportant. I refer to the size of the bottle. It has frequently happened that visitors to Australia hare said to me, "I should very much like--indeed, I am anxious--to try your Australian wines; but unfortunately I cannot drink a whole bottle at table, and I am unable to obtain less." Now, this is undoubtedly a grievance, and should be overcome in some way; either by putting up a portion of our wines in smaller bottles, or else by making some arrangement so that a smaller quantity may be obtained. Since these lines were written, however, it is very pleasing to record the fact that one enterprising firm in Sydney has taken a highly commendable step in this very direction; and already smaller bottles of Australian wine may be obtained for the low prices of 6d. and 9d.

Up to this point I have made no remarks with regard to the knowledge of wine possessed by the majority of Australians, and yet in many respects it is the most important of all. They are not called upon to pronounce an opinion upon a wine, such as would be looked for from an expert. But I do think it is very desirable that they should know, at least, the kind of wine that is suitable for Australian use. Once this is accomplished, and it is by no means difficult to learn, a great deal will have been achieved. It is quite a mistake to imagine that the value of a wine increases with its strength, and that the stronger a wine is, the more valuable it becomes. Even in Europe itself strong wines are going out of fashion, and lighter ones are taking their place. People much prefer a light wine, of which they can take a fair amount and quench their thirst, in preference to a strong wine of the port or sherry type, of which they can only take a small wineglassful. But in Australia, the very place where one would expect a demand for all lighter wines, the taste for strong wines as the rule. This is another striking example of the same antagonism to climatic environment which is found all through our food habits. A light wine is the wine above all others which should be most sought after. What Australia requires as a national beverage is a wine of low alcoholic strength. It should be so cheap as to come within the easy every-day reach of all classes. And finally, it should take the place of all other liquids, since it is essentially wholesome, hygienic, restorative, and cheering.

The reputation of Australian wines in the English market has hitherto been damaged to a considerable extent by the practices which have been followed on the part of some of the large buyers. But before referring to these proceedings, to which Mr. Hans Irvine, of the Great Western Vineyard, in Victoria, has so properly and powerfully drawn attention, it must be distinctly understood that any subsequent remarks do not apply to all the London wine-merchants. On the contrary, there are many whose characters are irreproachable, and whose integrity is above suspicion. By clearing the ground in this way one is enabled to protest against the treatment which Australian wine receives in London, without levelling charges against estimable men, who command respect, and who deserve the gratitude of all Australians for their fair dealings.

Well then, most of our wines purchased by English buyers have been those of full-bodied, crude, and coarse young wines, containing a great amount of alcohol. Two reasons have been assigned for this proceeding; the first being that Australian wines would not bear the voyage unless they were sufficiently strong; and the second, that in England the demand was more particularly for such a class of wine. But many of these firms are utterly ignorant of any special knowledge as to treating the finer and more delicate wines. It has suited these buyers to deal only with the stronger wines, as they are the more secured from any loss or trouble. For the fact is, these wines, while being of a greater alcoholic strength, are really of most excellent character and quality. And besides this, they release certain customers, whose idea of a good wine--even at the present time--is a wine of great body and strength, and not so much one with that delicacy of character and bouquet which the finer wines possess.

Some of the merchants, having but little bother with the heavier wines, have encouraged their sale to as great an extent as possible. From this it follows that those who prefer and habitually drink a better class of wine have never had the opportunity of becoming acquainted with the magnificent wines which Australia can supply. As Mr. Irvine tells us, the higher types of fine, light, delicate, dry wines, with a richness of bouquet, such as most districts in Australia are capable of producing, are the kinds of wine we must look forward to for establishing a name and fame for our produce. It is not too much to assert that before very long Australia will be able to supply wines whose quality will rival the choicest vintages of the most famous vineyards of Europe. Even as it is, the delicacy of bouquet and excellent characters of many of the Australian red and white wines have fairly astonished connoisseurs on being submitted to them.

It seems a thousand pities, then, that such misconception should exist with regard to our wines. And quite undeservedly so, for as a matter of fact these lighter wines are most unfairly neglected. They simply require to be properly fined and carefully attended to. The casks in which they are shipped should be thoroughly cleansed and treated before being filled, in order to take out any taint of spirits they may contain; or any excess of tannin, which is always present in Dew wood. If these different matters be looked to they will improve to a wonderful extent on the voyage, and after being allowed a week or fortnight's rest on arrival, they will be found in a highly satisfactory condition. After this time these delicate wines of a low alcoholic strength require to be duly cared for. But they are worth a little extra attention, for it is absolutely certain that through them, and through them alone, will our Australian wines be accorded the merit and the appreciation which they so undoubtedly deserve.

It must not be imagined, however, that the foregoing is the only handicap which Australian wine has to carry. In other cases there are many reprehensible proceedings adopted, which irretrievably injure the reputation of our wines in the English market. Some of the inferior wines are shipped home and "restored," by blending them with full, heavy, rich wines from warmer districts. When "clothed" in this way, their imperfections are for a time hidden, but the bad soon contaminates the whole. It is true that a good, sound, and well-made wine improves with age. But with these "restored" and "clothed" wines the reverse happens, and they become worse and worse by keeping.

Then again, many of the widely advertised Australian wines in the old country are sold too young; and unfortunately these young wines constitute the bulk of the trade done with England. They are bottled when too green and crude, and have not been given a sufficient time in cask to develop into high-class wines. They must be allowed to acquire a proper amount of cask ripeness, and if they were stored and attended to for twelve months before being bottled they would vastly improve. In some cases, also, wines are shipped from Australia before they are twelve months old, and as they are usually fined, bottled, and sold as soon as possible after arrival, it has actually happened that the British public have repeatedly drunk wines that are hardly one year old. Indeed, the wines are frequently bottled when in a state of fermentation, consequently secondary fermentation goes on in the bottle, and the bottles are often shattered by an explosion. And more than this, they are often badly blended; they do not receive sufficient care and attention; and they are not uncommonly in the hands of a few men whose sole object is to make money.

There is still something further which is greatly prejudicial to the fair name of Australian wine, and it is this: Many of the wine merchants hold very small stocks, so that any one supply soon runs out and is no longer obtainable. As a result it is urged against the wines that they are not constant, and that it is impossible to procure the same wine twice running. With larger stocks, too, there would be some certainty that the wine was matured, as for example with a merchant holding a three years' supply. In this case, also, the consumer would be enabled to obtain a continued supply of any particular wine to which he might have become attached.

My own belief, however, is that the most powerful impetus to our wine industry will arise from the Australians themselves taking an interest in all that concerns this great source of health, wealth, and employment. I have said so before, and take this opportunity of saying so again. Let our people take an active interest in every detail connected with the growing of the grape, and with the making of the wine! Let a light, wholesome wine, also, enter into the daily dietary of the whole people! For the national drink for Australian use is unquestionably a wine of low alcoholic strength; a wine of a sufficient age to be free from any reproach of newness; and a wine possessing those qualities which render it wholesome, beneficial, hygienic, cheering, and restorative.

There are two other matters which require to be noticed before leaping the whole subject of Australian wine. The first of these is a reference to the establishment of Viticultural Colleges, and it is one of very great importance, because it has much to do with the development of the wine industry. Now, I am not one of those who look to the State for everything, but it seems to me that if you recognise the necessity of State education, you must at least equally recognise the necessity of affording the youthful population of Australia the opportunity of learning that which must eventually develop into the one distinctive industry of this land. France at the present day, even with her unrivalled reputation as the wine-growing country of the world, avails herself of the advantages of Viticultural Colleges. Italy, also, by means of their help is making strides in a manner actually bordering on the miraculous. If these countries, then, in which vine-growing and winemaking have been carried on for centuries find Viticultural Colleges indispensable, how much more must a young country, with its wine industry quite undeveloped, need them!

It must with confidence be said, therefore, that Australia cannot do without these Viticultural Colleges. Something has already been done by the establishment of Agricultural Colleges, and this is most commendable. But what I believe is this, that a wine-grower must be a wine-grower and nothing else. To know everything connected with the growth of the grape and cellar management thoroughly is quite enough for any ordinary man to attempt to master. Therefore viticulture must either be made a distinctly separate course at the Agricultural

Colleges; or, what if better still, Viticultural Colleges must be established for the purpose alone.

At Montpellier, in France, the course of viticultural education is elaborately comprehensive, and includes the study of the anatomy of the vine, its flowers, leaves, seeds, &c. The pupils become thoroughly acquainted with every variety of wine in practical form; they see it grow, learn the art of pruning, and of everything pertaining to the growth of the vine. They also master all the details connected with grafting, the laying out of vineyards, the diseases to which the vine is liable, and the remedies which are most effectual. And, in addition, there is minute instruction in every step in cellar management and the after care and treatment of the wine itself, from the start to the finish. In this way the subject is studied from a thoroughly scientific standpoint, with a result that influences for good the whole of French viticulture.

But if the benefits derived from the establishment of Viticultural Colleges in France are thus remarkable, those which have followed their introduction into Italy are nothing less than wonderful. The School of Viticulture at Conegliano has been the means of increasing the wine production of Italy to an incredible extent. In 1870 Italy exported only 4,000,000 gallons of wine; yet in 1890, in the short space of twenty years, this had risen to 88,000,000 gallons. This school has taught the people to make good wine; it has induced people who had never dreamt of it to plant vineyards; it hag led people to plant them properly, since they were shown the way on a rational principle; and lastly, they have thus learnt how to make wine on a scientific basis. The course of study there is extremely severe, and as a result all those who receive diplomas from it thoroughly understand the cultivation of the vine and the management of the cellar. This School of Viticulture has been such a phenomenal success that other provinces of Italy brought pressure upon the Government. As a consequence therefrom, secondary schools have been established at many places, notably Gioia del Colle, Pozzuolo, Tmola, Avellino, Alda, Catania, &c.

In conclusion, there is that other most important matter to which I should like to draw attention. It is to advocate the establishment of an Australian Wine-Growers' Association on a federal basis. The advantage resulting from the formation of a strong Association, with a numerically powerful membership roll, would be very great. Such an organization would be well able to conduct a weekly paper of its own, with contributors from all the different colonies. There would be no dearth of literary material, for the whole subject is one teeming with interest. Even now a substantial beginning has been made, and THE AUSTRALIAN VIGNERON AND FRUIT-GROWERS JOURNAL is well deserving of
success, and is already doing good work in this very direction. And besides the foregoing, an Intercolonial Wine-Growers' Congress should meet annually at the different Australian metropolitan centres (Sydney, Melbourne, Adelaide, Brisbane, &c.), in rotation, where there would be the opportunity of discussing theoretical questions, and of tasting practical results. In all these many ways public interest in the Australian wine industry would be continually sustained; and, rising from its unfairly neglected position, it would speedily attain to that pride of place which is manifestly its destiny.

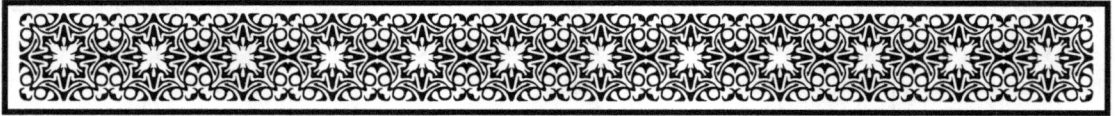

PART II.
AUSTRALIAN COOKERY RECIPES AND ACCESSORY KITCHEN INFORMATION.

MRS. H. WICKEN.
Diplomee of the National Training School for Cookery, London; Lecturer on Cookery to the Technical College, Sydney.

CHAPTER XIII. THE KITCHEN

Furnishing the kitchen is often looked upon as quite of secondary importance; but, instead of being last and least, it ought to be first and foremost, for a cook cannot be expected to send up a good dinner without proper utensils, any more than a carpenter can turn out a piece of furniture without proper tools. It is no doubt a great mistake to have many things in use, for a bad servant will have every one dirty before she begins to wash up, and a good servant will have a lot of work in keeping them clean and in good order. There are a few utensils, not at all expensive, which are a great aid to the cook and a saving of time too, and yet from some cause or other are seldom found in an ordinary kitchen. Before glancing at these we might consider what is the best covering for the floor. There is no doubt that deal boards well scrubbed look nicer than anything else, but to keep them spotless involves a lot of labour, and as this is not always to be had, perhaps the wisest plan is to cover it with oilcloth or linoleum; a good medium quality can be bought for 3s. 3d. a square yard, and if properly laid will last for years. By the way, it should not be washed, but only rubbed with a damp cloth first and then with a piece of flannel dipped in oil soda and scrubbing will ruin it very quickly. If the cupboard accommodation is scanty the dresser should be bought with cupboards underneath; in this case it will cost about three pounds, but if without cupboards one pound ten shillings. A deal table is the best, and this must be kept white with constant scrubbing; while the cookery is going on a piece of oil baize might be laid over it. Pearson's carbolic sand soap will remove any grease spots very quickly; the paste board and rolling pin can also be kept white in the same way. It will be found an advantage to have two or three French or butchers' knives for cooking purposes, instead of using the dinner knives. These can be bought from 1s. 6d. each; they are stronger and take a better edge than ordinary knives. Wooden and iron spoons will be found cheaper and better than using table spoons as these latter are soon ruined if used for stirring; cookery spoons cost about 3d. each; two of each would be found sufficient. A conical strainer is more convenient and useful than the round ones so generally used. For mixing bowls the agate iron are the best; they are a little more expensive in the first place than the yellow earthenware, but they are unbreakable, and therefore cheaper in the end; they cost about 4s. 6d. each. A small sausage machine is very necessary, for by means of this useful contrivance many scraps of meat and bread can be utilized; the cost of one is 10s. 6d. A pestle and mortar, too, will be found of great use in making up odds and ends into dainty tit-bits; these, too, cost about 10s. 6d. Wire and hair sieves are invaluable for preparing soups and many other dishes; sieves with a wooden rim will be found the most durable; they cost 2s. 6d. Each. Agate iron saucepans are light and durable and very easy to keep clean; they are much better than the blue enamelled ware, as they do not burn so readily or chip so soon. Frying pans are nice, too, of the same ware. A set each of wire and metal dish-covers must not be forgotten;

the latter should be of plain blocked tin, and as the fluted ones soon get shabby, these should be well washed inside and out with scouring soap and polished with Goddard's plate powder. A French fryer is invaluable; it will cost 7s. 6d. Three or four pounds of dripping clarified should be put at first; this will require straining. After being used once or twice, the fryer should then be washed out with soda water, well dried, and the fat put back; it can be renewed from time to time with some fresh fat, and it will keep good for weeks. When it looks very dark throw it away and start with a fresh lot of fat; it can be used for fish, rissoles, fritters, &c., and one can never tell that anything has been fried in it before, if it attains the right heat before the FRITURE is put in. It should be between boiling water heat (212 degrees) and boiling fat (600 degrees), 385 degrees being exactly right, and can be tested by dropping in a small piece of bred. If it browns instantly it is ready; whatever is put into it will fry in two or three minutes. Food cooked in this way will not be so greasy and indigestible as it often is if cooked in a frying pan.

And now, last and most important of all, the stove; for although we may do without a great many things which are nice and useful to have, without a stove it is impossible to cook well. It may be for gas, wood, or coal, but it must act well. Gas stoves are extremely simple, clean, and easy to use, there are no flues to get choked, and in towns where gas is cheap it is no doubt the easiest and pleasantest heat to use. To keep them clean and sweet they should be well washed inside and out with soda and water at least once a week and polished with a little Electric black lead. The flues of wood and coal stoves should be thoroughly cleansed out once a week, and the oven cleansed with soap and soda; this is very necessary work, for if the ovens are not clean whatever is cooked in them will be spoilt. A little thoughtful care in these matters will often prevent much trouble when cooking. Let a housekeeper, therefore, thoroughly master her stove first, and understand the flues and dampers, for only in this way will she be able to successfully cook the dishes she has skilfully prepared. Cleanliness and care in respect of the stove and kitchen utensils generally are as necessary to success as knowing the right materials to use and how to put them together, and every one who can cook a dinner should also know how to clean and keep in good order the stove and all culinary utensils. Order and neatness must reign in the kitchen as well as in the drawing-room, and it will help greatly to bring about this desirable state of affairs if all utensils are cleansed and put away immediately they are finished with, for it is much easier to wash them then than if left dirty for some time. As soon as the contents of a saucepan have been dished, fill it with cold water, add a lump of soda, and stand it on the stove till hot; it can then be washed up in a few minutes. Plates and dishes should at once be put into a bowl of hot or cold water; treat spoons and forks in the same way. Knives, wipe at once, and clean as soon as possible. A damp cloth rubbed with Monkey soap will do wonders in removing stains and dust; these, if left for a time, are hard to get off, and the kitchen, which ought to be bright and cheerful, soon has a greasy, dirty look.

Some of us can call to mind delightful old kitchens in country houses, which were a pleasure and a joy to both mistress and maids, where bright copper stewpans reflected the blazing fire on all sides, and metal covers shone like mirrors; while as for "eating off the floor," one might certainly do it if so inclined, without the "peck of dirt" at once.

How cosy and delightful everything seems in a kitchen like this, and what visions can we not see of home-made bread and cakes, well-cooked joints, succulent vegetables, delicious puddings, dainty dishes of all kinds concocted with skilful fingers! And why should not these visions turn into substantial realities? They will do so if women will consider it a pleasure, instead of a degradation, to "look well to the ways of her household," and establish a system of order and neatness from cellar to garret. When this happy time comes she will be "emancipated" from many cares and have more leisure to cultivate her intellect than she has now. Surely "a study which helps" to make cheerful homes and healthy, well-conducted, "prosperous citizens is worth at least a trial."

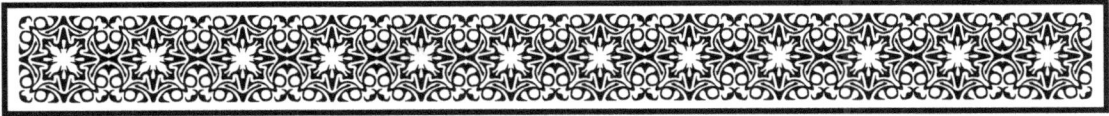

CHAPTER XIV.
THE ICE CHEST

"An ice chest!" someone exclaims. "I should like to know how I am to get that." Well, very easily indeed, if there is a will to have one, for then the way is plain. A refrigerator years ago was perhaps only obtainable by the wealthy, and regarded rightly by others as a not-to-be-thought-of-luxury; but, thanks to the rapid development of scientific knowledge, both ice and refrigerators are now within the means of nearly all. The Americans in this led the way, and those in the Central States would no more dream of being without ice during the hot season, than they would of failure to take daily supplies of bread and milk. In almost every home through bright and sunny Australia we find a piano and a sewing machine, and yet either of these costs far more than an ice chest, and perhaps as much to keep in repair as the ice to fill it. Looking at it from many points of view, it ought to be considered an indispensable article of furniture, and it has this great advantage over many "household gods," that the first expense is the last; for it never gets out of order, and lasts a lifetime; and this cannot be said of many other pieces of furniture, which perhaps cost more and yet are not so useful. In such a warm climate as this, where for six months in the year our one desire is to keep cool, it must certainly be worth while to secure a simple and inexpensive article which will help us to attain this object. Looking at the matter from the Domestic Economy point of view, we shall certainly decide at once in favour of the purchase. Housekeepers, both young and experienced, know how much food has to be thrown away because it will not keep sweet for even a few hours in the hot season. All this waste is at an end if there is ice about, as it will keep perishable food cool and pleasant and ready for a second meal. Many odds and ends of vegetables, fish, and meat can be turned into a dainty salad with the ice chest which must have been thrown away without it. Thus the expense, not only of the ice, but also of the chest, is soon saved, to say nothing of the pleasure and enjoyment of the said salad, which one would so infinitely rather have had than the chops and steaks so universally served. Delicious little breakfast dishes can be concocted over night from the remains of fish and meat served at tea and put down into the ice all night. These are cooked in a few minutes in the morning, and form such a pleasant change to the standing dish of eggs and bacon; and how proud a good house-keeper will feel when her little dishes are enjoyed, and she knows that they have cost nothing!--for the food would not have kept, and must therefore have been thrown away if she had not possessed an ice chest. This is only one instance of what may be accomplished, but in the daily routine of work many more will be found. Think, for a moment, of the state of the butter without ice on a hot day. Who does not dread the sight of the liquid or greasy fat usually seen in the butter-dish, and what a remote chance there is of enjoying a slice of bread and butter with bread as hard and dry as a brickbat, and butter running to oil? Put both into a refrigerator and note the difference. Look at it, also, from the hygenic standpoint. Most people, save the very strong and robust, lose their appetite during the hot season, and therefore feel languid and weak. Give them dry bread and liquid butter, and they can't touch a morsel; but with fresh bread, hard butter, and some dainty tit-bit, kept in the ice also, placed before them, a good meal is often enjoyed. Again, in cases of illness ice becomes at once a necessity; and if it is at hand in the house and ready for use much time and trouble will be saved, and suffering too, as the poor invalid waits with what patience he can for the relief which is so often brought with ice.

And now we come to the practical question of how we are to get it, and how to keep it. There are several companies who undertake to deliver a daily supply of ice in town and country at a very moderate price, about sixpence a block of 10 lbs.; but when there is a larger demand for it, it will very soon be supplied at even a cheaper rate. There is a very simple little American invention which makes ice very quickly. It is not by any means expensive, about 2l. 2s. 0d., and is invaluable in country districts away from the railway. Then for a refrigerator there are several very simple chests which require only a small quantity of ice to keep them charged. The smallest and cheapest is the Baldwin, costing from 30s., and another is the Iceberg, which acts splendidly. Unlike other machines, which are liable from their complicated structure to get out of order, these are so simple that they require no repairs, but only strict cleanliness to keep them in good order. They should be well washed out with soap and soda at least once a week, and care taken that no little bits of food are left in when the plate containing the main part is removed, for these morsels will cause an unpleasant smell and quickly taint anything that may be put in afterwards. It is better not to break the ice up, but to put the whole block in the refrigerator, and when once it is in to close the lid securely and keep it closed. It is a good plan to put a piece of newspaper over the block, as that forces the cold air down into the lower chamber. The larger blocks will be found almost as cheap as the small ones, as if carefully used they last much longer. No doubt, as the desire for ice increases, smaller blocks, costing perhaps 2d., or 3d., will be made, or the present prices reduced to that figure. This, to a great extent, is in the hands of the consumers, for as soon as there is a more spirited demand some energetic firm will arise and supply the want, and we shall have, not only cheaper ice, but cheaper ice-chests too. Dr. Muskett has pointed out some of the advantages of ice in his work on THE HEALTH AND DIET OF CHILDREN IN AUSTRALIA, as will be seen from the following paragraph:--

"In our semi-tropical climate a dislike is often taken to butter, when it is presented at breakfast in the form of semi-liquid grease. It would require a person with the stomach of an ostrich to digest, to say nothing of relish, such an oleaginous composition during our summer months. But if this necessary and all-important article of diet can be presented in an appetising form, what a desirable result is achieved! The mass of the people--I am not referring to those who are well endowed with wordly gifts--are apt to look upon the Ice Chest as a luxury which is altogether beyond their means. But I am firmly persuaded that if the price of ice were brought down to one halfpenny per pound, and that if a company were formed to deliver such a small quantity as six pounds per day, or every second day, it would be a great boon, and, moreover, a wonderfully profitable speculation. A very small and suitable Ice Chest could be constructed solely to preserve the butter in a congealed and therefore palatable state, both to children and to adults. The former would take it with great avidity, and the benefit to health resulting therefrom would be incalculable. Even in some of the better-class houses Ice is looked upon too much as a luxury, and not as it should be, a necessity; indeed, the money saved from gas during the summer months might well be expended on Ice."

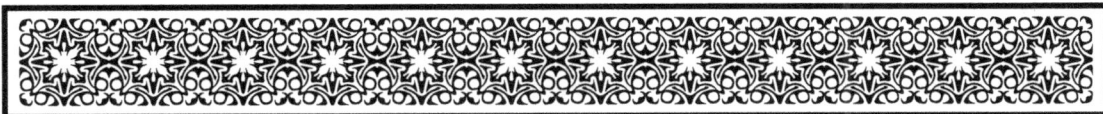

CHAPTER XV.
THE STOCK POT.

The stock pot is indispensable to good cooking, and although many soups and sauces can be made with water as a foundation, nearly all of them are improved by using stock, and no cook who desires to achieve good results should be without a basin of stock when she commences operations in the morning. There are saucepans now called digesters, which are most useful as stock pots, but any good-sized saucepan or boiler will do very well indeed. This should be put on fresh every morning with everything the larder contains that is suitable--such, for instance, as the bones of fresh or cooked meat, poultry, or rabbits. Never put in fat, as this can be rendered down for pastry and frying, and only makes the stock greasy; always cover the bones with cold water, but regulate the quantity by the material used. Put in cold water with a teaspoonful of salt, and when it boils up, skim well; when skimming, take an iron spoon and a basin of water, and dip the spoon in the water each time the scum is removed; then put in the peppercorns and vegetables. In very hot weather put peppercorns and a fagot of herbs only, as the vegetables cause the stock to turn sour very soon; peppercorns should always be used, as they impart a much pleasanter flavour to soup than pepper. A fagot of herbs is made with a bay or peach leaf, a sprig each of parsley, thyme, and marjoram tied together with a piece of cotton. These herbs can be grown so easily if one has a small garden, or even in a box, with very little care; they impart such a pleasant flavour to soups and gravies. Leeks cut up with the green

tops and put into the stock pot instead of onions are very good.
Part of the onion skin left on makes a good colour, but it can
be coloured by burning half a teaspoonful of sugar in an old spoon, or
by a few drops of caramel--the recipe for which is given elsewhere.
All fresh meat and bones should be carefully trimmed and wiped with a
warm damp cloth before putting into the pot; when the stock has boiled,
stand the saucepan at the back of the stove and simmer slowly for at
least five or six hours. If strong stock is desired, leave the lid off
the saucepan for the last hour; the water will then evaporate and make
the stock richer. The stock should be strained through a hair sieve or
a colander, and should stand in a cool place till the next day. If it
has been carefully made it will be in a jelly; the fat can very easily
be removed with a spoon. It should finally be wiped with a damp cloth.
Removing the fat thoroughly is a most important item, for greasy soups
and sauces are most indigestible and unwholesome. If the stock has to
be used at once, remove the fat first with a spoon, and then pass
pieces of this paper lightly across the surface; these will absorb the
fat. A small piece of charcoal laid on top of the stock will prevent it
turning sour in the hot weather. With this basin of stock to work on,
many dainty tit-bits are possible which could not be made without it.
How often has the cookery book been searched for "something nice" and
laid down with a sigh when half a pint of gravy has been found
necessary to concoct the desired dainty! But with a basin of stock on
hand, all these things are procurable, and it certainly does not take
more than ten minutes to break up the bones, skim the pot, and strain
it, and last of all it costs nothing. In cases of sudden emergency,
when stock is wanted and is not to be had, the recipe for Quick Beef
Tea answers very well, using one quart of water instead of one pint,
and by adding a few vegetables; this is made in five minutes.
White soup is looked upon as quite a high-class soup, but it is just as
easy to make as any other kind. A piece of stewed veal or mutton, or a
boiled chicken, gives the stock at once, or the bones of mutton, veal,
or pork alone will form the foundation. Never throw away the water in

which carrots, parsnips, celery, or even cauliflowers have been boiled.
Vegetables contain a great deal of potash, which is a valuable food for
the blood. A great deal of this potash comes out in the water during
the process of cooking; if this liquor is used as a foundation for
soup, we utilize this. For this reason vegetable soups, and stews
containing plenty of vegetables, are such a good diet for anyone
suffering from or subject to diseases of the blood and bones. These
simple facts seem to be overlooked; but if Australia is to become in
the future, as we all hope it may, a power in the world second to none,
the wives and mothers of her husbands and sons must understand the
necessity of providing them with a diet which shall make them strong
and brave, and root out what now seems to be the curse of the land--
dyspepsia--brought on in a great measure by badly cooked and therefore
indigestible food. The remedy for this is in the hands of the women of
Australia, and if they will rise to their position and importance and
do their work with a high and holy motive, they will not find it the
drudgery it is often supposed to be. What does Owen Meredith say?--

"We may live without poetry, music, and art,
We may live without conscience, and live without heart,
We may live without friends, we may live without books,
But civilised man cannot live without cooks.
He may live without books--what is knowledge but grieving?
He may live without hope--what is hope but deceiving?
He may live without love--what is passion but pining?
But where is the man that can live without dining?"

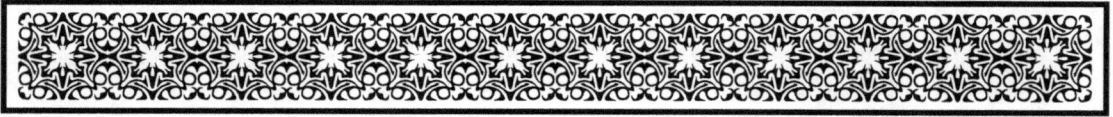

CHAPTER XVI.
SOUP

Soup is a much neglected food; there are many excuses made for this--
one says it is "expensive", another it is "too much trouble" and "quite
unnecessary".

When once the principle of the stock pot is understood the first excuse
falls through, for in any ordinary households the stock can be made
from bones and trimmings of meat, and costs nothing. Neither does the
excuse of too much trouble hold good. Some little time must be devoted
to cooking, and soup will almost cook itself while other preparations
are going on, and it can be made at any time and just boiled up when
required. As for being unnecessary, that is quite a mistake. To give
the greatest amount of nourishment with the least trouble to the
digestive organs should be the study of every housekeeper, and soup is
a valuable aid in this respect. For weakly and delicate constitutions,
for the young and the aged, there is no better food, and for the busy
workers it is invaluable, for immediately after work the digestive
organs are not in a proper state to do hard work, and little soup
prepares the stomach for the more solid food to follow. It is quite a
mistake to suppose that a rich, heavy soup is necessary, and that a
large quantity must be taken. In either case, the effect would be to
take away the appetite, instead of which it is to stimulate and
encourage the appetite that the soup should be given.

Soup is a splendid restorative, and if given to any one suffering from exhaustion or over fatigue will quickly restore strength, and be found far better than any stimulant. Soup is often disliked because it is greasy and served lukewarm; if the directions given in the paragraph on the stock pot for removing the fat be carried out, it will never be greasy, and if it is boiled up just before serving, it will be hot. Allow half a pint of soup for each guest, have a warm tureen and hot plates, and "try the effect".

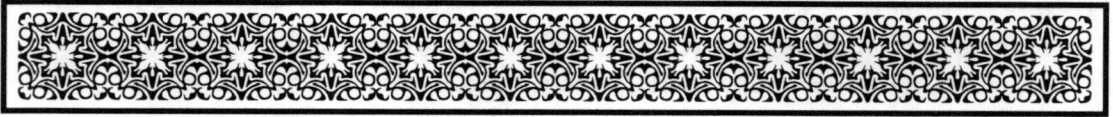

CHAPTER XVII.
FIFTY RECIPES FOR SOUPS.

STOCK FROM BONES (FRESH BONES).

* Bones--3d.
*
* Vegetables--1d.
*
* Total Cost--4d.
*

Beef bones are the best for this stock; break them up very small with a chopper, put them into a large saucepan and cover well with cold water, add two teaspoonsful of salt, and when it boils up remove the scum carefully, and put in one onion, one carrot, half a turnip, a little

piece of the outside stalk of celery, and one dozen peppercorns. Boil steadily for six hours, or longer, then strain off through a colander or sieve, and stand in a cool place till the next day. Carefully remove the fat by directions given elsewhere, and it is ready for use.

This stock is a good foundation for all soups, gravies, and sauces. In very hot weather omit all the vegetables.

STOCK FROM BONES (NO. 2)

The bones from all joints of meat, whether roasted or boiled, make excellent stock. Beef bones are the best, but very good stock can be made from mutton and veal bones. The bones and trimmings of all kinds of poultry, game, and rabbits are also excellent, particularly for soups that require a special flavour. To make this stock successfully care must be taken to remove all pieces that may be burnt, as these give the stock an unpleasant flavour. The bones must be chopped very small, and well covered with cold water. When the pot boils put in a teaspoonful of salt and skim well, then boil steadily for six hours or longer; strain off and remove the fat, and it is ready for use, but it is much better to let it stand till the next day before converting it into soup or gravy.

FISH STOCK

Vegetables and Peppercorns--1d.

Fish for nearly all dishes is better if boned before cooking; it is also economy to do this, as the bones can then be used for stock for fish soups. These soups, although not well known here at present, are a valuable food; they are easy to make, wholesome, and nourishing. After the fillets of fish have been removed, directions for which are given amongst the fish recipes, take the bones, wash them well in cold water, and cut away any black substance that may be adhering to them. Break them up and put into a saucepan with a teaspoonful of salt; when it boils remove the scum and put in one dozen white peppercorns, a fagot of herbs, one onion, and one carrot; boil steadily for two hours or longer, strain through a sieve into a basin, and it is ready for use.

POT BOILINGS

Water in which meat of fish has been boiled should never be thrown away, as it forms an excellent foundation for many soups and sauces which might otherwise have to be made with water.

If a large quantity of water has been used, the boilings will be poor; therefore, when the meat has been taken up, leave the pot on the fire and let it boil quickly, without the lid, for an hour or so, then strain off for use.

The water in which corned beef or pork has been cooked is generally too salt for soups, but it should be stood away till cold, when a thick cake of fat will be found on the top. Put this into a basin and pour over it some boiling water; when it is cold again it can be used for cakes and pastry. It makes an excellent and wholesome substitute for butter in cooking.

VEAL STOCK

* Knuckle of Veal
*
* Peppercorns and Vegetables
*
* Total Cost--10d.
*

The butcher should chop the bones very small. Cut the meat across in several places, lay it in a very clean stock pot, cover well with cold water, and bring to the boil slowly; put in a dessertspoonful of salt, and skim very carefully; draw away from the fire, place it where it will boil steadily, put in 2 dozen white peppercorns, one onion stuck with six cloves, and a fagot of herbs. This is made with a sprig each of parsley, marjoram, and thyme, tied up with a bay or peach leaf; boil steadily for six hours, and strain off.

This is the foundation for the best white soups and sauces; it is also a very nutritious broth for invalids. The meat can be made hot again in about half a pint of the stock and served with parsley butter sauce. A recipe for this is given with the sauces.

BEEF STOCK

* Leg of Beef--9d.
*
* Vegetables--1d.
*
* Total Cost--10d.
*

The bone in this meat should be chopped small by the butcher. Remove the marrow from the bones, and cut the meat into small pieces; put all together into a stock pot or digester, cover well with cold water, and bring it to the boil; add a dessertspoonful of salt; this will throw up the scum, which must be carefully removed. When this has been done put in 2 dozen peppercorns, an onion, and two carrots, draw away from the fire and let it boil steadily for five or six hours or longer, then strain off through a colander and stand away in a cool place.

This is the foundation for nearly all good brown soups. The bones boiled again will make second stock, and the meat does very well for brawn, a recipe for which is given amongst the meat dishes.

BEEF TEA--NO. 1

* 1 lb. Gravy Beef
*

* 1 pint water
*

* 3d.
*

Remove all fat and skin from the meat and put it twice through a sausage machine or scrape it into a pulp with a sharp knife, pour over the cold water, and let it stand for an hour. Pour it into a brown baking jar and put it into a cool oven, and keep it below boiling point for an hour or longer, according to the heat of the oven. It should look brown, thick, and rich, when sufficiently cooked. Strain through a colander, add salt to taste, and it is ready to serve.

QUICK BEEF TEA--NO. 2

* 1 lb Gravy Beef
*

* 1 pint water
*

* 3d.
*

Pass the meat twice through a sausage machine, put it into a saucepan, pour over the cold water, and stand on the stove; stir constantly until it comes to boiling point, but do not allow it to boil. As soon as it changes colour from red to brown strain through a colander, add salt to taste, and it is ready to serve.

RAW BEEF TEA.

1/4 lb Gravy Beef and 1 gill of Water

Scrape the meat to a pulp with a sharp knife, pour over it with water; cover over and stand away for an hour. Strain off, and it is ready. As this is given to an invalid in small quantities, very little should be made at a time.

BEEF ESSENCE.

1 lb Gravy Beef--3d.

Mince the meat very small, put it into a brown baking jar, and cover down with a closely-fitting lid or with brown paper. Stand in a saucepan of boiling water for one hour, pour off the essence, add a little salt, and it is ready.

MUTTON BROTH

4 or 5 scrags of Mutton and Shank Bones--6d

Carefully trim the scrags of mutton, remove the pith from the bones, and wipe with a damp cloth; break these and the shank bones into very small pieces; put them into an enamelled saucepan, well covered with cold water; add a teaspoonful of salt, stand on the stove, and when it boils up remove the scum very carefully. Add 1 dozen peppercorns, and an onion and carrot, if vegetables are allowed the patient. Boil steadily for eight or nine hours; the liquor should then be reduced to one quart. Strain off, and, if possible, let it stand till quite cold; it should then be in a jelly, and can be made hot as required. When serving this to a convalescent a spoonful of rice or pearl barley well washed in cold water and boiled in either stock or milk may be added.

COCK-A-LEEKIE SOUP

* 9 Leeks--3d.
*
* 1 set of Giblets
*
* 2 oz. Beef Dripping
*
* 3 quarts Water or Pot Boilings
*
* Salt and Peppercorns--4d.
*
* Total Cost--7d.

Wash and slice up the leeks into pieces about one inch long, put them into a saucepan with the butter or dripping made thoroughly hot; cover over and let them cook for half an hour, stirring occasionally. While they are cooking clean the giblets thoroughly, washing them first in hot and then in cold water. Cut open the gizzard, remove the stones, and cleanse well. Cut them all up into small pieces and put them into the saucepan with the leeks, pour over the boiling water or liquor, put in the peppercorns tied in a piece of muslin, and a piece of bacon rind if there is any in the larder. Let it simmer slowly for three hours; if not brown enough add a few drops of caramel, take out the peppercorns and bacon rind, season to taste, pour into a hot tureen and serve.

CABBAGE AND BACON SOUP

* 1 Cabbage--3d.
*
* 1 lb. Bacon--9d.
*
* 1 doz. Peppercorns
*
* 2 Turnips
*
* 1 Carrot
*
* 1 Onion
*
* Pieces of Stale Bread--1d.
*
* Total Cost--1s. 1d.
*

* Time--Three Hours and a Half
*

This soup is not as expensive as it appears, for the bacon is served as a dish of meat, either after the soup or cold for breakfast or tea. Put two quarts of water into a saucepan; when it boils put in a pound of bacon neither too lean nor too fat. Let it boil slowly for one hour. The bacon must be well washed and scraped before cooking, and when it boils skim the pot thoroughly. Well wash the cabbage and soak it in hot water for half an hour. Take all the water away and put the cabbage into the saucepan with the bacon and vegetables cut up, and the peppercorns tied in a piece of muslin; let them simmer together for two and a half hours, take up the cabbage, and cut it into quarters. Take one quarter and cut it into small pieces and put it into a soup tureen. Cut some stale pieces of bread into thin slices and lay on the top, pour over the boiling liquor, and serve. Dish the bacon, pull off the rind, and put the rest of the cabbage round the dish.

ITALIAN SOUP

* 2 oz. Macaroni--1 1/2d.
*

* 2 quarts Water or Pot Boilings
*

* 2 Tomatoes
*

* 1 oz. Butter
*

* 2 oz. Cheese Rind--1 1/2d.
*

* Total Cost--3 d.
*

* Time--Half an Hour.
*

Put the water or stock on to boil, and when it boils put in the macaroni and boil from twenty-five to thirty minutes. While it is boiling grate up a dry piece of cheese. Put the tomatoes into boiling water and remove the skin, slice them up and put them into a saucepan with the butter and some pepper and salt, and cook them for a few minutes. When the macaroni is soft, cut it into pieces one inch long, put a layer of tomatoes at the bottom of the soup tureen, then a layer of grated cheese, then one of macaroni; repeat this until all the materials are used up, pour over it boiling the liquor in which the macaroni has been cooked, cover down for a few minutes, and serve.

POT-AU-FEU

* 3 lbs. Leg of Beef--6d.
*

* 2 quarts Water
*

* 1 fagot of Herbs
*

* Salt and Pepper
*

* 2 Onions
*

* 2 Carrots
*

* 2 Turnips
*

* 1 doz. Peppercorns--1 1/2d.
*

* Total Cost--7 1/2 d.
*

* Time--Five Hours
*

Pot-au-feu is the national dish of France; it is cheap, nourishing and palatable, and very simple to make. The slower it is cooked the better it is; in fact, in this lies the whole secret of success, for if it boils instead of simmering it is spoilt. Tie the meat up into a nice shape with a piece of tape, put it into cold water, bring slowly to the boil, and very carefully remove the scum; peel and slice up the vegetables, and put them in with the fagot of herbs and the peppercorns tied in a piece of muslin; bring to simmering point, and keep it so for five hours. The liquor can then be served as a soup with part of the vegetables and some sippets of toast. Take the tapes off the meat, and serve with the rest of the vegetables round the dish as a border or garnish. The remains of the beef can be pressed between heavy weights till cold, or put into a brawn tin and served cold with a salad.

VERMICELLI SOUP

* 1 oz. Vermicelli--1d.
*

* Vegetables and Saffron
*

* 2 quarts Bone Stock--1d.
*

* Total Cost--2 d.
*

* Time--One Hour
*

The stock for this soup should be good and in a strong jelly when cold.

Put it into a saucepan with three or four threads of saffron, an onion or leek stuck with six cloves, 1 dozen white peppercorns and some salt, and boil all together for half an hour; then strain out the vegetables and put it back into the saucepan. It should be of a bright straw colour; if it is not, a thread more saffron may be added before straining. Put in the vermicelli broken small, and simmer for twenty minutes; it is then ready to serve.

MULLIGATAWNY SOUP

* 2 quarts Stock
*
* 1 Apple
*
* 1 Onion
*
* 1 Carrot--1d.
*
* 1/2 oz. Curry Powder
*
* 1 oz. Flour--1d.
*
* 1 oz. Butter--1d.
*
* Total Cost--3d.
*
* Time--One Hour
*

The liquor in which poultry or a rabbit has been boiled is the best for this soup. Slice up the apple, onion, and carrot, and fry them in the butter; sprinkle over the curry powder and flour and brown that too; pour over the boiling stock and stir until it boils up, simmer gently for one hour, then rub through a sieve and return to the saucepan. Bring to the boil, flavour with salt and lemon juice. Pour into a warm tureen and serve. Send well-boiled rice to the table with this soup.

FRENCH SOUP

* 3 Potatoes
*
* 3 Carrots
*
* 2 Turnips--1 1/2d.
*
* 2 quarts Bone Stock
*
* Pepper
*
* 2 Onions
*
* 1/2 stalk Celery--1d.
*
* 1 oz. Butter--1d.
*
* 1 teaspoonful Sugar
*
* Salt--1/2d.
*
* Total Cost--4d.
*
* Time--One Hour.

Peel and slice up the vegetables and sprinkle them with the sugar and salt, and put them into a saucepan with the butter, and sweat for five minutes. Pour over the boiling stock and stir until it boils; boil slowly for an hour, then rub through a sieve. If it is too thick, reduce it with a little more stock or milk, return to a saucepan, and bring to the boil. When tomatoes are in season slice up two with the other vegetables; these will make the soup a good colour and improve the flavour.

SAGO SOUP

* 3 oz. Sago--1d.
*
* 1 pint Milk--2 1/2d.
*
* 2 quarts Bone Stock
*
* 1 Leek
*
* Salt and Pepper--1/2d.
*
* Total Cost--4d.
*
* Time--Half an Hour.
*

Wash the sago in cold water, boil the leek in the stock for ten minutes, take it out and stir in the sago; continue stirring until the sago is transparent and the stock quite thick, then pour in the milk and bring up to the boil. Season with salt and pepper, and serve.

CELERY SOUP

* 2 heads of Celery--2d.
*
* 2 quarts Pot Boilings
*
* 1 pint of Milk--2 1/2d.
*
* 1 oz. Sago--1/2d.
*
* Total Cost--5d.
*
* Time--One Hour
*

If vegetables have been boiled with the meat the stock will be sufficiently flavoured; if not, boil an onion and carrot in it and strain out. Wash the celery thoroughly and cut it into pieces one inch long, put it into the boiling stock and boil for half an hour, then sprinkle in 1 oz of sago and stir until it is transparent. Pour in the milk and bring to boiling point; it is then ready to serve. This is an excellent soup for any one suffering from or subject to rheumatism or gout.

TURNIP AND RICE SOUP

* 4 Turnips--2d.
*
* 1/4 lb. Rice--1d.

* 2 quarts Water
*

* 1 pint Milk--2 1/2d.
*

* Onion and Salt--1/2d.
*

* Total Cost--6d.
*

* Time--One Hour and a Quarter
*

Peel and slice up the turnips, wash the rice and put into a saucepan with the onion and 1 dozen white peppercorns. Pour over the water and boil for an hour, rub through a sieve and return to the saucepan, with the milk and a seasoning of salt and pepper; stir until it boils, then pour into a warm tureen and sprinkle some chopped parsley on top. This soup is much improved by putting one ounce of butter into the water in which the rice and turnips are boiled.

TAPIOCA SOUP

* 2 oz. Tapioca--1d.
*

* 1 Onion
*

* 1 Carrot
*

* 3 quarts Bone Stock--1/2d.
*

Boil the onion and carrot in the stock for twenty minutes. If the stock is not a good colour put in half a teaspoonful of burnt sugar. Strain out the vegetables, wash the tapioca in cold water and stir it in;

continue stirring until the tapioca is quite clear, flavour with salt and lemon juice, and serve very hot. This soup should be quite transparent and of a bright brown colour.

WATER SOUCHET

* 6 Small Fish--1s.6d.
*
* Vegetables
*
* Salt and Pepper
*
* Lemon Juice--1d.
*
* Total Cost--1s. 7d.
*
* Time--One Hour and a Half.
*

Choose small fish of different kinds and fillet them. As only half the fillets are wanted for the souchet, the rest may be dressed in another way. Wash the bones in cold water and remove the black substance from them, put them into two quarts of cold water with a teaspoonful of salt, and when it boils remove the scum and add 1 dozen peppercorns, one carrot, one small turnip, one onion, a small piece of celery, and a fagot of herbs. Put the vegetables in whole. Boil this together for one hour, then strain off through a hair sieve and return to the saucepan; wash the vegetables that have been boiled in it, slice them up and put them into the liquor. Cut the fillets of fish into small pieces and put them in; simmer for half an hour, then put in a little lemon juice, pour into a tureen, and sprinkle a little chopped parsley on the top. Send brown bread and butter to table with it and a lemon.

OYSTER SOUP

* 1 bottle Oysters--1s.
*

* 1 pint of Milk--2 1/2d.
*

* Cornflour and Vegetables
*

* 2 quarts Fish Stock--1d.
*

* Total Cost--1 s. 3 1/2 d.
*

* Time--One Hour.
*

If there is no fish stock, use pot boilings. As this is a white soup a special saucepan must be used. Put the stock and the liquor from the bottle of oysters into this stewpan with an onion stuck with six cloves, 2 dozen white peppercorns, and a fagot of herbs, and boil together for half an hour, then strain off and return to the saucepan with the milk. When nearly boiling thicken with a tablespoonful of cornflour and boil two or three minutes; put in the oysters and simmer for five minutes. Flavour with a little lemon juice, nutmeg, and salt. Pour into a warm tureen, and send fried bread to table with it.

BROWN MACARONI SOUP

* 1 1/2 oz. Macaroni--1 1/2d.
*

* 1 oz. Butter--1d.
*

* Vegetables--1d.
*

* Cornflour
*

* 2 quarts Bone Stock--1/2d.
*

* Total Cost--4d.
*

* Time--One Hour and a Quarter.
*

Slice up the onions or leeks, one carrot, and make a fagot of herbs;
fry them in the butter with 1 dozen peppercorns till they are quite
brown, but not burnt. Sprinkle over a tablespoonful of cornflour, and
when brown pour over the boiling stock and stir till it boils up; let
it simmer for an hour. If it is not brown enough, burn a little
sugar in a spoon and stir it in. If half a teaspoonful of sugar is
sprinkled over the vegetables when they are frying they will brown much
quicker. When the vegetables are soft rub the soup through a wire sieve
and return to the saucepan. Boil the macaroni in salt and water for
twenty minutes, strain off, and cut into pieces one inch long; put
these into the soup and simmer for a quarter of an hour. Flavour with a
little salt and pepper if necessary, and pour into a hot tureen.

HARICOT BEAN SOUP

* 1 lb. Haricot Beans--4d.
*
* 2 Onions
*
* 1/2 pint of Milk
*
* 2 quarts Bone Stock--1 1/2d.
*
* Total Cost--5 1/2 d.
*
* Time--Four Hours
*

Soak the haricot beans for an hour or two, then put them into a saucepan with the stock or water, the onions, and 1 dozen white peppercorns; boil for four hours and then rub through a sieve, return to the saucepan with the milk and seasoning of pepper and salt, stir until it boils. It is then ready to serve. An ounce of butter stirred in just before it is finished is a great improvement.

This is one of the most nourishing soups that can be made. It is an excellent food for outdoor workers. When butter is dear, sweat the haricots in 1 oz. of beef dripping.

MILK SOUP

* 2 lbs. Potatoes--2d.
*
* 1 oz. Butter--1d.
*
* 1 Onion
*
* 1/2 pint of Milk
*
* 3 pints of Water--1 1/2d.
*
* Total Cost--4 1/2 d.
*
* Time--Half an Hour
*

Peel, wash, and slice up the potatoes and onions and put them into a saucepan with the butter, and stir them about till all the butter is dissolved and worked into the potatoes, but they must not get brown. Pour over the boiling water and boil until they are of a pulp, then rub them through a sieve, return to the saucepan, add the milk and seasoning, and stir till it boils. Pour into a hot tureen, and serve with fried bread.

ONION SOUP

* 4 Onions--1d.
*
* 1 oz. Butter--1d.
*
* 1 1/2 oz. Flour
*
* 1 gill of Milk
*
* 2 quarts of Stock
*
* Salt and Pepper--1d.
*
* Total Cost--3d.
*
* Time--One Hour.
*

Peel and slice up the onions and fry them in the butter till they are a good brown colour. Sprinkle over the flour and brown that too. Pour on the boiling stock and boil steadily till the onions are very soft, then rub through a sieve. If there is any fat on it remove it carefully, pour back into the saucepan, add the milk, pepper, and salt, and boil up.

Just before serving put in a few drops of lemon juice. Send fried bread to table with it.

PUMPKIN SOUP

* 1 small Pumpkin--4d.
*

* 2 oz. Butter--2d.
*

* 1/2 pint of Milk--1d.
*

* 2 Onions, 1 Carrot
*

* 2 quarts of Water--1d.
*

* Total Cost--8d.
*

* Time--One Hour and a Half.
*

Peel and slice up the pumpkin, onions, and carrot, put them into a saucepan with half the butter, and sweat the vegetables in it for five minutes, then pour over the boiling water and boil until the vegetables are very soft. Rub through a sieve and return to the saucepan with the milk and some pepper and salt; stir until it boils up.

Just before serving, stir in, in tiny pieces, the rest of the butter and a little lemon juice.

VEGETABLE SOUP

* 2 lbs. Mixed Vegetables--4d.
*
* 2 oz. Butter--2d.
*
* 1/4 lb Haricot Beans--1d.
*
* Peppercorns, Salt, and Sugar
*
* 4 quarts of Water--1/2d.
*
* Total Cost--7 1/2 d.
*
* Time--One Hour and a Half.
*

Take any vegetables that may be in season, such as carrots, turnips, leeks, onions, and celery, and slice them up; put them into a saucepan with the haricot beans and the butter, and turn them all about till the butter is all absorbed; sprinkle over them a teaspoonful each of salt and sugar, add the peppercorns and the water, and boil until the vegetables are very soft.

Rub them through a sieve, return to the saucepan and make thoroughly hot, and it is ready to serve.

SEMOLINA SOUP

* 2 oz. Semolina--2d.
*
* 1/2 pint of Milk
*
* 3 pints Bone Stock
*
* Salt and Pepper--1d.
*
* Total Cost--3d.
*
* Time--One Hour.
*

If the stock has been made without vegetables, as it must often be in hot weather, boil an onion, carrot, fagot of herbs, and a dozen peppercorns in it for half an hour, then strain the stock and put it back in the saucepan. Sprinkle in the semolina and stir until it boils; simmer till the semolina thickens, then add the milk, pepper, and salt, and boil up. Pour into a warm tureen, and send fried bread to table with it.

CARROT SOUP

* 6 Carrots--2d.
*
* 1 oz. Butter--1d.
*
* Sugar, Salt, and Pepper

* 3 quarts Bone Stock--1/2d.
*

* Total Cost--3 1/2 d.
*

* Time--One Hour.
*

Scrape and slice up the carrots and put them into a saucepan with the butter. Sprinkle over a teaspoonful each of salt and sugar and a quarter of a teaspoonful of pepper; turn them about in butter for five minutes, pour over the boiling stock and boil for an our. Rub through a sieve, return to the saucepan and boil up, season to taste, and serve very hot.

TOMATO SOUP

* 1 doz. Tomatoes--4d.
*

* 1 oz. Butter--1d.
*

* 2 Onions, 1 Carrot
*

* 2 oz. Flour
*

* Salt and 1 teaspoonful Sugar
*

* 2 doz. Peppercorns
*

* 3 quarts Bone Stock--1 1/2d.
*

* Total Cost--6 1/2 d.

* Time--One Hour.

Slice up the onions and carrot, and fry them in the butter with the peppercorns and sugar. Sprinkle over the flour and mix well together. Cut up the tomatoes and put them in, then pour over the boiling stock and stir until it boils. Simmer slowly for an hour. Rub through a sieve, return to the saucepan and make thoroughly hot, pour into a warm tureen, and serve with fried bread.

JERSEY SOUP

* 2 quarts White Stock--6d.
*

* 1 pint Milk--2 1/2d.
*

* 1 oz. Sage
*

* 1 Leek
*

* 1 Fagot of Herbs
*

* 1 doz. White Peppercorn
*

* Salt--1 1/2d.
*

* Total Cost--10d.
*

* Time--One Hour.
*

Put the stock into a stewpan; slice in the leek and add the fagot of herbs and the peppercorns. Boil them together for half an hour, strain out the vegetables and return to the saucepan; stir in the sage and continue stirring until it is clear and the soup is thick; pour in the boiling milk, boil up and pour into a tureen. Sprinkle finely chopped parsley on the top before serving.

SCOTCH BROTH

* 2 quarts of the Liquor in which Mutton has been cooked
*
* Salt
*
* 1 oz. Rice
*
* 1 Carrot
*
* 1/2 Turnip, and Stalk of Celery
*
* Total Cost--1 1/2 d.
*
* Time--One Hour.
*

Carefully remove all the fat from the liquor; put it into a saucepan. Wash the rice and cut all the vegetables into dice; stir them in, and simmer by the side of the fire for an hour. It must be cooked very slowly and without the lid. Add salt to taste, and pour it into a tureen. Pearl barley may be used instead of rice.

LENTIL SOUP

* 1 lb. Split Lentils--2d.
*
* 1/2 oz. Butter--1d.
*
* 3 Onions and 2 doz. Peppercorns
*
* 1 teaspoonful Sugar
*
* 3 quarts Water
*
* Salt--1d.
*
* Total Cost--4 d.
*
* Time--Four Hours.
*

Wash the lentils well in two or three waters and put them into a saucepan with the onions, peppercorns, sugar, salt, and half the butter, and sweat them for five minutes. Pour over the boiling water and boil steadily for four hours. If the soup gets too thick, pour in a little more water or stock. Rub through a sieve and return to the saucepan; stir in the butter, salt, and pepper to taste. Boil up and serve.

Lentil soup is one of the most nourishing of all soups, and particularly nice during the winter months.

PEA SOUP

* 1 lb. Split Peas--3d.
*
* 2 Onions and 1/4 Head of Celery--1d.
*
* 1 oz. Butter or Dripping--1d.
*
* 2 Carrots
*
* 2 doz. Peppercorns
*
* 3 quarts Water--1d.
*
* Total Cost--6d.
*
* Time--Four Hours.
*

Wash the peas well in cold water, and put them into a saucepan with the vegetables sliced up, the peppercorns and the water. Bring to the boil and boil steadily for four hours, then rub through a sieve and return to the saucepan. Season well with salt, and stir in 1 oz butter or dripping. Bring to the boil and pour into a warm tureen. Send some dried mint and fried bread to table with it. This is a very nourishing soup, particularly if it is made with stock instead of water; it is very suitable for the cold season.

VEGETABLE MARROW AND TOMATO SOUP

* 1 doz. Tomatoes--3d.
*
* 1 Vegetable Marrow--2d.
*
* 9 Onions
*
* 1 oz. Butter
*
* 2 doz. Peppercorns
*
* 1 teaspoonful Sugar
*
* 3 pints Stock
*
* Salt--2d.
*
* Total Cost--7d.
*
* Time--One Hour.
*

Peel the vegetable marrow, slice it up, and take out the seeds; slice
up the tomatoes and put them, with the marrow, into the saucepan with
the butter, sugar, salt, and peppercorns; sweat them for five minutes.
Pour over the boiling water or stock, and simmer for one hour. Rub
through a sieve and return to the saucepan. Add more salt, if
necessary, bring it to the boil, pour into a tureen, and serve.

KIDNEY SOUP

* 1 Ox Kidney--4d.
*
* 2 Onions--1/2d.
*
* 1 oz. Butter--1d.
*
* 1 oz. Cornflour--1/2d.
*
* Salt, Lemon Juice, and parsley
*
* 2 quarts Stock--1/2d.
*
* Total Cost--6 1/2 d.
*
* Time--One Hour.
*

Slice up the onions and fry them in the butter, strain them out and return the butter to the saucepan. Stir in the cornflour, and when well mixed pour over the stock and stir until it boils. Slice the kidney up into small pieces, and put it in; simmer very gently for one hour. Just before serving, season with salt and a little lemon juice; pour into a tureen and sprinkle a little chopped parsley on top.

This soup must be cooked very slowly, or the kidney will be hard and tough.

EGG SOUP

* 1 quart White Stock
*
* 1 pint of Milk--2 1/2d.
*
* 3 Yolks of Eggs--3d.
*
* 1 oz. Sago--1/2d.
*
* 1 Onion--1/2d.
*
* Salt and Pepper--1/2d.
*
* Total Cost--7d.
*
* Time--Half an Hour
*

Boil the sago, stock, and onion together till the sago is clear; then take out the onion and season the soup with salt and pepper.

Beat the yolks of the eggs in a basin, pour over the boiling milk, strain into the stock. Put over the fire and whisk till it comes to boiling point, but do not let it boil, or it may curdle. Pour into a tureen, sprinkle with chopped parsley, and send some fried bread to table with it.

WHITE MACARONI SOUP

* 1 1/2 oz. Macaroni--1d.
*
* 1 pint Milk--2 1/2d.
*
* 1 oz. Butter--1d.
*
* 3 pints Bone Stock
*
* Vegetables and Flour--1d.
*
* Total Cost--5 1/2 d.
*
* Time--One Hour.
*

The stock made from veal or mutton bones is the best for this soup, as it must be white. Nothing is nicer than the liquor in which a piece of veal has been stewed. If plenty of vegetables have been boiled in it none need be added when the soup is made. If not, boil an onion or leek, a slice of turnip, and a small piece of celery stalk in the stock for twenty minuets, and strain them out. Put the butter into a stewpan, and when it is melted stir in a tablespoonful of cornflour, pour over the milk and stock, and stir until it boils. Boil the macaroni in salt and water for twenty minutes, strain off the water, and cut it into pieces about 1 inch long; put these into the soup, and simmer for ten minutes. Just before serving, flavour with salt, a dust of white pepper, and a few drops of lemon juice.

LOBSTER SOUP

* 1 Lobster, Crayfish, or Tin of Lobster--1s.
*

* 2 quarts Fish Stock
*

* 1/2 pint of Milk--1d.
*

* 1 oz. Cornflour--1/2d.
*

* Lemon Juice, Salt, and Pepper--1/2d.
*

* Total Cost--1s. 2d.
*

* Time--One Hour
*

The fish stock for this soup should be well flavoured with vegetables. If a crayfish be used, remove all the white meat and boil the shells in the stock for half an hour and strain them out; thicken with the cornflour, pour in the milk, and boil up. Cut the lobster into small pieces and put into the soup; simmer for ten minutes. Flavour with lemon juice and salt, pour into a warm tureen, and serve with fried bread. Wash the shells well in cold water before putting them into the soup.

FISH SOUP

* 3 pints Fish Stock
*
* 1 pint Milk--2 1/2d.
*
* Cornflour--1/2d.
*
* Vegetables--1d.
*
* Fish--6d.
*
* Total Cost--10d.
*
* Time--Half an Hour
*

Remove all the fat from the fish stock and put it into a saucepan with six white peppercorns, an onion, one slice of turnip, a fagot of herbs, and some carrot. Boil this together for twenty minutes, then strain out the vegetables and pour back into the saucepan. Mix a tablespoonful of cornflour smoothly with the milk and stir it in; continue stirring till it boils. Skin and fillet the fish and cut it into dice, put these pieces of fish into the soup, and simmer for ten minutes. Just before serving add a few drops of lemon juice, and salt to taste. Pour into a tureen and sprinkle a little chopped parsley on top.

CABBAGE SOUP

* 1 Cabbage--3d.
*

* 2 oz. Butter--1 1/2d.
*

* 1 pint Milk
*

* Pepper, Salt, and Bread--3d.
*

* Total Cost--7 1/2 d.
*

* Time--One Hour
*

Wash and strain the cabbage well, and cut it up into slices; throw it into boiling salt and water, and cook for five minutes; strain all the water off and put it into a saucepan with the salt, pepper, and two quarts of boiling water, and boil for one hour. Add the milk and let it boil up again, toast the slice of bread and cut it up into dice. Put it into a warm soup tureen and pour the boiling soup over it.

SYDNEY SOUP

* 1/2 doz. Tomatoes--2d.
*

* 1 Carrot
*

* 2 Small Onions
*

* 12 Peppercorns
*

* 1 fagot Herbs
*

* 1/2 teaspoon Salt
*

* 2 quarts Stock--1 1/2d.
*

* 1 oz. Butter--1d.
*

* 1 oz. Cornflour and 1/2 oz. Tapioca--1d.
*

* 1 cup of Green Peas--2d.
*

* Curry Powder
*

* 1/2 teaspoonful of Sugar--1/2d.
*

* Total Cost--8d.
*

* Time--One Hour.
*

Put the butter into a saucepan, slice up the onions and carrot and fry them in it with the herbs, peppercorns, and a good pinch of curry powder. Mix the cornflour with a little stock and pour it over. Slice up the tomatoes and add them to the boiling stock; stir until it boils, and then simmer slowly for an hour. Rub through a sieve and return to the saucepan. Add the salt, sugar, and the tapioca; stir until this becomes transparent and thickens the soup. Put in a cupful of cold boiled peas; boil up and serve.

WHITE ONION SOUP

(SOUBISE BLANCHE.)

* 1 pint of Milk--2d.
*
* 1 oz. Butter--1d.
*
* 4 Onions
*
* Salt and Pepper
*
* 1 pint White Bone Stock
*
* Dry Crusts--1d.
*
* Total Cost--4d.
*
* Time--One Hour.
*

Peel and slice up the onions and put them into a saucepan with the butter; make them very hot, and then cover them down and leave them to cook by the side of the fire for an hour, but they must not get any colour. Break in some dry, hard pieces of bread; it should be crust only for this soup. Boil the milk and stock together, pour it over the onions and bread, and let it simmer very slowly, closely covered, for an hour; rub through a sieve, season with salt and pepper and a few drops of lemon juice. Boil up and serve with fried bread.

CRECY SOUP

* 6 Carrots--2d.
*
* 2 oz. Butter--2d.
*
* 1 Onion
*
* 1/2 teaspoonful Sugar
*
* 1/2 teaspoonful Salt
*
* 1 Turnip
*
* 1 stalk of Celery
*
* 3 pints of Boiling Water--1/2d.
*
* Total Cost--4 1/2 d.
*
* Time--Two Hours.
*

Slice up the carrots and vegetables, put them into boiling water, and cook for half-an-hour; strain them out of the water, which must be saved, and put them into a saucepan with the butter and a few scraps of bacon, if any are in the larder. Sprinkle over the sugar, make very hot, and cover down closely until the vegetables are very soft. Rub them through a sieve and pour on by degrees the water in which the vegetables were boiled; mix well together, return to a saucepan, and boil slowly for an hour. Stir in a small piece of butter and it is ready to serve. This soup should be perfectly smooth if properly made. A hair sieve should be used for the vegetables, and the soup should be cooked very slowly.

LENTEN SOUP

* 6 Onions--1 1/2d.
*
* 2 oz. Butter or Beef Dripping
*
* 2 quarts of Water or Pot Liquor
*
* Crusts of Bread
*
* Salt and Pepper--2d.
*
* Total Cost, with Butter--3 1/2 d.
*
* Time--Two Hours.
*

Peel and slice up the onions and put them into a sauce--pan
with the butter or dripping, and brown them. Then let them cook,
covered over, for an hour. Break in some brown dry crusts of bread.
Pour over the boiling liquor the water in which some vegetables, such
as carrots, turnips, or cauliflowers, have been boiled, stir it well
and boil for an hour; rub through a sieve. If it is not thick enough,
let it boil again without the lid for ten minutes. Season well with
pepper and salt, and serve.

SOUP MAIGRE

* 1/2 lb. Rice--1d.
*
* 2 oz. Butter--2d.
*
* 1 gill Milk--1/2d.
*
* Salt
*
* 2 Eggs
*
* 1 Carrot
*
* 1 Onion--2 1/2d.
*
* Total Cost--6d.
*
* Time--Half an Hour
*

Wash the rice well in two waters, put into a saucepan with 2 1/2 pints of cold water and the onion and carrot whole. As the rice begins to swell add some more boiling water, until it is about the right consistency. Take out the onion and carrot and stir in the butter, a small piece at a time. Beat the yolks of the eggs in a basin, stir them quickly in, and bring again to boiling point, but do not let it boil; season with salt, and serve at once, with tiny rusks of bread. Make these by cutting up a dry crust into small pieces, dipping them in water, and baking until crisp in a moderate oven.

ARTICHOKE SOUP

* 2 lbs. Artichokes--3d.
*
* 2 Onions--1/2d.
*
* 1 1/2 pints Milk--4d.
*
* 2 quarts Bone Stock (White)
*
* 1 tablespoonful Vinegar
*
* 1 tablespoonful Lemon Juice
*
* 1 doz. White Peppercorns--1d.
*
* Total Cost--8 1/2 d
*
* Time--One Hour and a Quarter.
*

Peel the artichokes and lay them in vinegar and water for an
hour; this will make them a good colour. Mix up half a pint of the milk
with the stock, and boil the artichokes, onions, and peppercorns in
this for an hour. Rub through a hair sieve with a wooden spoon. Stir in
the milk and some salt, pour back into the saucepan and stir until it
boils. If the artichokes do not thicken the soup sufficiently, sprinkle
in a little sago or semolina when it is returned to the saucepan. Serve
with fried bread.

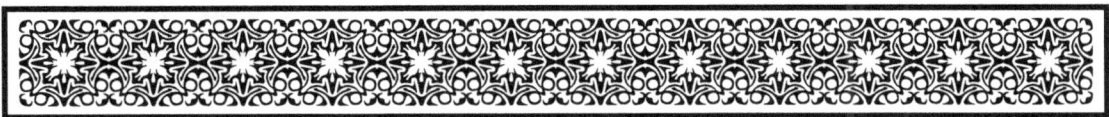

CHAPTER XVIII.
FIFTY RECIPES FOR FISH.

The consumption of fish as a daily article of food is not nearly so large as it ought to be if we studied our health. It must be admitted that it is much more expensive than meat, and cannot be bought so readily. Then again, ordinary plain cooks only know how to fry and boil it, so that very little variety can be obtained; and even these two methods are often so badly followed as to take away rather than tempt the appetite. Not one cook in a hundred knows how to boil fish properly. If a little more time and attention were given to fish-cooking we should not have so many complaints, and fish, instead of being a neglected food, would be a much desired one. It has one or two advantages over meat. It is easier of digestion, for one thing. It is therefore an invaluable food for people obliged to be indoors a great deal, or for those engaged in literary work, for it contains, besides other good things, a good proportion of phosphorus, and this is excellent food for the brain and organs of the chest. It is, however, with the cooking of fish that we have to deal. In the first place, be sure that it is perfectly fresh. The flesh should be firm and hard; if soft and leaving the mark of the finger if pressed, it must be rejected. It must also smell sweet; again, it must be thoroughly cooked. It is a matter of taste whether we like well or underdone meat, but underdone fish is the most unwholesome as it is the most repulsive food that can be offered to us, and in no process of cooking is more judgement required than in the cooking of fish. Fillets of fish of all kinds, either boiled, steamed, or baked, look transparent when raw, but are milk white when cooked sufficiently. If the French method of frying is practised, the large quantity of fat cooks it very quickly, and as soon as it is brown it is done. In boiling and steaming large fish so much depends upon the quantity of water or steam used. Never leave fish in the water after it is cooked. Put it on to a hot dish and cover with a cloth, and stand over a saucepan of hot water till required; if left in the water it soon becomes insipid and watery. In all dishes of dressed fish much depends upon the sauce served with it. Very simple directions for making several fish sauces will be found amongst the sauce recipes, and if these are carefully studied, the art will be easily acquired. In country districts where fish can be had for the catching, it should form the chief item in at least one meal during the day; and if variety in dressing it is studied, it will not be found monotonous, as it sometimes is if only fried and boiled. The ice chest will be found invaluable for keeping fish good and sweet.

FISH CAKES

* 1/2 lb. Cold Boiled Fish--5d.
*
* 1/2 lb. Cold Boiled Potatoes--1d.
*
* Pepper and Salt
*
* Frying Fat
*
* 1 oz. Butter--1d.
*
* 1 Egg--1d.
*

* 1 tablespoonful of Milk, Bread Crumbs--1d.
*
* Total Cost--9d.
*
* Time--5 minutes.
*

Free the fish from skin and bone and flake it up; mash the potatoes smoothly, mix together and season with pepper and salt. Put the milk and butter into a saucepan, and when it is quite hot put in the fish and the potatoes. Beat up the egg, and put half in, and mix together till hot through; spread on to a plate and stand away to cool.
Add a teaspoonful each of water and oil to the egg. Make some bread crumbs on a sieve, and put them on to a piece of paper. Shape the fish mixture into cakes about one inch high and two inches across; brush them over with the egg, and toss them into the crumbs. Shape again and fry in very hot fat, arrange in the form of a wheel on a dish paper, garnish with fresh or fried parsley, and serve hot.

BAKED BREAM AND EGG SAUCE

* 1 Bream--6d.
*
* 1/2 pint White Sauce--2 1/2d.
*
* 1 Egg--1d.
*
* Parsley, Lemon Juice--1/2d.
*
* Total Cost--10d.
*
* Time--20 minutes

Wash the bream, rub some dripping on to a baking sheet, lay on it the fish, squeeze over a few drops of lemon juice; cover with a piece of paper well rubbed with dripping, and bake in a moderate oven for about twenty minutes or longer, if the fish is large. Remove the skin and fins, and put them on the dish; pour over the white sauce, which should be just thick enough to coat the fish. Chop the parsley finely, and boil the egg hard, cut it in half, and either chop the yolk or rub it through a sieve, and chop the white. Arrange these in alternate rows all over the fish, and garnish with a few lemon slices.

FISH A LA MAITRE D'HOTEL

* 2 Bream--8d.
*

* 1/2 pint White Sauce--2 1/1d.
*

* Lemon, Parsley, Pepper and Salt--1/2d.
*

* Total Cost--11d.
*

* Time--20 minutes
*

Fillet the fish, wash and trim them, roll them lightly up with the skin inside. Rub a baking sheet with some butter or dripping. Put on the rolls of fish close together. Squeeze over them some lemon juice, cover with a piece of buttered paper, and bake in the oven for twenty minutes or until they look milk white. Dish them carefully, make the white sauce by recipe given, season it with pepper, salt, and half a teaspoonful of lemon juice. Chop half a teaspoonful of parsley very finely and stir it in, pour over the fish, and serve.

FISH AND TOMATO SAUCE

* 2 Bream--8d.
*
* 1/2 pint of Tomato Sauce
*
* Salt, Pepper, and Parsley--3d.
*
* Total Cost--11d.
*
* Time--20 minutes
*

Fillet the bream; cut each fillet into two pieces, wash and trim them. Make some tomato sauce by recipe given. Butter a pie dish, lay in the fillets, and season them; pour over the sauce, and bake in a moderate oven for twenty minutes. Garnish with a little chopped parsley, and serve in the dish in which they were cooked.

OYSTER STEW

* 1 bottle Oysters--1s.
*
* 1 oz. Butter--1d.
*
* 1/2 pint Milk
*
* 1/2 oz. Flour--1d.
*

* Pepper, Salt, and Lemon Juice--1/2d.
*
* Total Cost--1s. 2 1/2 d.
*
* Time--5 Minutes
*

Make a sauce by directions given, using a little of the oyster liquor mixed with the milk; flavour with salt and pepper, and a little nutmeg and lemon juice. Stir in the oysters and simmer for five minutes, it is then ready to serve.

AMERICAN OYSTERS

* 1 bottle of Oysters--1s.
*
* 1/2 pint of Milk--1d.
*
* 6 Soda Biscuits
*
* 1 oz. Butter
*
* Pepper and Salt--1 1/2d
*
* Total Cost--1s. 2 1/2 d.
*
* Time--5 Minutes
*

Put the milk and butter into a saucepan; when it boils put in the oysters and simmer for five minutes. Season with pepper and salt; break up the biscuits and throw them it. Boil up and pour into a deep dish, and it is ready to serve.

FISH AND BUTTER SAUCE

* 3 Whiting or Bream--1s.
*
* 1 1/2 oz. Butter
*
* 1 teaspoonful Parsley, Pepper and Salt 1 1/2d.
*
* Total Cost--1s 1 1/2d.
*
* Time--Three-quarters of an Hour.
*

Fillet the fish and cut them into strips, wash them well in cold water and dry in a cloth; twist them round, and lay in a buttered soup plate, sprinkle with white pepper and salt, and chopped parsley. Put in the rest of the butter, cover with another soup plate, and stand over a saucepan of boiling water for three-quarters of an hour; reserve the plates once while it is cooking, place in a hot dish, and pour over it the butter and parsley in which it was cooked.

This is a nice delicate way of cooking fish for an invalid.

FISH PATTIES

* 1 Small Bream--4d.
*

* 1 oz. Butter--1d.
*

* 1 oz. Flour
*

* 1 teaspoonful Anchovy Sauce
*

* 1 gill Milk
*

* Pepper, Salt and Lemon Juice
*

* Flaky Pastry--6 1/2d.
*

* Total Cost--11 1/2 d.
*

* Time--20 minutes
*

Bake the fish in the oven, unless there is cold fish in the larder, which will do just as well; take away the skin and bone, and flake it up. Make a sauce of the butter, flour, and milk; season with anchovy, pepper, salt, and lemon juice; stir in the fish and mix well. Line some small patty pans with flaky pastry, put a spoonful of the mixture in the centre, cover with a round of pastry, press the edges together, and trim into a neat shape; make a small hole in the centre with a skewer, brush over with egg or milk, put into a quick oven, and bake for about twenty minutes. Dish on a fancy paper, and garnish each patty with a tiny sprig of parsley.

FISH, TO FRY

Fish requires careful preparation for successful frying; it may be filleted or fried whole, but in either case it must be well washed in cold water, but not soaked; dry in a cloth. Mix on a plate a spoonful of flour, pepper, and salt. Beat on another plate an egg, with a spoonful each of water and oil, and have plenty of dry fine crumbs on a sheet of paper; when these things are all ready, dip the fish in the flour and dust off again; put at once into the egg and cover well; then drop into the crumbs, shake them all over it; next toss in the hands to shake all the loose crumbs off; lay on a plate separately, and either fry at once or leave in a cool place for an hour or two. Plunge into plenty of hot fat and fry till crisp and brown; drain for a few minutes on kitchen paper; pile on a dish, and garnish with either fresh or fried parsley.

CURRIED FISH

* 3 Bream--1s.
*
* 1/2 pint Curry Sauce--3d.
*
* 1/4 lb. Rice--1d.
*
* Total Cost--1s 4d.
*
* Time--One Hour
*

Make the curry sauce by recipe given elsewhere. Fillet the fish and cut each fillet in two pieces, butter a saucepan and lay in the fish; pour over the sauce, bring it up to the boil, and cook on the stove very slowly for an hour. Just before serving, season with salt and lemon juice to taste. Boil the rice and dry thoroughly; press into little cups or moulds. Dish the fish carefully and pour the sauce over it; garnish with the moulds of rice.

SCALLOPED FISH

* 1/2 lb. Cold Fish
*

* 2 oz. Bread Crumbs--4d.
*

* 1 gill Cold Fish Sauce, Pepper, and Salt--2d.
*

* 1 oz. Butter--1d.
*

* Total Cost--7d.
*

* Time--20 minutes.
*

Flake up the fish, butter a small dish, and sprinkle well with bread crumbs; put in a layer of fish, a little sauce and seasoning, and some bread crumbs. Continue this in layers until all the fish is used up. Put plenty of crumbs on top and the rest of the butter in small pieces. Bake in a moderate oven for 20 minutes. Garnish with a sprig of parsley, and serve.

FISH PUDDING

* 1/2 lb. Blue Cod--5d.
*
* 1 lb. Potatoes--1d.
*
* 1 oz. Butter--1d.
*
* 1 Egg
*
* Pepper and Salt--1d.
*
* Total Cost--8d.
*
* Time--Half an Hour
*

Use cold fish and potatoes, if there are any in the larder; if not, boil a piece of blue smoked cod in some water for five minutes. Flake it up free from skin and bone and put it into a basin; mash up the potatoes and mix them in with the pepper and salt. Bind into a paste with an egg; rub some dripping on a baking sheet, turn the mixture on to it and shape into the letter S, brush over with egg or milk, and bake till brown. Slip it off on to a hot dish, and garnish with parsley.

FISH PIE

* 2 or 3 Bream--1s.
*
* 1 gill Milk or Melted Butter--1d.
*
* Short Pastry, Pepper and Salt
*
* Parsley--3d.
*
* Total Cost--1s. 4d.
*
* Time--Three-quarters of an Hour.
*

Cold fish will do very well for this dish. If fresh is used, fillet it and cut into small pieces; if cooked, flake up into small pieces. Lay in a buttered pie-dish, season with pepper, salt, and chopped parsley; pour over the sauce and cover with a short pastry made with 1/2 lb flour and 1/4 lb dripping. Brush over with egg or milk, and bake for three-quarters of an hour; garnish with parsley, and serve.

FISH IN BATTER

* 2 Mullet--8d.
*
* Frying Batter
*
* Hot Fat--2d.

* Total Cost--10d.
*

* Time--5 Minutes.
*

Fillet the mullet and cut into small pieces; dip in flour seasoned with salt and pepper. Cover with French frying batter, the recipe for which is given elsewhere. Plunge into plenty of hot fat and fry until a good colour; drain for a few minutes on kitchen paper. Pile high on a dish, garnish with parsley, and serve hot.

FISH AU GRATIN

* 1 Sole--9d.
*

* 1 teaspoonful of Parsley
*

* 4 teaspoonful Bread Crumbs--1/2d.
*

* 1/2 Small Onion
*

* 1 oz. Butter
*

* 1 gill Good Gravy
*

* 1/2 oz. Fat Bacon--1 1/2d.
*

* Total Cost--11d.
*

* Time--20 minutes.

Mince the onion, parsley, and bacon very finely, and put them into a basin with the seasoning and crumbs, and mix thoroughly. Butter a dish in which the fish can be both cooked and served. Spread half the seasoning on it, wash and dry the fish and lay it on this bed of seasoning; spread the rest of the seasoning on the top, pour over gently the gravy. Cover with a few raspings and put the butter on in tiny pieces. Put it into a quick oven and bake from 15 to 20 minutes, according to the thickness of the fish. Pin a paper collar round the dish, and serve at once.

FISH HASH

* 1/2 lb. Cold Boiled Fish--4d.
*
* 1/2 lb. Cold Boiled Potatoes
*
* 1/4 of an Onion--1d.
*
* 2 oz. Fat Bacon--1d.
*
* 1 teaspoonful Parsley
*
* 1 oz. Butter
*
* 1 gill Milk or Gravy
*
* Pepper and Salt--1d.
*
* Total Cost--7d
*
* Time--10 Minutes

Flake up the fish free from skin and bone, mash the potatoes and mix them together; season with half the parsley, pepper and salt. Mince the bacon and onion very finely; put them into a frying pan with the butter and fry for a few minutes. Stir in the fish and potatoes and turn about until thoroughly hot through. Pour over the gravy or milk and again make thoroughly hot. Heap on to a dish, and garnish with the rest of the parsley. Serve very hot.

FISH BALLS

* 1/2 lb. Cold Fish--4d.
*
* 1 gill Thick Sauce--1 1/2d.
*
* 1 teaspoonful Anchovy--1/2d.
*
* 1/2 pint Melted Butter--1 1/2d.
*
* 2 oz. Fat Bacon
*
* 1 teaspoonful Parsley--1d.
*
* 1 Egg and Pepper and Salt--1 1/2d.
*
* Total Cost--10d.
*
* Time--10 Minutes
*

Chop the fish, bacon, and parsley finely, and mix them together with the seasoning. Make a thick sauce with 1 gill water, 1 oz flour, and 1 oz butter; flavour with anchovy and stir the fish in. Simmer for a few minutes, stir in the yolk of the egg, and turn on to a plate to cool. Make up into small balls, fill a frying pan with boiling water, put in the balls. Cover over and simmer gently for ten minutes. Dish the balls in a circle and pour over the melted butter, which has been nicely flavoured with anchovy; garnish with parsley, and serve.

FISH A LA CREME

* 4 Whiting or Schnapper--1s.
*

* 1 gill Milk--1d.
*

* 1 oz. Butter
*

* 1/2 oz. Flour, and Lemon Juice
*

* Pepper and Salt--1d.
*

* Total Cost--1s. 2d.
*

* Time--One Hour
*

Fillet the fish, wash the bones, and put them into half a pint of white stock, and boil them for half an hour. Strain out and mix with 1 gill of milk. Wash the fillets and roll them up, stand them in a stewpan and cook them in this liquor, covering them with a piece of buttered paper; they will take about 20 minutes.
Dish them carefully, strain the liquor, and make a sauce of it with the butter and flour by directions given. Season and flavour this and pour it over the fillets; garnish with chopped parsley and red bread crumbs, and serve hot.

FILLETS OF FISH AND CHEESE SAUCE.

* 3 Mullet or Bream--1s.
*
* 1/2 pint Cheese Sauce--4d.
*
* 1 oz. Dry Cheese
*
* 1 oz. Butter
*
* Lemon Juice
*
* Salt and Pepper--1 1/2d.
*
* Total Cost--1s. 51/2 d.
*
* Time--25 Minutes.
*

Fillet the fish, wash and dry them; put them on to a baking sheet, sprinkle with lemon juice. Put a few little pieces of butter over them; cover with buttered paper and bake from 20 minutes to half an hour, according to the thickness of the fillets. Place them carefully on the dish in which they are to be served, pour over them the cheese sauce nicely flavoured with pepper, salt, and parsley. Sprinkle over them some dry cheese, brown in front of the fire, or under the grill if using a gas stove, and serve hot.

COLLARED EELS

* 2 Eels--1s. 5d.
*

* 1 Egg--1d.
*

* 1/2 oz. Gelatine--1 1/2d.
*

* 1 fagot of Herbs
*

* 1 Onion
*

* 1 Carrot
*

* 1 spoonful Vinegar
*

* Pepper and Salt--1d.
*

* Total Cost--1s. 81/2 d.
*

* Time--One Hour and a Half
*

Clean the eels, cut them into pieces 2 inches long; put them in cold water well seasoned with salt, 2 dozen peppercorns and the vegetables, and a spoonful of vinegar. Bring to the boil, and skim well; then boil steadily for an hour, or longer if the eels are large. Take out the fish, slip out the bones, and cut the meat into small pieces. Put back the bones and boil the liquor quickly without the lid for half an hour, then strain off.

Dissolve the gelatine in a little cold water or gravy and stir in. If a very special dish is desired, the liquor can be clarified with the white of an egg in the same way as jelly. Rinse a mould in cold water, arrange in it the pieces of eel and a hard boiled egg cut into slices with a few sprigs of parsley. Strain the liquor over and stand away till cold. Turn out and serve with a salad.

STUFFED FLATHEAD

* 1 Flathead--9d.
*
* 2 oz. Forcemeat--2d.
*
* 1 gill Gravy
*
* 1 oz. Dripping--1d.
*
* Total Cost--1s.
*
* Time--Half an Hour
*

Take a little veal forcemeat and season nicely. Sew this into the flathead and truss it into the shape of the letter S. Rub some dripping on to a baking sheet, which should only be just large enough to take the fish. Put some dripping on the top, and bake in a moderate oven for half-an-hour, or longer if large. Slip it on to a hot dish, draw out the trussing string carefully, flavour and boil up the gravy and pour round it. Serve very hot.

OYSTERS AND BACON

* 1 doz. Large Oysters--6d.
*
* 3 Rashers Bacon
*
* Pepper, Salt and Lime Juice--3d.
*
* Total Cost--9d.
*
* Time--10 Minutes.
*

Mix some pepper, salt, and lemon juice together, and lay oysters in this. The bacon should be cut very thin, and then into strips about 1 inch broad and 3 inches long. Roll these up, and thread on a skewer first a roll of bacon and then an oyster, until the skewer is full; lay on a baking sheet and cook in the oven for about ten minutes. Have ready a hot dish, slip the bacon and oysters off the skewers on to this, and serve hot.

SCALLOPED OYSTERS

* 1 bottle Oysters--1s.
*
* 3 oz. Bread Crumbs--1d.
*
* 2 oz. Butter
*
* Lemon Juice, Pepper and Salt--2d.

* Total Cost--1 s. 3 d.
*

* Time--20 Minutes
*

Strain the liquor from the oysters, boil it up and pour over them, cover down for five minutes, and strain off again. Melt the butter, season with lemon juice, pepper, and salt.

Butter a dish, put in a layer of crumbs, then one of oysters; moisten with the butter, then more crumbs, and continue in layers till the dish is full. Pour over all the rest of the butter, and bake for a quarter of an hour. Serve at once.

TO COOK DRIED FISH

Put it into hot water, and boil gently for five minutes or longer if the fish is very thick. Take it out of water and put it on to a hot dish, rub a small piece of cold butter over it and cook for a few minutes either in the oven or in front of the fire. One or two soft boiled eggs broken over it is a nice way of serving it, or a few very thin slices of bacon well cooked may be placed round the dish as a garnish.

FRIED CRAYFISH

* 1 Crayfish--1s.
*
* French Frying Batter--2d.
*
* 1 teaspoonful Anchovy
*
* Frying Fat--1/2d.
*
* Total Cost--1s. 21/2 d.
*
* Time--3 Minutes
*

Pick all the white meat from a crayfish, and cut it into pieces about two inches long and one inch broad. Make a frying batter by recipe given elsewhere, and season with anchovy, lemon juice, pepper, and salt. Dip the pieces of crayfish into this and plunge into plenty of very hot fat; fry a good colour, drain on kitchen paper for a few minutes, pile high on a dish, and garnish with fried parsley.

BREAM PUDDING

* 2 Bream--8d.
*
* 1 gill Melted Butter--1d.
*
* 1/2 lb. Suet--1d.

* 1/2 teaspoonful Parsley
*

* Pepper and Salt
*

* 1/2 lb. Flour--1d.
*

* Total Cost--11 d.
*

* Time--One Hour and a Half.
*

Skin and fillet the fish and cut into small pieces; make a dry crust of the suet, and flour and line a pudding basin with it. Lay the fish in lightly, and season with the parsley, pepper, and salt. Pour over the melted butter; this should be made with 1/2 oz butter, 1/2 oz flour, and 1 gill of water. Cover the top of the pudding with crust, tie down securely with a cloth and string, and plunge into plenty of boiling water. Boil for one hour and a half, turn out of the basin, and sprinkle with chopped parsley. Serve hot.

FISH RISSOLES

* 1/2 lb. Cold Fish--4d.
*

* 1 oz. Butter--1d.
*

* 1 gill Milk--1d.
*

* Bread Crumbs
*

* Hot Fat

* 1 oz. Flour
*

* 1 teaspoonful of Anchovy
*

* 1/2 teaspoonful of Parsley
*

* Pepper and Salt--2d.
*

* Total Cost--8d.
*

* Time--5 Minutes
*

Pick the fish free from skin and bone, and chop it up. Make a smooth thick sauce with the flour, butter, and water, by directions given elsewhere. Flavour it with anchovy, parsley, pepper, and salt; stir in the fish, and mix well. Turn on to a plate till cold. Make up into small balls, cover with egg and bread crumbs, and fry in hot fat; drain for a few minutes on kitchen paper, arrange carefully on a dish, and garnish with parsley.

FISH A LA SAUMAREZ

* 2 Bream--1s.
*

* 2 Tomatoes--1/2d.
*

* 1 oz. Butter--1d.
*

* 1 fagot of Herbs
*

* 1 Carrot

* 1 oz. Flour
*

* Pepper and Salt
*

* 1 Onion
*

* 1 doz. Peppercorns
*

* Lemon Juice--1 1/2d.
*

* Total Cost--1s. 3d.
*

* Time--One Hour
*

Fillet the fish, put the bones in a saucepan, and just cover them with
water. When they boil, skim well, and add the tomatoes sliced up, the
peppercorns and vegetables; boil quickly without the lid for
half an hour, then strain, rubbing the pulp of the tomatoes through
with the liquor. Make a smooth sauce with half a pint of this liquor,
the butter, and the flour; if the colour is not good add a few drops of
cochineal. Fold the fillets of fish neatly, and bake in the oven with a
little lemon juice, and covered with a buttered paper. Arrange them on
a dish and pour the sauce over. Serve hot.

KEDGEREE.

* 1/2 lb. Gold Fish--4d.
*

* 1/4 lb. Boiled Rice--1d.
*

* 2 Hard Boiled Eggs--2d.

* 1 oz. Butter
*
* Pepper and Salt--1d.
*
* Total Cost--8d.
*
* Time--5 Minutes
*

Flake up the fish and mix it with the rice; shell the eggs and cut them in half, put the yolks on one side. Chop the whites and mix them with the rice and fish; season nicely and put into a saucepan with the butter, and stir until thoroughly hot. Pile on a dish, and either chop the yolks and sprinkle them over, or hold a sieve over the kedgeree and rub them lightly through. Serve hot.

FISH BAKED IN VINEGAR

* 2 Mullet--6d.
*
* 1/2 pint Vinegar--2d.
*
* 1 gill Water
*
* 1 fagot of Herbs
*
* 1 doz. Peppercorns
*
* Salt--1/2d.
*
* Total Cost--81/2 d.
* Time--One Hour

Wash the fish, dry them on a cloth, and rub them with a little salt.
Lay them in a deep dish, put in the herbs and peppercorns, pour over
the vinegar and water. Cover with a tin, and stand in a cool
oven, and bake very slowly for an hour. Take them out and let them get
quite cold in the vinegar, then lay them in a dish, and strain the
sauce over. Garnish with sprigs of parsley.

STUFFED CONGER EEL.

* 1 Eel--1s.
*
* 3 oz. Veal Seasoning--2d.
*
* 1 1/2 oz. Flour
*
* Pepper and Salt--1/2d.
*
* 1 1/2 oz. Butter--1d.
*
* Total Cost--1s. 31/2 d.
*
* Time--One Hour
*

Make the veal seasoning by recipe given elsewhere; sew it into the eel
and put it into a deep dish. Just cover it with water, and bake it in a
good oven for about one hour. Take it up and keep hot, strain the
liquor in which it has been cooked; take about one pint and make into a
brown sauce with the butter and flour. Colour it with a few drops of
caramel, let it boil for a few minutes, season with salt, pepper, and
lemon juice; pour over the fish, and serve very hot.

EEL AND TOMATO SAUCE.

* 1 Eel--1s.
*
* 6 Tomatoes--2d.
*
* 2 oz. Veal Seasoning--2d.
*
* 1 oz. Butter
*
* 1 oz. Flour
*
* Pepper and Salt--1d.
*
* Total Cost--1 s. 5d.
*
* Time--One Hour
*

Stuff and cook the eel as in the preceding recipe, and strain off the liquor. Rub the tomatoes through a sieve; mix with half a pint of the liquor in which the fish was cooked. Make a sauce of this of this with butte and flour, season with pepper and salt, and pour it over the fish. Garnish with parsley, and serve.

FRIED ROES

* 3 Roes--6d.
*
* Frying Batter
*
* Hot Fat
*
* Salt and Pepper--1d.
*
* Total Cost--7d
*
* Time--35 Minutes
*

Put the roes on in cold water and boil for about half an hour. Take
them up and let them get quite cold, then cut into slices. Make some
frying batter by recipe given elsewhere. Season it with salt and
pepper, dip in the slices, and fry a good colour. Pile high on a dish
and garnish with fried parsley. Roes may also be fried in egg and bread
crumbs; they are prepared just in the same way, only covered with egg
and crumbs instead of batter.

CODS' ROES IN TOMATO SAUCE

* 2 Roes--4d.
*
* 1 gill Tomato Sauce--2d.
*
* Cayenne

* 3 slices Toast
*
* 1 Egg
*
* Nutmeg and Salt--2d.
*
* Total Cost--8d.
*
* Time--40 Minutes.
*

Cods' roes are the best for this dish, but any roes will do. Wash them well, cover with cold water seasoned with salt, and boil for half an hour, or longer if the roes are large. Take them up and stand away till cold, then cut into slices about half an inch thick. Make some tomato sauce by recipe given elsewhere; when it is boiling, season with cayenne, nutmeg, and salt; stir in the yolk of an egg, lay in the slices of roe, cover down until hot through. Cut the toast into as many pieces as there are slices of roe, stand them in a dish, and put on each some roe. Make the sauce very hot, pour it over, and serve at once.

MULLET AND TOMATOES

* 2 Mullet--8d.
*
* 6 Tomatoes
*
* Bread Crumbs
*
* 1 teaspoonful Parsley

* Salt and Pepper--2d.
*

* 1 oz. Butter--1d.
*

* Total Cost--11d.
*

* Time--30 Minutes
*

Fillet and slice up the mullet, season each slice with parsley, pepper, and salt. Dip the tomatoes in boiling water, skim and slice them up. Butter a pie-dish, lay in the slices of fish and tomatoes alternately. Cover the top with bread crumbs and little pieces of butter. Cover the buttered paper and bake in a moderate oven for half an hour; take off the paper, and serve hot.

AMERICAN FISH

* 1 Flathead--1s.
*

* 1/2 pint Brown Sauce--1d.
*

* 3 oz. Fish Forcemeat
*

* 1 oz. Dripping--4d.
*

* Total Cost--1s. 5d.
*

* Time--30 Minutes.
*

Make a forcemeat and sew it into the fish. Rub some dripping over a baking sheet, truss the fish into shape, and lay it on. Rub the rest of the dripping on to a piece of paper, cover the fish carefully, bake in rather a hot oven for half an hour or longer, according to size; take of the paper, dish it, and pour round a nice brown sauce. A fish forcemeat is made with 2 oz cold fish, 1 oz suet, 1 oz bread crumbs well mixed together, with some seasoning and an egg.

COLD FISH AU GRATIN

Any scraps of cold fish may be served in this way. If any fish sauce is left, nothing is nicer to warm it in; if not, make a little with 1 gill of milk or water, 1 oz of butter, and 1 oz of flour. Flake the fish up, butter a plate, put the fish in and pour the sauce over. Sprinkle with brown bread crumbs, and bake in the oven for a quarter of an hour.

SMALL FISH

Any kind of small fish will do for this dish. Wash and dry them; well butter a sheet of stiff writing paper, lay the fish in, sprinkle them with a little very finely chopped onion or shallot, parsley, pepper, and salt. Squeeze over a few drops of lemon juice, and put a few little pieces of butter about them; wrap them up in the paper and bake for twenty minutes. Serve in the paper in which they were cooked.

BAKED FISH

* 4 Mullet or Jew-fish--1s.
*
* 2 oz. Bread Crumbs--1/2d.
*
* 1 oz. Butter--1d.
*
* Pepper and Salt
*
* 1 teaspoonful Parsley
*
* 1 teaspoonful Sweet Herbs
*
* 1/2 lemon
*
* 2 oz. Suet--2 1/2d.
*
* Total Cost--1 s. 4 d.
*
* Time--30 Minutes.
*

Split open the fish and remove the head and backbone, wash well in cold water and dry in a cloth. Chop the parsley, herbs, and suet, and mix these together; add half the crumbs, the rind of half a lemon, and pepper and salt. Butter a baking tin, lay on a fish skin downwards. On this place a layer of seasoning, a little lemon juice, and a few pieces of butter; on this another fish with the cut part next the seasoning. Do the rest in the same way, piling one on top of another; over all put the rest of the crumbs and butter, bake in a moderate oven for half an hour. Slip into a hot dish, and serve.

CODFISH AND POTATOES-
-BOUILLABAISSE OF COD.

* 2 lbs. Murray Cod--1s.
*
* 1 lb. Potatoes--1d.
*
* Slices of Roll
*
* 1 quart Water
*
* 1 fagot of Herbs
*
* 2 Leeks or 1 Onion
*
* Pinch of Saffron
*
* 1 1/2 oz. Butter--3 1/2d.
*
* Total Cost--1s. 41/2 d.
*
* Time--One Hour.

Put the butter into a saucepan, and when it is hot add the leeks or onion chopped small, and let them get a good colour without burning; then add a quart of water, the fagot of herbs, the saffron tied in a piece of muslin, and the potatoes peeled. Bring up to the boil, and when they are nearly cooked cut the cod into slices and lay it in. Cook slowly for twenty minutes, take up the fish, and put it in a hot dish and lay the potatoes round. Season and flavour the liquor, and boil up. Cut the bread into slices, put it into a hot dish, and strain the liquor over; serve with the fish.

BUTTERED WHITING

* 3 Whiting--1s.
*

* Pepper and Salt
*

* 1 1/2 oz. Butter
*

* 1 Lemon--2d.
*

* Total Cost--1s. 2d.
*

* Time--20 Minutes
*

Wash the whiting, dry them in a cloth, mix a little flour, pepper, and salt together, cover the fish thoroughly with this. Butter a thin dish, lay the whiting in and put the rest of the butter over them in small pieces, and put them into a hot oven; baste constantly with the butter. This must not be allowed to get black; it should be brown. When the whiting are done, which will be in from fifteen to twenty minutes, according to the thickness of the fish, place them in a hot dish and pour the butter in which they have been cooked over them.

BROILED FISH

* 2 Mullet--8d.
*
* 2 teaspoonful Oil
*
* Pepper
*
* Salt--1/2d.
*
* Total Cost--81/2 d.
*
* Time--10 Minutes.
*

Split the mullet open and wash away the black substance from the bones, dry on a cloth, rub with oil and sprinkle them with pepper and salt, and leave them in a cool place for an hour. Rub a gridiron with a piece of suet, and when it is quite hot put on the fish and broil it carefully, turning it two or three times whilst cooking. Lay on a hot dish and rub over with a little butter.

To broil successfully a very clear fire is required, and it should be made up some time before it is wanted. Broiling on a gas-stove is equivalent to broiling over a fire.

BOILED FISH

To boil fish properly it must never really boil; and in this lies the
secret of success. If it boils it has a watery, insipid flavour, and
drops of pieces very often when it is taken out of the water. The water
must boil well before the fish is put in, and be seasoned with salt and
a teaspoonful of vinegar or lemon juice; lay the fish carefully in, and
bring the water to the boil again. Then draw it away from the fire,
cover down closely, and keep it just below the boil. The time it takes
to cook depends so much on the size and thickness of the fish that no
hard and fast rule can be given; about ten minutes to every lb., will
be sufficient. It is always done when it begins to leave the
bone. Take it out of the water directly it is cooked, and if it is not
wanted just at the time, cover it with a cloth and keep it hot. Any
kind of fish sauce can be served with it, such as plain melted butter,
parsley, or egg sauce.

SALT FISH

To cook salt fish it should be soaked in cold water for twelve hours,
then well washed in fresh water, scraped and cleaned. Lay it in a
fish-kettle, cover with cold water, then simmer very gently indeed for one
hour and a half, according to the thickness of the fish. It should be
dished on a serviette, and garnished with sprigs of parsley and slices
of lemon. Send it to table with boiled parsnips and egg sauce.

DEVILLED SARDINES

* 1 tin Sardines--6d.
*
* 1/2 oz. Mustard--1/2d.
*
* Buttered Toast
*
* Cayenne--1d.
*
* Total Cost--71/2 d.
*
* Time--5 Minutes
*

Make the mustard with vinegar instead of water, and stir into it some cayenne and salt. Rub the sardines over with this, and either fry them in a little dripping or grill them. Cut the toast into fingers, lay a sardine on each piece, and serve hot. Sardines are also very good dipped in French batter and fried and served with fried parsley.

FISH A L'AURORE

* 1 Jew-fish--9d.
*
* 1/2 Small Onion
*
* 1/2 teaspoonful Parsley
*
* 1 Egg

* 1/2 pint White Sauce
*

* Pepper and Salt--3d.
*

* Total Cost--1s.
*

* Time--30 Minutes.
*

Put some dripping on a tin dish, lay the fish in it, and cover
with a buttered paper and bake in the oven for twenty minutes. Take it
out, split open and take out the centre bone; sprinkle the inside of
the fish with finely chopped onion and parsley, pepper, and salt. Put
back the upper fillet, trim away some of the bones, pour over the
melted butter or white sauce, and put back into the oven for ten
minutes. Boil the egg hard, remove the shell, take out the yolk and
either chop it or rub it through a sieve, cut the white into shapes.
Take the fish from the oven and decorate the top with the yolk and
white of egg; serve hot.

FILLETS A LA ORLY

* 2 Bream--8d.
*

* Lemon Juice
*

* Parsley
*

* Half an Onion
*

* 1/2 pint Tomato Sauce

* Pepper and Salt--3d.
*

* Total Cost--11d.
*

* Time--5 Minutes
*

Fillet the fish and lay them in a dish; sprinkle them well with lemon juice, pepper, salt and parsley. Lay over them some slices of onion and leave them for an hour, then fry them either in batter or flour. Drain them for a few moments on kitchen paper, and serve on a dish very hot with some good thick tomato sauce in a sauce-boat.

SCANDINAVIAN PUDDING

* 2 Bream--8d.
*

* 2 Eggs--2d.
*

* 1/2 pint Milk--1d.
*

* 1/2 lb. Flour
*

* Pepper and Salt
*

* 1/2 pint Fish Sauce--2d.
*

* Total Cost--1s. 1d.
*

* Time--One Hour.
*

Fillet the fish, skin and chop very find; sift the flour into a basin,

drop in the eggs, and make into a batter with the milk. Season
with salt and pepper, and stir in the chopped fish. Butter a basin,
pour in the mixture and boil for one hour; turn out of the basin and
serve with melted butter sauce, flavoured with anchovy, or with any
other fish-sauce that may be preferred.

OYSTERS AND POTATOES

* 1 bottle Oysters--1s.
*
* 4 Cold Potatoes--1d.
*
* 1 Egg--1d.
*
* 2 oz. Flour
*
* Pepper and Salt--1/2d.
*
* Total Cost--1s. 21/2 d.
*
* Time--20 Minutes.
*

Mash the potatoes and make them into a paste with the flour and egg,
roll out and cut into small pieces. Season the oysters with lemon
juice, pepper, and salt; put three of four into each piece of potato
crust. Roll it up, brush over with milk, and bake for twenty minutes.
Pile high on a dish, and serve hot.

STEWED FISH

* 2 Fish--9d.
*
* 1/2 pint Stock
*
* 1 blade of Mace
*
* 2 Cloves
*
* 1/2 oz. Flour--1/2d.
*
* 2 tablespoonful Ketchup
*
* 1 Onion--1d.
*
* 1 Egg--1d.
*
* Bread Crumbs
*
* 1 doz. Peppercorns--1/2d.
*
* Total Cost--1s.
*
* Time--One Hour and a Quarter
*

Fillet the fish and fry them in egg and bread crumbs; slice and fry the onion, lay this and the fish in a tin dish. Cover with stock, put in the cloves, peppercorns, and mace, cover over, and put into a moderate oven for an hour. Mix the flour and ketchup together and stir it in; put back into the oven for ten minutes. Dish the fish and strain the sauce over it.

OYSTERS AND MACARONI

* 2 oz. Macaroni--1 1/2d.
*
* 1 bottle Oysters--1s.
*
* 1 gill Milk or Melted Butter Sauce--1d.
*
* Cayenne
*
* Salt
*
* Bread Crumbs--1d.
*
* Total Cost--1s. 31/2 d.
*
* Time--Half an Hour.
*

Boil the macaroni in the oyster liquor or in weak stock till quite soft. Rub a little butter on a dish, cut the macaroni into pieces two inches long and lay it at the bottom. On this place the oysters, and season them with cayenne, salt, and a little lemon juice or nutmeg. Pour over the milk or sauce, cover with bread crumbs, and brown it in a quick oven. A few little pieces of butter laid on top of the crumbs make a richer dish. It must be served very hot.

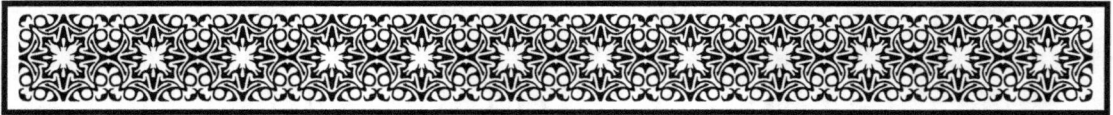

CHAPTER XIX.
FIFTY RECIPES FOR MEAT DISHES

COOKERY OF MEAT.

The principal methods of cooking meat are roasting, baking, boiling, stewing, broiling, braising, and frying. Of these methods roasting and baking are conducted on the same principle--dry heat; boiling and stewing are often spoken of as if they were the same, but this is quite a mistake. When we boil a joint we plunge it into boiling water, and this water should cover it completely; but when meat is stewed it must be cooked in a very small quantity of water, and never allowed to boil. Water boils at 212, but simmering heat is 180, and meat cannot be properly stewed if it is cooked quicker than this. One of the great faults of English cooks is that they cook too quickly, and it is particularly necessary in stewing to cook slowly, because we want to extract and blend all the different flavours of the various substances, which are necessary for a good and savoury stew. When boiling meat for table plunge it into boiling water, and then reduce the heat; but when broth or soup is to be made it must be put into cold water, so that the goodness may be drawn from it. Corned beef or pork should also be placed in cold water and heated gradually, so that some of the salt is drawn out. The frying-pan should be discarded from the kitchen, at least as far as steaks and chops are concerned; grilling or broiling is by far the best method of cooking them. Meat unless it is very carefully fried is tough and greasy, yet the same piece of meat if grilled or stewed would be tender and nutritious. There is often a prejudice against meat twice cooked, but the most delicate ENTREES that are so highly esteemed by many are only re-cooked meat. It is the time and care expended on it that makes it so delicious. Even in plain cooking there is no reason why the homely dish of hash should not be appetizing and wholesome. I trust that the following recipes, if carefully carried out, will prove this to be true.

STEAK AND KIDNEY PIE

* 2 lbs. Steak--5d.
*
* 2 Kidneys--1 1/2d.
*
* 1 lb. Flour
*
* 1/2 lb. Dripping
*
* 1 gill Water
*
* Pepper and Salt--2d.
*
* Total Cost--81/2 d.
*
* Time--One Hour and a Half
*

Mix a teaspoonful of flour in a plate with some pepper and salt, slice up the meat into pieces about three inches long by two broad, dip each piece lightly in the flour; skin and slice up the kidneys, and cut the fat into small pieces. Roll a piece of kidney and a piece of fat alternatively in the slices of meat, pile high in a dish, and pour in a gill of water or stock. Make a short crust by directions given for short pastry, wet the edge of the dish and line it with a strip of the paste, wet this strip again with water and cover the dish with paste; trim off the edge, cut a small piece out of the centre of the pie, and ornament it with a few leaves cut out of the paste trimmings. Brush over with water and bake in a moderate oven for one hour and a half. As soon as the crust has acquired some colour, cover with a piece of paper well rubbed with dripping.

STEAK AND KIDNEY PUDDING

* 2 lbs. Steak--5d.
*
* 2 Kidneys--1 1/2d.
*
* 1 lb. Flour--2d.
*
* 1/2 lb. Suet
*
* 1/2 pint Water
*
* Pepper and Salt--1 1/2d.
*
* Total Cost--10d.
*
* Time--Three Hours
*

Make a dry crust, by directions given elsewhere, of the flour, suet, and butter. Rub the pudding basin well with dripping, roll out the crust, take two-thirds and line the basin, well pressing the crust in.

Slice up the meat and kidney, season with pepper and salt, pile lightly in the basin, pour in half a gill of water, wet the edge of the crust. Roll out the piece left, and cover the pudding securely. Dip a cloth in boiling water, put it over the top, tie it round with string, and pin or tie the ends of the cloth over the top. Plunge into plenty of boiling water, and boil for three hours. Take it up, take off the cloth, turn it out of the basin on to a hot dish, and serve hot.

STEWED KIDNEYS AND MACARONI

* 6 Kidneys--6d.
*
* 1 gill Stock
*
* 1 oz. Butter
*
* 2 oz. Macaroni
*
* Parsley, Pepper, and Salt--2 1/2d.
*
* Total Cost--81/2 d.
*
* Time--25 Minutes
*

Put the Macaroni into boiling water seasoned with salt, and boil for about twenty minutes, or until quite soft, but not broken. When it is boiling, skin and cut the kidneys in half, put them into a frying-pan with the butter, and toss them over the fire for two or three minutes. Sprinkle with parsley, pepper, and salt, pour over the stock or water.

Bring it to the boil, then cover down by the side of the fire for five minutes. Place carefully in the centre of a hot dish, boil up the gravy and pour over. Arrange the macaroni round the dish as a border, and serve hot.

STEWED STEAK AND WALNUTS

* 2 lbs. Steak--5d.
*
* 1/2 pint Water or Stock
*
* 3 Pickled Walnuts
*
* 1 teaspoonful Vinegar
*
* 1 teaspoonful Cornflour
*
* Salt and Pepper
*
* Total Cost--6d.--1d.
*
* Time--Three Hours
*

Cut the steak into neat pieces, put it into hot water and bring to the boil, then keep it below boiling point, but simmering very gently for two hours and a half. Mix the cornflour with a tablespoonful of the vinegar from the walnuts and stir it in, add salt to taste and a small pinch of pepper. Cut up three walnuts and put them in, bring to simmering point again, and cook for at least another half-hour, then dish neatly. Boil up the gravy and pour over it.

STEAK AND MACARONI

* 2 lbs. Steak--5d.
*
* 2 oz. Macaroni--1 1/2d.
*
* 1 oz. Dripping
*
* 1/2 pint Stock
*
* 1 Onion
*
* 1 doz. Peppercorns
*
* Salt--1/2d.
*
* Total Cost--7d.
*
* Time--Three Hours
*

Cut the steak into neat pieces, put the butter or dripping into a
saucepan and fry the steak quickly; take it out, shred the onion and
put it in with the peppercorns, and let it get quite brown.
Pour over the stock and stir until it boils, then put back the steak
and let it simmer very gently for three hours. While it is cooking,
boil the macaroni in weak stock or water for twenty-five minutes, and
if it is ready before it is wanted keep it in hot water. When the steak
is done, dish it neatly, flavour the gravy, boil it up and pour over.
Cut the macaroni into short pieces and place it round the dish as a
garnish.

MUTTON CHOPS IN BATTER

* 2 Eggs--2d.
*
* 2 lbs. Chops--5.
*
* 1 pint Milk--2 1/2d.
*
* 3/4 lb. Flour
*
* Salt and Pepper--1/2d.
*
* Total Cost--10d.
*
* Time--One Hour and a Quarter
*

Break the eggs into a basin, beat in the flour with a fork, then add gradually the milk, season with a little pepper and salt. Rub some dripping on a baking dish, pour in the batter, lay in the chops. Put into a moderate oven and bake for about one hour and a quarter. Serve hot.

TOMATO PIE

* 3 or 4 Tomatoes--2d.
*
* 1 lb. Chops--2 1/2d.
*
* 1 oz. Butter--1d.

* 4 Cold Potatoes--1d.
*

* Pepper and Salt
*

* 1 tablespoonful Milk--1/2d.
*

* Total Cost--7d.
*

* Time--One Hour and a Quarter
*

Skin and slice up the tomatoes, put a layer at the bottom of a pie-dish,
then lay in the chops. Season with pepper and salt, and cover
with the rest of the tomatoes; mash up the potatoes until ver smooth.
Warm the butter and milk and pour it over them and make into a paste.
Cover the dish with this crust, brush the top over with a
little milk, put into the oven and bake for about one hour and a
quarter.

KABOBS

* 1 1/2 lbs. of Steak--4d.
*

* 1 dessertspoonful Curry Powder
*

* 1 dessertspoonful Worcester Sauce
*

* 1 dessertspoonful Vinegar--1 1/2d.
*

* 1/2 pint Stock
*

* 1 tablespoonful Flour

* 1 tablespoonful Chutney
*

* 1/4 lb. Rice
*

* Salt--2d.
*

* Total Cost--71/2 d.
*

* Time--One Hour and a Half
*

Slice up the steak into pieces about three inches long and two broad. Mix the curry powder, sauce, vinegar, flour and chutney together and spread this over the steak; roll up and thread a small wooden skewers. These skewers should be made from a very small splint of wood, just large enough to hold one or at most two of the rolls; lay them in a saucepan, pour over the stock, bring to the boil and simmer one hour and a half. While they are cooking, well wash the rice in cold water and let it soak for half an hour, throw it into boiling water for three minutes and strain off. Put a pinch of saffron in some fresh water, season with salt, and finish cooking in this. Strain off and dry in the saucepan. Pile this on a dish and lay the kabobs over it; boil up the gravy, season and flavour, and strain round the dish.

SCOTCH COLLOPS

* 1 lb. Lean Steak--2 1/2d.
*

* 1 gill Stock
*

* Pepper and Salt
*

* 1 oz. Butter--1d.
*

* Quarter of an Onion
*

* Small Sippets of Toast--1d.
*

* Total Cost--41/2 d.
*

* Time--One Hour
*

Remove all the fat, and cut the meat into very thin and small dice, mince up the onion very finely. Mix together, season with some pepper and salt, and put into a saucepan with the butter. Stir it about for five minutes, then pour on the stock, bring to the boil, and simmer for one hour. Arrange neatly on a hot dish, and put the sippets of toast round.

POOR MAN'S DISH

* 1/2 pint Poor Man's Sauce--1/2d.
*

* Slice of Toast
*

* Slices of Cold Meat--2d.
*

* Total Cost--21/2 d.
*

* Time--Half an Hour
*

Make the sauce by directions given elsewhere, pour it into a pie dish, lay in some slices of underdone beef or mutton; cover over and stand in the oven for a quarter of an hour. Cut the slice of toast into sippets, lay them round, and serve.

BREAST OF MUTTON AND PEAS

* 2 Breasts of Mutton--4d.
*
* 2 Onions
*
* 1 Carrot--1/2d.
*
* 1 Egg--1d.
*
* Bread Crumbs--1/2d.
*
* 1 fagot of Herbs
*
* 1 pint Peas
*
* Salt and Pepper
*
* Hot Fat
*
* 12 Peppercorns--7d.
*
* Total Cost--1s. 1d.
*
* Time--Two Hours
*

Wipe the meat with a warm damp cloth, and put it into a saucepan with the vegetables; bring to the boil and stew very gently for two hours.

Take it up and remove all the bones, put it between two boards and stand some heavy weights on it till quite cold. Then cut into neat-shaped pieces, egg and bread crumb them; fry a good colour. Boil the peas by recipe given elsewhere. Pile the mutton on a dish and put the peas round. A breast of lamb is exceedingly nice done in this way; it may be cut off before the quarter is roasted. The liquor in which the meat was cooked makes excellent soup.

TRIPE AND TOMATOES

* 2 lbs. Tripe--5d.
*
* 1 doz. Tomatoes--3d.
*
* 1/2 pint Water or Stock
*
* 1 oz. Cornflour--1/2d.
*
* 1 Onion
*
* Pepper and Salt--1/2d.
*
* Total Cost--9d
*
* Time--Four Hours
*

Cut the tripe into neat pieces, put it on in cold water and bring to the boil; let it boil for five minutes, put it into cold water, and wash and scrape it well. Slice up the tomatoes and rub them through a sieve; mix them with the stock or water, and season with pepper and salt. Pour this into a saucepan, slice in the onion, put in the tripe, and let it boil up. Simmer gently for four hours, mix the cornflour smoothly with a little water or stock, and pour it in; stir until it boils, dish the tripe carefully, season and flavour the sauce to taste, and pour it over. Tripe is more easily digested than any other animal food, and is therefore good for people suffering with dyspepsia.

TRIPE IN MILK

* 2 lbs. Tripe--5d.
*
* 1 pint Milk--2d.
*
* Pepper and Salt
*
* 2 Onions
*
* 1 oz. Flour
*
* 1/2 pint Water--1/2d.
*
* Total Cost--71/2 d.
*
* Time--Four Hours
*

Prepare the tripe as in the preceding recipe. Mix the milk and water together, pour it into a saucepan; lay in the tripe, slice in the onions, bring to the boil, and let it simmer slowly for four hours. Season with pepper and salt, thicken with the flour; after adding the flour let it cook for fifteen minutes, then dish the tripe carefully and pour the sauce over it.

TOMATOES AND MINCE

* 8 Tomatoes--3d.
*
* 8 pieces Toast
*
* 1/4 lb. Minced Meat
*
* Parsley--1d.
*
* Total Cost--4d.
*
* Time--10 Minutes.
*

Take any remains of cold mince or hash, add more flavouring if necessary, and make it hot in the saucepan. Wipe the tomatoes and scrape out the centre, fill it up with the mince, and stand in the oven for ten minutes. Have ready some rounds of toast about the same size as the tomatoes. When the tomatoes are cooked enough, stand them on the toast, and serve.

BREAKFAST MEAT

* 1 lb. Cold Meat--3d.
*
* 2 oz. Macaroni--1 1/2d.
*
* Pepper and Salt
*

* 3 Tomatoes
*

* 1/2 gill Stock
*

* Bread Crumbs--1d.
*

* Total Cost--51/2 d.
*

* Time--Half an Hour
*

Mince up the meat, or any remains of cold hash or mince will do. If there is any cold macaroni it can be used; if not, boil some by directions given, and slice up the tomatoes. Butter a dish in which it can be cooked and served. Place at the bottom a layer of meat, then one of macaroni, then one of tomatoes, season with pepper and salt, and continue this in layers until all the materials are used up.
Sprinkle a few bread crumbs on the top, put into the oven, and bake for half an hour. Serve hot.

RISSOLES

* 2 lb. Cold Meat--3d.
*

* 1 oz. Butter--1d.
*

* 1 1/2 oz. Flour
*

* 1 Egg
*

* Bread Crumbs
*

* 1/2 pint Stock
*

* Quarter of an Onion
*

* Parsley
*

* Pepper and Salt
*

* Hot Fat--2d.
*

* Total Cost--6d.
*

* Time--5 Minutes.
*

Mince up the meat and mix in some chopped parsley, pepper and salt; put the butter into a stewpan, and when it is dissolved mince up the pieces of onion very finely and fry that for two minutes, then stir in the flour. Pour in the gravy and stir until it boils; mix in the meat and let it get thoroughly hot. Turn it out on to a plate, spread it over, and leave until quite cold. Make up into balls, cover with egg and bread crumbs, and fry in hot fat; arrange in a circle and garnish with fried parsley.

KIDNEY FRITTERS

* 6 Kidneys--6d.
*

* 1 teaspoonful Minced Herbs--1/2d.
*

* Hot Fat
*

* 1 teaspoonful Onion
*

* Frying Batter
*

* Pepper and Salt--1d.
*

* Total Cost--71/2 d.
*

* Time--5 Minutes
*

Skin the kidneys and cut up each one into three or four slices. Make a frying batter by directions given elsewhere; stir in the minced onions and herbs, and season with pepper and salt. Dip the slices of kidney into this and plunge into very hot fat. Fry a good colour, pile high on a dish, garnish with fried parsley, and serve very hot. Slices of cold beef or mutton are very nice done in this way.

KIDNEY TOAST

* 2 Kidneys--1 1/2d.
*

* 1/2 oz. Butter--1/2d.
*

* 1 Slice Toast
*

* Parsley
*

* Pepper and Salt--1/2d.
*

* Total Cost--21/2 d.
*

* Time--5 Minutes.
*

Skin and chop the kidneys small, put into a saucepan with the butter, and cook for two or three minutes; season with pepper and salt. Spread it on the toast, sprinkle over some chopped parsley, and serve.

BEEF TRIFLES

* 1 lb. Cold Roast Beef--3d.
*

* 4 oz. Bread Crumbs
*

* Pepper and Salt--1d.
*

* 1 teaspoonful Onion
*

* 1 Egg
*

* 1 teaspoonful Parsley or Horse-radish--1 1/2d.
*

* Total Cost--51/2 d
*

* Time--Half and Hour
*

Mince the beef and onion very finely, and mix it with the bread crumbs, pepper, and salt. Add either some chopped parsley or finely scraped horse-radish; mix thoroughly. Moisten with an egg well beaten, and if very dry a spoonful of gravy or milk. Butter some small cups or moulds, fill them with this mixture, and bake for about half an hour.
Garnish with sprigs of parsley, and serve with them some horse-radish sauce or brown gravy.

HASHED BEEF AND TOMATO SAUCE

* 1 lb. Cold Roast Beef--3d.
*

* 8 tomatoes--3d.
*

* 1 fagot of Herbs
*

* Salt and Pepper--1/2d.
*

* 1 gill Gravy
*

* 1 oz. Butter
*

* 1/2 teaspoonful Sugar
*

* Toast--1 1/2d.
*

* Total Cost--8d.
*

* Time--Half an Hour
*

Slice up the tomatoes and put them into a saucepan with the butter, herbs, pepper, salt, sugar, and gravy. Stir about until it becomes quite a pulp; then rub through a sieve, season to taste, and let it get quite cold. Cut the beef into thin slices and lay it in a saucepan, pour over the cold sauce and let it get hot through, very slowly. Arrange on a hot dish, and garnish with fried sippets of bread or toast.

STEWED CHOPS

* 1 lb. Chops--2 1/2d.
*
* 1 oz. Butter--1d.
*
* Pepper and Salt
*
* 1/2 oz. Flour
*
* 1 gill Gravy--1/2d.
*
* Total Cost--4d.
*
* Time--One Hour
*

Trim some of the fat from the chops, put the butter into a saucepan, and when it is melted stir in the flour. Mix well, and pour in the gravy; stir until it boils, lay in the chops, and simmer very gently for one hour. Dish the chops in a circle, boil up and season the gravy, and pour over the stew.

BAKED CHOP

* 1 Chop
*
* Pepper and Salt
*
* Total Cost--1d

* Time--One Hour
*

Choose a nice loin chop with an undercut. Rub a little butter in a soup plate, lay in the chop, cover with another plate, and stand in a cool oven for an hour. Put on a very hot plate and pour over the gravy which has run from it. Serve very hot.

RICE CUTLETS

* 1/2 lb. Cold Meat--1 1/2d.
*

* 2 oz. Rice
*

* Pepper and Salt--1/2d.
*

* 1 Egg--1d.
*

* Bread Crumbs
*

* Hot Fat--1/2d.
*

* Total Cost--31/2 d.
*

* Time--5 Minutes
*

Mince the meat finely; if there is any cold rice in the larder it will do; if not, boil some. Mix the rice and meat well together, season and flavour with a little nutmeg or lemon peel; if the meat is very lean add 2 oz fat or beef suet. Shape into cutlets, egg and bread crumb them, and fry in hot fat; dish in a circle and garnish with fried parsley.

POTATO SAUSAGES

* 3 Cold Potatoes--1/2d.
*
* 1/4 lb. Cold Meat--1d.
*
* Nutmeg, Pepper, and Salt
*
* 1 Egg
*
* Bread Crumbs
*
* Hot Fat--1 1/2d.
*
* Total Cost--3d.
*
* Time--5 Minutes.
*

Mash up the potatoes, and mince the meat; mix together,

season nicely, and mix into a paste with half the egg. Roll into
sausages, egg and bread crumb, and fry in hot fat. Dish in a pyramid,
and garnish with fried parsley.

BRAZILIAN STEW

* 2 lbs. Leg of Beef--5d.
*
* 1 Onion
*
* 1 Carrot
*
* 1 tablespoonful Vinegar
*
* 1 doz. Peppercorns--1/2d.
*
* Total Cost--51/2 d.
*
* Time--Three Hours
*

Cut the beef up in small pieces, dip them in the vinegar, and lay in a jar. Slice in the vegetables, add the peppercorns, and tie a paper over the top of the jar. Stand in a saucepan of boiling water for three hours; dish up the meat, garnish with the carrot, strain the gravy, season and flavour, boil up and pour over. Serve hot.

BEEF OLIVES

* 2 lbs. Rump Steak--10d.
*
* 1/4 lb. Veal Seasoning--2d.
*
* 12 Peppercorns

* 1/2 pint Stock
*

* 1 Onion
*

* 1 Carrot--1/2d.
*

* Total Cost--1s. O1/2 d.
*

* Time--One Hour and a Quarter
*

Cut up the steak into thin slices about three inches long and two broad, shape the seasoning into small corks, roll a piece up in each slice of steak, thread them on a skewer and lay them in a saucepan. Pour in the stock, add the peppercorns and vegetables, bring to the boil, simmer very gently for one hour and a half. Place the olives on a hot dish and draw out the skewers, remove the fat, boil up the gravy, season and flavour to taste, and pour round. Serve hot.

MACARONI PUDDING

* 3 oz. Macaroni--2d.
*

* 1/2 lb. Cold Meat--2d.
*

* Pepper and Salt
*

* 1/2 pint Gravy
*

* 2 Eggs
*

* 1/2 pint Milk

* 1 teaspoonful Parsley--3d.
*

* Total Cost--7d.
*

* Time--One Hour
*

Boil the macaroni in stock or water. Mince the meat finely, and season with parsley, pepper, and salt. Rub a pudding basin or mould with butter, put the macaroni and meat in in layers, and season nicely. Beat up the eggs and milk and pour them over, cover with buttered paper, and steam for one hour. Turn out of the basin carefully, and pour round it a little nice brown gravy or white sauce.

SHEEP'S TONGUES IN TOMATO SAUCE

* 6 Tongues--1s.
*

* 1/2 pint Tomato Sauce--2 1/2d.
*

* 1 doz. Peppercorns
*

* 1 Onion
*

* 1 fagot Herbs
*

* 1 Carrot--1d.
*

* Total Cost--1s. 31/2 d.
*

* Time--Three Hours.
*

Wash the tongues in cold water, put them into a saucepan, cover them with cold water or stock, and bring to the boil, then skim well. Either corned or fresh tongues will do for this dish. If corned, no salt is required; but if fresh ones are used, put in a dessertspoonful of salt. Put in the vegetables and peppercorns and simmer gently for two hours, then take them up, plunge them into cold water and remove the skin. Trim them off and cut in half. Make some tomato sauce by recipe given elsewhere. The liquor in which the tongues were boiled may be used for this if it is not too salt. Lay the tongues in and simmer for another hour; dish carefully, boil up the sauce and pour over. Garnish with chopped parsley.

BROWN MINCE

* 1 lb. Cold Roast Beef--4d.
*
* 1/2 lb. Bread Crumbs--1d.
*
* Pepper and Salt
*
* 1 Egg
*
* 1/2 pint Gravy
*
* Nutmeg--1d.
*
* Total Cost--6d.
*
* Time--One Hour
*

Mince up the beef finely and mix it with the bread crumbs; season with

pepper, salt, nutmeg, or parsley. Beat up the egg, mix it with the
gravy, and pour over the meat and crumbs. Butter a basin, sprinkle well
with brown bread crumbs, put in the mince. Cover over with a plate and
bake for an hour, then turn on to a hot dish and pour a little nice
gravy round it.

STEAK A LA JARDINIERE

* 1 lbs. Steak--5d.
*
* 1 gill Green Peas--2d.
*
* 1 gill French Beans--1d.
*
* 1/2 oz. Flour
*
* 1 oz. Butter
*
* 1 Carrot
*
* 1 Turnip
*
* 1/2 pint Gravy
*
* Salt--1 1/2d.
*
* Total Cost--91/2 d.
*
* Time--Three Hours
*

Cut the steak into neat pieces and fry very quickly in the butter; take it out, put in the flour, and when quite smooth pour on the gravy and stir until it boils. Put back the steak, and simmer very gently for three hours. Cut the carrot and turnip up into thin strips, and put them in when the steak has been cooking for two hours. Boil the peas and beans separately, and add them to the stew five minutes before serving. Arrange the steak on a hot dish, put the vegetables round, and pour over the gravy. The greater the variety of vegetables used the nicer this dish will be.

KROMSKIES

* 1/2 lb. Cold Meat--2d.
*
* 2 Rashers Fat Bacon--2d.
*
* 1 oz. Butter--1d.
*
* Frying Butter--1d.
*
* 1/2 gill Stock
*
* 1 oz. Flour
*
* Parsley, Pepper, and Salt
*
* Hot Fat--1/2d.
*
* Total Cost--61/2 d.
*
* Time--5 Minutes

Mince the meat finely or put it through the sausage machine, season with parsley, pepper, and salt; put the butter into a saucepan, and when it is melted stir in the flour and the stock. Stir until it boils, then add the meat and mix thoroughly. Turn on to a plate to cool. When cold make up into pieces about the size of a cork. Take some very thin rashers of fat bacon and cut into strips about half an inch wide by two inches long. Roll the meat in this, dip in frying batter, and fry in very hot fat; drain for a few minutes on kitchen paper, pile high on a dish, garnish with fried parsley, and serve very hot.

KOTTBULLAR

* 2 lbs. Fillet or Beef--10d.
*

* 1/2 lb. Suet--1d.
*

* Salt and Pepper
*

* Hot Fat
*

* 1/2 pint Milk--1d.
*

* 2 Eggs--2d.
*

* Nutmeg
*

* Soda Biscuit
*

* Total Cost--1s. 21/2 d.
*

* Time--10 Minutes

Mince the lean of the meat very small with about a quarter of a pound of the suet which surrounds it; season with pepper, salt, and nutmeg. Make a little boiled custard by recipe given elsewhere, pour it over the biscuit, which must be made into fine crumbs, then stir in the meat and let it get quite cold. Roll into small balls with a little flour. Put three ounces of dripping into a frying pan, and when very hot drop in the balls and fry a good colour; drain for a few minutes on kitchen paper, and dish in a circle. Serve hot.

BRAISED LEG OF MUTTON

* 1 Leg of Mutton--1s. 3d.
*
* 1 Rasher of Ham--2d.
*
* 1 fagot of Herbs
*
* 20 Peppercorns--1/2d.
*
* 1 1/2 oz. Butter--1d.
*
* 2 Carrots
*
* 1 Turnip
*
* 1 Onion
*
* 1 quart Stock--1d.
*
* Total Cost--1s. 71/2 d.

* Time--Four Hours.
*

Put the butter into a saucepan, and when it is dissolved put in the mutton and brown it all over; then lay the ham and vegetables round it, pour in the stock, and bring it to the boil. Cover down closely, and stand the saucepan in a moderate oven where it will cook slowly. If the braising is being done by a coal fire the lid of the stewpan may be reversed and some hot coals placed in it; these will want renewing f rom time to time. In any case cook very slowly, then dish the meat, strain the gravy, remove the fat carefully, and boil to a sort of half glaze; pour round the dish, serve with Julienne or plain vegetables.

PRESSED BEEF

* 10 lbs. Thick Brisket of Beef, Corned or Fresh--1s. 6d.
*

* 1 fagot of Herbs
*

* 1 stalk Celery--1/2d.
*

* 1 Onion
*

* 2 Carrots
*

* 1 Turnip
*

* 40 Peppercorns--1 1/2d.
*

* Total Cost--1s. 8d.
*

* Time--Four Hours

Bind the beef with tapes to keep it a good shape. If it is corned, put it on in cold water; if fresh, in hot stock or water, and bring to the boil, then skim carefully and put in the vegetables and peppercorns. Simmer very gently indeed for four hours, then take it up. Take off the tapes, slip out the bones, and put it into a dish; place a piece of board on the top and some heavy weights and leave till the next day, then turn out and serve with a salad. If fresh meat is used for this dish the liquor may be used for soup, or the bones may be put back when removed from the meat and boiled without the lid very quickly for an hour. Then strain off and stand away till the next day; it should then be in a strong jelly. This may be cut into blocks and put round the meat.

CURRIED CHOPS

* 2 lbs. Chops--5d.
*

* 1/2 oz. Curry Powder--1d.
*

* 1 oz. Butter--1d.
*

* Lemon Juice
*

* 1/4 lb. Rice
*

* 1/2 pint Gravy or Water--1d.
*

* 1/2 oz. Flour
*

* 1 Apple

* 1 Onion
*

* Salt--1d.
*

* Total Cost--9d.
*

* Time--Three Hours.
*

Trim some of the fat away from the chops. Put the butter into a
stewpan, put in the chops and brown them quickly; take out,
chop up the apple and onion, and fry that too. Sprinkle with the curry
powder and flour, pour in the stock or water and stir until it boils,
then put back the chops, bring to the boil, and simmer very gently for
three hours. Dish carefully, boil up the gravy, and if it is not thick
enough boil quickly without the lid for some minutes. Season with salt
and lemon juice and pour over the chops. Boil the rice by directions
given elsewhere; rinse out a small mould or cup in cold water, press
the rice into it, and turn out. Serve this in a separate dish, but send
it to the table with the curry.

BEEF A LA MODE

* 6 lbs. Leg of Beef or Silverside--9d.
*

* 1 Calf's Foot--4d.
*

* 2 Onions
*

* 2 Carrots
*

* 1 Turnip--1d.

* 1 fagot of Herbs
*
* 40 Peppercorns
*
* 1 blade of Mace
*
* 6 Cloves
*
* Salt--1d.
*
* Total Cost--1s. 3d.
*
* Time--Five Hours.
*

Have the foot well chopped up, put it on in cold water, bring it to the boil. Let it boil for five minutes, then take it up and scrape and wash it well, lay it in a stewpan with the beef cut into pieces. Cover with cold water and bring to the boil, put in the spices tied in a piece of muslin, and let it simmer very gently for three hours.

Slice up the vegetables and put them in, and continue simmering altogether for about five hours. Take up the foot, take out all the bones, and cut into pieces; put back the meat of the foot into the saucepan, take out the spices, season with salt, remove the fat, boil up, and serve. This dish is always better for being made the day before it is wanted, as the fat can be more easily removed.

BEEFSTEAK ROLLS

* 1 lb. Of Beefsteak--2d.
*
* Bread and Butter--1d.
*
* 2 Cloves
*
* 1 Onion
*
* Stalk of Celery--1/2d.
*
* 1/2 pint Gravy
*
* 1 oz. Butter
*
* 1/2 oz. Flour
*
* Salt--1d.
*
* Total Cost--41/2 d.
*
* Time--Two Hours
*

Take a thick steak and split it open, cut it into strips five inches
wide by three long. Cut some very thin bread and butter the same size
seasoned with pepper and salt, lay it on the steak and roll it up,
thread on a skewer and dust with flour. Put the butter into a frying-pan,
and when it is hot put in the rolls and fry them quickly; take out
and lay in a saucepan, cut up the onion and fry in the same butter as
the rolls were fried in. Shake in a teaspoonful of flour and pour in
the gravy; stir until it boils, then pour over the rolls. Put in the

celery and cloves, and simmer very gently for two hours; take up the
rolls on a hot dish and slip off the skewers, boil up and flavour the
gravy. Remove the fat and pour round the meat. Veal or mutton is also
very good prepared in this way.

BEEFSTEAK STUFFED

* 1 1/2 lbs. Of Beefsteak--4d.
*
* 1/2 lb. Potatoes
*
* 2 oz. Dripping
*
* Salt and Pepper--1d.
*
* 1 oz. Butter
*
* 1 tablespoonful Milk
*
* 1 Onion
*
* 1/2 teaspoonful Sage--1 1/2d.
*
* Total Cost--61/2 d.
*
* Time--One Hour
*

Boil and mash the potatoes with the butter, milk, and salt (if
there are any cold ones they will do as well); lay the steak flat and
spread the potatoes over it. Chop the onion very fine and powder the
sage, and sprinkle over the potatoes; roll up and tie with a tape or

string. Rub some dripping over a baking sheet, put in the steak, and plenty of dripping on the top. Put into a moderate oven and bake for an hour, basting frequently. Put on to a hot dish, take off the tapes, and pour round it some nice gravy. Send mashed potatoes to table with it.

FRICASSEE OF LIVER

* Half a Calf's Liver--3d.
*
* 1 1/2 oz. Butter--1 1/2d.
*
* 1 Carrot
*
* Lemon Juice--1/2d.
*
* 1 Onion
*
* 1 oz. Flour
*
* 1 pint of Gravy
*
* Parsley
*
* Pepper and Salt--1d.
*
* Total Cost--6d.
*
* Time--One Hour
*

Wash and slice up the liver, and dip in the flour; fry very lightly and quickly in the butter and lay in a saucepan. Slice up the carrot and fry in the same butter. Stir in the gravy, boil up, and pour over the liver; simmer very gently for one hour, then dish carefully. Season the gravy with salt, pepper, and lemon juice; boil up and pour over it. Serve hot.

STEWED SWEETBREADS

* 1 pair Sweetbreads--4d.
*
* 1 pint Gravy
*
* Salt and Pepper
*
* 1/2 Onion--1/2d.
*
* 1 oz. Butter
*
* 1/2 oz. Flour
*
* 1 Carrot--1d.
*
* Total Cost--51/2 d.
*
* Time--One Hour.
*

Put the sweetbreads in cold water, bring to the boil, strain away the water, scrape and clean them and remove the pieces of skin. Put the butter into a stewpan and flour the sweetbreads; dry very lightly and quickly, take them out. Slice up and fry the onion and carrot, stir in the flour and gravy, and bring to the boil. Lay in the sweetbreads and simmer very gently for one hour; take them up on a hot dish, season and flavour the gravy, remove the fat, boil up and pour round them. Serve hot. Sweetbreads are very nice served with tomato sauce.

ROULADES OF BEEF

* 1/2 lb. Fillet of Beef--9d.
*
* 1/2 lb. Cold Boiled Bacon--4d.
*
* 1 Egg--1d.
*
* 1 1/2 oz. Dripping
*
* 1/2 pint Gravy
*
* Pepper and Mustard
*
* 2 oz. Crumbs--1d.
*
* Total Cost--1s. 3d.
*
* Time--10 Minutes

Trim away the fat from the fillet and cut it into very small thin slices, and cut the bacon also into thin slices, but smaller. Spread the side of the beef with mustard and pepper, cover with bacon, and roll up as lightly as possible. When all are rolled beat up an egg, mix it with a spoonful of water, brush over the rolls; cover them with crumbs and thread on a small skewer. Put the dripping into a frying-pan, and when quite hot lay in the rolls and fry until a good colour.

Place on a hot dish and slip out the skewers. Make the gravy hot, season and flavour, and pour boiling round the roulades. Should there be any brown sauce in the larder it is nicer than gravy.

VEAL SHAPE

* 2 lbs. Neck of Veal--8d.
*

* 1 Lemon
*

* Pepper and Salt--1/2d.
*

* 1/4 lb. Ham or Bacon--2d.
*

* 3 Eggs
*

* 1/2 pint Stock--3d.
*

* Total Cost--1s. 11/2 d.
*

* Time--Three Hours
*

Put the meat into a saucepan with the rind of the lemon cut very thinly, pour in the stock and simmer very gently for three hours; if the bacon is not cooked put it in and stew it for the last half-hour, then take up the meat and ham, cut it off the bones, and put these back in the saucepan and let them boil quickly without the lid. Boil the eggs hard and cut them in slices and arrange in a plain mould or dish, then lay in the veal and ham, and season with pepper and salt. Strain and flavour the gravy, add the lemon juice, and pour it over the meat. Set aside until quite cold, then turn out. This is a very nice breakfast or luncheon dish.

SWISS PATES

* Cold Roast Veal, Fowl, or Lamb--6d.
*
* Half a Stale Loaf--1 1/2d.
*
* Sweet Herbs or Parsley--1d.
*
* 1 Egg--1d.
*
* 1 gill Melted Butter
*
* Pepper and Salt
*
* Hot Fat--1d.
*
* Total Cost--101/2 d.
*
* Time--5 Minutes.
*

Mince the meat very finely, season with any forcemeat that may be left, or else some grated lemon peel, parsley and sweet herbs, pepper and salt. Make one gill of melted butter by recipe given elsewhere, stir in the meat and let it simmer for a few minutes; cut some slices of bread about an inch and a half thick, stamp them out with a round cutter about two inches across. Remove the centre for about half way through with a smaller cutter, brush them over with a raw egg beaten up, and cover them with fine crumbs. Fry in hot fat till a good colour, drain away the fat from them on kitchen paper. Fill these with the mince, garnish with sprigs of parsley, and serve.

DEVILLED MEAT

* 1 teaspoonful Mustard
*
* 1 teaspoonful Worcester Sauce
*
* 2 teaspoonful Vinegar
*
* 1/2 oz. Butter
*
* 1 teaspoonful Oil
*
* 1 teaspoonful Lemon Juice
*
* 1/2 teaspoonful Curry Powder--2 1/2d.
*
* Mashed Potatoes
*
* 1/2 gill Gravy
*
* Slices of Cold Meat--1d.
*
* Total Cost--31/2 d.
*
* Time--10 Minutes
*

Put the mustard, made with vinegar instead of water, into a basin; add gradually the oil and butter, curry powder, sauce, vinegar, and lemon juice, and mix very thoroughly, then pour in the gravy. Cut some slices of underdone meat and lay them in a pie dish, pour over the mixture, cover with a plate, and stand in a hot oven for ten minutes; stir frequently. Serve with mashed potatoes.

JUGGED RABBITS

* 2 Rabbits--1s.
*
* 1/2 lb. Pickled Pork--3d.
*
* 1 Onion
*
* 1 fagot of Herbs--1/2d.
*
* 1 pint Gravy
*
* 1/2 oz. Flour
*
* 1 tablespoonful Red Currant Jelly--1d.
*
* Total Cost--1s. 41/2 d.
*
* Time--Two Hours
*

Wash and joint up the rabbits and cut the pork into slices; lay some of
the pork over the bottom of a baking jar, and on this some
joints of rabbit; continue in layers until all the meat is in, then put
in the onion, sliced up, the fagot of herbs, and a few peppercorns.
Cover down closely, stand in a moderate oven, and cook for two hours.
Take up the meat and arrange nicely on a hot dish, strain the gravy
into a saucepan, thicken with the flour, and when it boils stir in the
jelly. Flavour to taste, pour it over the rabbits, and serve.

BREAKFAST DISH OF BEEF

* Slices of Cold Roast Beef (underdone)--4d.
*
* 1/2 gill Melted Butter Sauce--1/2d.
*
* 1/2 gill Gravy or Water
*
* Salt and Pepper
*
* 1 tablespoonful Walnut Ketchup or Vinegar--1/2d.
*
* 1 tablespoonful Red Currant Jelly--1d.
*
* Total Cost--6d.
*
* Time--Half an Hour
*

Cut some thin slices of beef and lay them in a saucepan or basin, mix the melted butter sauce, gravy, jelly, and ketchup together, and pour over them. Cover down closely and stand the saucepan in a larger one, half full of boiling water, and steam for half an hour. Put the meat into a dish and pour the sauce over it.

SOUBISE CUTLETS

* 1 lbs. Neck Chops--5d.
*
* 1 1/2 oz. Butter--1 1/2d.

*

* 1 oz. Flour

*

* 3 Onions

*

* 1 gill Milk

*

* Pepper, Salt, and Lemon Juice--1d.

*

* Total Cost--71/2 d.

*

* Time--20 Minutes

*

Trim off the cutlets, lay them in a tin dish, cover with buttered paper, and bake in the oven from fifteen to twenty minutes, according to thickness, turning once while cooking. Peel the onions, put them into cold water, bring to the boil, throw away the water. Put them on again in cold water and boil until rather soft, then strain all the water away, put in the butter, let it get quite hot, then cover down and finish cooking the onions in this, but do not brown them. Stir in the flour and pour over the milk, stir until it boils, let it boil two or three minutes, then rub through a sieve; season with salt, pepper, and lemon juice. Dish the cutlets in a circle, pour away some of the fat, and rinse the tin with a spoonful of gravy. Pour this round the dish and put the soubise sauce in the centre. Serve hot.

ROMAN RAGOUT

* 1 1/2 lbs. Gravy Beef--4d.

*

* 2 oz. Fat Bacon--1 1/2d.

* 2 oz. Onion--1/2d.
*

* 1 pint Milk
*

* 3 Tomatoes
*

* 1/2 pint Gravy
*

* 1 1/2 oz. Semolina
*

* 1 oz. Dry Cheese--6d.
*

* Total Cost--1s.
*

* Time--Three Hours
*

Mince the onion and bacon very fine indeed, put them into a saucepan and fry a good brown, then add half the gravy, and stir until a sort of half glaze. Rub the tomatoes through a sieve and stir them in with the rest of the gravy, bring to the boil. Cut the meat into strips and put it in with a little salt and pepper, and simmer very gently for about three hours. While it is cooking put the milk on to boil, mix the semolina with a little cold milk, and stir it in; cook it until the spoon will come out quite clean, then turn it on to a dish till cold. Cut it into squares and lay some in a deep dish, sprinkle with grated cheese, then more semolina and more cheese. Pour over this some of the gravy in which the meat is cooking, and put it in the oven to get hot. Dish up the meat and pour the sauce over it. Send the two dishes to table together, quite hot.

MUTTON OR HAM BONE AND POTATOES

* 1 Bone of Mutton or Ham
*

* 1 Onion
*

* 1 oz. Butter
*

* 1 oz. Flour
*

* 1/2 pint Water or Stock--1 1/2d.
*

* 1 lb. Potatoes--1d.
*

* Total Cost--21/2 d.
*

* Time--One Hour.
*

Put the butter into a saucepan, and when it is hot put in the flour; mix together smoothly, pour in the water of stock, and stir until it boils. Joint up a mutton or ham bone and lay it in; if it is mutton, add a little salt. Bring it to the boil, put in the onion whole stuck with two cloves, and simmer for half an hour or longer; then peel the potatoes, cut them in half and put them in, and cook until they are soft. Take out the bones and place on a dish, put the potatoes round, and pour the sauce over. This is a very homely dish, but a very savoury and economical one. A little meat goes a long way, and it is nourishing, too, as all the goodness of the bone and potatoes is in the stew.

VEAL IN WHITE SAUCE

* 2 lbs. Neck of Veal--10d.
*
* 2 oz. Butter--1 1/2d.
*
* 1 oz. Flour
*
* Salt and Pepper
*
* 1 Egg--1d.
*
* 3/4 pint Milk--2d.
*
* 1 Onion
*
* 1 fagot of Herbs
*
* 1 dozen Peppercorns
*
* Lemon Juice--1d.
*
* Total Cost--1s. 31/2 d.
*
* Time--One Hour and a Half.
*

Put the butter into a saucepan, and when it is melted stir in
the flour and cook well, but do not brown. Boil the onion, herbs, and
peppercorns in the milk, strain them out, pour the milk over the butter
and flour, and stir till it boils. Cut the meat into cutlets, lay them
in and simmer very gently till the meat is tender, then take it up and
arrange nicely on a dish. Beat up an egg with a drop or two of lemon

juice and a spoonful of gravy or milk. Pour into the sauce in which the meat was cooked, and stir briskly over the fire until it thickens; strain over the meat, and serve.

A few very small fat rashers of bacon rolled up and fried are a great improvement to this dish.

CHAPTER XX.
FIFTY RECIPES FOR VEGETABLES

TOMATOES STUFFED

* 6 Tomatoes--2d.
*

* 1/4 lb. Veal Forcemeat--2d.
*

* 1 oz. Cheese--1 1/2d.
*

* 6 pieces Fried Bread--1/2d.
*

* Total Cost--6d.
*

* Time--10 Minutes
*

Choose tomatoes of a good colour, and all about the same size; scoop out the centre. Grate up the cheese and mix it with the forcemeat, put this into the tomatoes; place on a buttered tin, and bake in the oven for ten minutes. Put each tomato on to a round of fried bread, and serve.

POTATOES IN WHITE SAUCE

* 1 lb. Potatoes--1d.
*
* 1/2 pint White Sauce
*
* Salt and Pepper--2d.
*
* Total Cost--3d.
*
* Time--Half an Hour
*

Peel and slice the potatoes, put them in water seasoned with salt, and boil for five minutes; strain off the water, make some white sauce by directions given elsewhere. Lay in the potatoes and simmer gently till they are soft, but not broken; place them on a hot dish and pour the sauce over.

TO BOIL POTATOES

To boil potatoes properly much care and judgement are required. They should be peeled thinly, and well washed in cold water, but not soaked; put them into a saucepan and kept for this vegetable only. Just cover them with cold water seasoned with salt, and bring to a boil. Then simmer very gently for about twenty minutes; test them with a fork, and if soft, strain off the water and toss them in a saucepan over the fire until they are dry. Some potatoes will not bear boiling as long as this, but begin to break soon after they boil up. When this is the case, pour off nearly all the water, leaving only one inch at the bottom of the saucepan. Cook the potatoes slowly in this and then strain off and dry. Potatoes that are very troublesome to boil often steam well; they must be allowed from an hour to one hour and a half, according to the quantity of water over which they are cooking.

TO BOIL NEW POTATOES

New potatoes may be either scraped while raw, or peeled after boiling; they are a better flavour if cooked in their skins. In either case they should be well washed in cold water, plunged into boiling water seasoned with salt and a sprig of mint, and boiled quickly until a fork will go through easily; then strain off the water, dry, and serve.

TO BOIL CABBAGE

The outer leaves of the cabbage should be removed, then cut it into quarters and cut out the salt; wash it well in salt and water, and leave in the water for half-an-hour. Then put it into a colander and shake all the water from it. Place on the fire a large saucepan of water, and when it boils, put in two teaspoonsful of salt and a quarter of a teaspoonful of carbonate of soda. Put in the cabbage and cover down till it boils up; then remove the lid and boil very quickly, pressing it down into the water from time to time. It will be done in from fifteen to twenty minutes; try it with a fork, and if soft turn into a colander, and very carefully press all the water from it. Slip into a vegetable dish and cut into neat pieces.

TO BOIL GREEN PEAS

Shell the peas and wash them well; just cover them with cold water, season it with a little salt, sugar, and mint. Bring quickly to the boil and cook for about twenty minutes. When soft, but not broken, strain off the water and put them into a vegetable dish.

TO BOIL FRENCH BEANS

Slice up the beans and wash in cold water, put them into plenty of boiling water, seasoned with salt and a quarter of a teaspoonful of carbonate of soda; boil quickly without the lid for about ten minutes or a quarter of an hour. When soft, strain off and shake the water out thoroughly; put into a hot dish, and serve plainly or with melted butter.

TO BOIL CAULIFLOWERS

Soak the cauliflowers in plenty of salt and water, with the flower downwards, then cook, in plenty of boiling water seasoned with salt, putting the flower to the bottom of the saucepan. Keep uncovered all the time of cooking; take up with a slice and strain in a colander. Turn carefully into a vegetable dish, and serve with or without sauce.

VEGETABLE MARROW

* 1 Marrow--3d.
*
* 1/2 pint White Sauce
*
* Salt--2d.
*
* Total Cost--5d.
*
* Time--15 Minutes
*

Peel the marrow, take out the seeds, and cut it into small pieces; put into boiling water nicely seasoned with salt, and boil gently for about fifteen minutes. Take up with a slice and strain in a colander, place in a hot dish, and pour over the sauce.

BEETROOT IN SAUCE

* 3 Beetroots--2d.
*
* 1/2 pint White Sauce--2d.
*
* Total Cost--4d.
*
* Time--Two Hours
*

Wash the beetroots, but do not cut them; put them in cold water, and boil till they feel soft if pressed--the time depends upon the size;

then take them up, peel and slice them. Make the sauce by directions given elsewhere. Put in the beetroot and simmer for about half an hour; dish the beets and pour the sauce over. It should be of a bright red colour.

STEWED CABBAGE

* 1 Cabbage--3d.
*

* Salt and Pepper
*

* 1 oz. Butter--1d.
*

* Total Cost--4d.
*

* Time--25 Minutes
*

Boil the cabbage as directed, and squeeze very dry; melt the butter in a saucepan, season with pepper, salt, and a drop or two of lemon juice. Put in the cabbage and cook in the butter for ten minutes, stirring frequently; arrange neatly in a hot dish, and serve.

BAKED TOMATOES

* 1 doz. Tomatoes--4d.
*

* 1 oz. Bread Crumbs--1/2d.

* 1 oz. Butter
*

* 1/2 teaspoonful Mustard--1d.
*

* Total Cost--51/2 d.
*

* Time--15 Minutes
*

Slice up the tomatoes, spread with a very little made mustard.
Season some brown bread crumbs with pepper and salt, and sprinkle the
slices well. Put into a buttered dish and bake till soft. Serve hot.

CURRIED TOMATOES

* 1 doz. Tomatoes--4d.
*

* 1 1/2 oz. Butter--1d.
*

* 1 gill Milk--1d.
*

* 1/2 oz. Flour
*

* 1/2 lb. Rice--1 1/2d.
*

* 1 Apple
*

* 1 Onion
*

* 1 dessertspoonful Curry Powder
*

* Salt--2d.

* Total Cost--91/2 d.
*
* Time--Half an Hour
*

Mince the onion and apple finely, and fry in the batter till a good colour; sprinkle over it the curry power and flour, and mix well. Pour in the milk and stir until it boils; slice the tomatoes and put them in and simmer very gently for half an hour. Season with salt, dish carefully and serve either in a border of rice, or with rice moulds on a separate dish.

CURRIED VEGETABLES

Take any vegetables in season, such as potatoes, peas, carrots, beans, and cauliflowers, very young vegetables are the best, and if there are any cold ones in the larder they will do as well as fresh. Slice up the potatoes and branch the cauliflowers, and, if they are not been boiled before, boil them in water seasoned with a little salt and sugar, for ten minutes, and strain off the water. Put one ounce or more of butter into a saucepan according to the quantity of vegetables, and when hot stir in half an ounce of flour, and the same of curry powder. Pour in half a pint of milk and stir till it boils. Then put in the vegetables and simmer very gently for about half an hour. They should not be broken, but quite soft, and all the liquor absorbed. Pile in a hot dish and serve with boiled rice.

BEETROOT AND ONION STEW

* 3 Beetroots--2d.
*
* 3 Onions--1d.
*
* 1 1/2 oz. Butter
*
* 1 teaspoonful Sugar
*
* 1/2 teaspoonful Salt--1 1/2d.
*
* 1/2 pint Milk--1d.
*
* 1 tablespoonful Vinegar
*
* 1/2 oz. Flour--1/2d.
*
* Mashed Potatoes--1 1/2d.
*
* Total Cost--71/2 d.
*
* Time--One Hour
*

Boil the beetroots by directions given and slice them up; peel and slice up the onions and fry in the butter, but do not let them brown. Stir in the flour and the milk and bring to the boil, and when it has boiled a few minutes stir in gradually the vinegar, salt, and sugar, then the beetroot. Simmer slowly for one hour; make a border of the potatoes on a hot dish, garnish with sprigs of parsley. Put the beetroot and onion in the centre, and serve hot.

SAUTE OF TURNIPS

* 6 Turnips--1 1/2d.
*

* 1 oz. Butter
*

* 1 gill Stock
*

* 1 teaspoonful Sugar
*

* 1 teaspoonful Salt--1d.
*

* Total Cost--21/2 d.
*

* Time--Half an Hour
*

Peel the turnips and cut them into pieces like the quarter of an
orange; put them into a small stewpan with the butter, sprinkle over
them the sugar and salt, and stir about till quite brown. Pour
on the stock, bring it to the boil, and simmer till soft but not
broken. Dish the turnips, season the gravy with salt and a few drops of
lemon juice, pour over, and serve.

CARROTS IN BUTTER

* 4 Carrots--1 1/2d.
*

* 1 oz. Butter

* 1 teaspoonful Parsley
*

* Pinch of Salt and Sugar--1d.
*

* Total Cost--21/2 d.
*

* Time--One Hour
*

Scrape the carrots and slice them up, put them into boiling water seasoned with salt and sugar, and boil for ten minutes. Strain off the water. Put the butter into a small saucepan, and when it is hot stir in the parsley and a few drops of lemon juice. Toss the carrots in this until they are thoroughly hot, then cover down and cook slowly till soft. Dish and pour over the butter in which they were cooked.

PARSNIPS AND PARSLEY BUTTER

* 4 or 5 Parsnips
*

* 1/2 oz. Flour
*

* 1 teaspoonful Parsley--2d.
*

* 1 oz. Butter
*

* 1 gill Milk
*

* Pepper and Salt--2d.
*

* Total Cost--4d.

* Time--One Hour
*

Scrape and cut up the parsnips (or cold ones will do). If raw, boil them in water seasoned with salt for three-quarters of an hour. Make the butter, flour, and milk into a sauce by directions given, and season nicely. Stir in the parsley, put in the parsnips, bring to the boil and simmer for ten minutes. Arrange them on a hot dish, pour the sauce over, and serve.

PARSNIPS FRIED

Cold boiled parsnips make a delicious breakfast dish if sliced up and fried either in bacon fat, dripping, or butter. Pile high on a dish and serve very hot.

POTATO BALLS

* 1 lb. Cold Boiled Potatoes
*

* Bread Crumbs--1d.
*

* 2 Eggs
*

* 1 oz. Butter
*

* Hot Fat--3d.
*

* Total Cost--4d.
*

* Time--5 Minutes.
*

Rub the potatoes through a sieve or mash them smoothly. Put the butter
into a saucepan, and, when melted, season with pepper and salt; put in
the potatoes and turn them about till hot through. Drop in the egg and
mix into a paste, turn on to a plate to cool, and roll into balls. Beat
up an egg and brush over the balls, cover well with crumbs, and fry in
hot fat. The yolks of eggs will do for this dish if the whites are
wanted for other purposes.

HARICOT BEANS

Soak the haricots over night, if possible; if not, at least for two or
three hours. Put them on in plenty of cold water seasoned with salt and
an onion, and boil them steadily for three hours. Strain the water off,
put them into a vegetable dish, and pour over them some parsley butter
sauce. Haricot beans are the most nutritious of all pulse foods, and
are a particularly good food for people who work in the open air. They
are very nice eaten alone or served with meat. They make an exceedingly
delicious dish if boiled for two hours and then put into a nice brown
gravy and simmered for about an hour. Serve in the gravy with roast
mutton.

POTATO AND TOMATO PIE

* 6 Tomatoes--2d.
*

* 6 Potatoes--1d.

* 1/2 lb. Short Pastry
*

* Dripping
*

* 1 teaspoonful Parsley
*

* 1 1/2 teaspoonful Sweet Herbs
*

* Salt and Pepper--1 1/2d.
*

* Total Cost--4 1/2 d.
*

* Time--One Hour
*

Peel and slice up the potatoes and tomatoes; lay them alternatively in a pie dish and sprinkle over them some parsley, herbs, salt, and pepper. When the dish is full, cover with a short pastry and bake for one hour; serve hot.

CAULIFLOWERS AND TOMATOES

* 2 Cauliflowers--4d.
*

* 1/2 pint Tomato Sauce--1d.
*

* Total Cost--5d.
*

* Time--20 Minutes
*

Boil the cauliflowers and make the sauce by directions given elsewhere. Dish the cauliflowers carefully and pour over them the sauce, leaving just the centre of the flowers clear. Put into the oven for five minutes, and serve.

STEWED CELERY

* 3 heads of Celery--3d.
*
* 1 oz. Butter--1d.
*
* 1/2 gill Milk
*
* 1 oz. Flour
*
* Pepper and Salt--1d.
*
* Total Cost--5d.
*
* Time--Half an Hour
*

Take only the white and best part of celery for this dish, pull it to pieces, wash well in salt and water, and tie in a bundle. Put it into boiling water seasoned with salt, and boil for about half an hour, or until the fork will go through easily. Take half a pint of the water in which it was boiled and mix it with the milk; make a sauce with this and the butter and flour by directions given for sauces. Dish the celery and pour the sauce over. This is an excellent food for anyone suffering from, or subject to, rheumatism or gout. Celery is also very nice stewed in broth or gravy and thickened with a little butter and flour.

LETTUCE STEWED

* 4 Lettuces--3d.
*
* 1 oz. Butter
*
* Nutmeg
*
* Pepper and Salt--1d.
*
* Total Cost--4d.
*
* Time--Half an Hour
*

Wash the lettuces very thoroughly and lay them in salt and water for half an hour. Plunge them into plenty of boiling water seasoned with salt and a quarter of a teaspoonful of carbonate of soda. Boil quickly without the lid from fifteen to twenty minutes, take up and squeeze all the water from them. Chop them up and put into a saucepan with some butter, nutmeg, pepper and salt, and a few drops of lemon juice; stir them about and cook for about five minutes. Turn into a hot dish and serve.

BAKED ONIONS

* 2 lbs. Onion--2d.
*
* 1/2 pint Thick Gravy

* 1/2 pint Water
*

* Pepper and Salt--1d.
*

* Total Cost--3d.
*

* Time--One Hour.
*

Peel the onions, put them on in cold water, and bring to the boil. Strain the water off, butter a baking dish, put in the onions, pour in the water, cover with a plate, and stand in a moderate oven. Stew until soft, place in a hot dish and pour over them, either a nice gravy thickened with a little butter and flour, or some plain melted butter. Serve hot.

CASSOLETTES OF VEGETABLES

Peel some turnips and scoop out the centre; boil them in salt and water till soft, but quite whole. If there are any cold vegetables in the larder, such as beans, peas, carrots, and parsnips, make them hot; if not, cut some into small pieces and boil separately. Stir them into any cold sauce that may be left, or toss them in a little butter. Fill the turnip cups with these, arranging them on a dish, alternately red and green. Serve hot.

VEGETABLE MARROW STUFFED

* 1 Vegetable Marrow--3d.
*
* 1/4 lb. Veal Forcemeat--2d.
*
* 1/2 pint Melted Butter Sauce--1 1/2d.
*
* Total Cost--61/2 d.
*
* Time--Half an Hour
*

Peel a marrow and cut it in half length-ways. Prepare some veal forcemeat by recipe given elsewhere, and make it hot in a saucepan. Remove the seeds from the marrow and put in their place the forcemeat; put the pieces together and bind round with tape. Have ready a fish kettle full of boiling water seasoned with salt; lay the marrow on the drainer and plunge into the water; boil gently for about twenty-five minutes. Slip the marrow carefully into a dish and pour over some melted butter sauce.

LYONNAISE POTATOES

* 1 lb. Potatoes--1d.
*
* 1/2 pint Onion Sauce--2d.
*
* Total Cost--3d.
*

* Time--Half an Hour
*

Peel and boil the potatoes in the usual way, slice them up and
put them into a hot dish; make some rather thin onion sauce by
directions given elsewhere, season with a few drops of lemon juice, and
pour over the potatoes; serve hot.

POTATOES SAUTE

Cut up any cold potatoes that may be left into strips, not too thin,
put some dripping into a frying pan, and when very hot put in the
potatoes and fry them a pale colour. Place them on a hot dish; melt one
ounce of butter in a saucepan; season with lemon juice, parsley,
pepper, and salt. Pour this over the potatoes, and serve very hot.

COLCANNON

Take any remains of cold boiled cabbage and potatoes, and cut them into
small pieces, season with pepper and salt. Put a small piece of butter
into a frying pan; put in the vegetables and fry them until they are
thoroughly hot through and well mixed. Turn them on to a hot dish, make
into a neat pile, and serve.

BAKED VEGETABLE MARROW

* 1 Vegetable Marrow
*
* 1/2 pint Gravy
*
* 1 oz. Dripping
*
* Total Cost--3d.
*
* Time--One Hour
*

Peel the marrow and cut into pieces, remove the seeds, put on to a baking sheet with some beef dripping, and bake till soft and rather brown. Thicken a little gravy with some flour, and season and flavour it nicely; dish the marrow and pour this sauce over.

STEWED LEEKS

* 1 bunch Leeks
*
* 1/2 pint Stock--2d.
*
* Pepper and Salt
*
* 1/2 oz. Butter
*
* 1/2 oz. Flour

* Lemon Juice--1/2d.
*
* Total Cost--2 1/2 d.
*
* Time--One Hour
*

Cut off the roots and green tops of the leeks and wash well. Put them into a saucepan with the stock and stew very gently till soft; take them up and put on to a hot dish. Put the butter into a saucepan, and when it is dissolved stir in the flour, mix well, and strain in the stock. Stir until it boils. Season with some pepper, salt, and a few drops of lemon juice. Pour over the leeks, and serve.

POTATOES A LA MAITRE D'HOTEL

* Cold Potatoes--1d.
*
* 1/2 pint Maitre d'Hotel Sauce--1 1/2d.
*
* Total Cost--21/2 d.
*
* Time--5 Minutes
*

Make the sauce by recipe given elsewhere, flavour nicely with lemon juice, pepper, and salt. Slice up the potatoes, and put them into it; simmer for five minutes, dish, and serve.

LENTILS, TO BOIL

Wash the lentils well in cold water, cover them with cold water seasoned with salt, and boil for one hour and a half. Strain all the water off, put them into a hot dish with about half an ounce of butter, and serve.

CURRIED LENTILS

Any cold lentils left make a very nice breakfast dish if they are curried. If there should be any curry gravy left,

put them into that and simmer for half an hour; serve with boiled rice. If there is no curry sauce, make a little by a recipe given elsewhere.

STEWED BEETROOT AND MASHED POTATOES

* 1 bunch Beetroot--2d.
*
* 2 Onions--1/2d.
*
* 1 oz. Flour
*
* Mashed Potatoes

* Pepper and Salt
*

* 1 1/2 oz. Butter
*

* 1/2 pint Milk
*

* 1 dessertspoonful Vinegar--3d.
*

* Total Cost--51/2 d.
*

* Time--Half an Hour.
*

Peel and cut the onions into dice, put them into a frying-pan with the butter, and fry, but do not let them brown; sprinkle in the flour, pour in the milk, and stir until it boils. Season with salt, pepper, and vinegar. Boil the beetroot carefully, and when cold, peel and slice up. Put it into the sauce and simmer for half an hour. Make the mashed potatoes into a border on a hot dish, and put the beetroot in the centre; boil up the sauce, pour it over, and serve.

CAULIFLOWERS AU GRATIN

* 1 Cauliflower--4d.
*

* 1/2 pint White Sauce--1 1/2d.
*

* 2 oz. Dry Grated Cheese
*

* Pepper and Salt--1/2d.
*

* Total Cost--6d.

* Time--15 Minutes.
*

Boil the cauliflower and make the sauce by directions already given. Put the cauliflower into a dish in which it can be served, put half the cheese into the white sauce, season with pepper and salt, make it hot and pour over. Sprinkle the rest of the cheese on the top, and put into the oven till quite brown; it is then ready to serve.

NEW POTATOES SAUTE

* 1 lb. New Potatoes--1d.
*

* 1 oz. Butter--1d.
*

* Pepper and Salt
*

* 1 teaspoonful Parsley
*

* Lemon Juice--1/2d.
*

* Total Cost--21/2 d.
*

* Time--Half an Hour.
*

Wash the potatoes and put them into boiling salt and water, and boil for ten minutes. Take up, peel and cut them in half. Melt the butter in a saucepan, and when quite hot, put in the potatoes and toss over the fire. Sprinkle over the parsley, pepper, salt, and a few drops of lemon juice; cover down and cook gently till the potatoes are soft but not broken. Put into a hot dish and serve.

POTATO PUFF

* 1/2 lb. Cold Potatoes--1d.
*
* 2 Eggs--2d.
*
* 1 oz. Butter
*
* 1 gill Milk--1d.
*
* Total Cost--4d.
*
* Time--Half an Hour
*

Mash the potatoes, beat the butter to a cream, then beat in the eggs, pepper, salt, and milk. Stir up the potatoes, pour into a buttered pie-dish, and bake for about half an hour. Serve hot.

POTATOES STUFFED

* 6 Large Potatoes--2d.
*
* 1/4 lb. Cold Meat--1/2d.
*
* 1/2 gill Gravy or Sauce
*
* Pepper, Salt, and Parsley--1/2d.
*
* Total Cost--3d.

* Time--One Hour and a Half.
*

Wash and scrub the potatoes, and bake them in the oven till quite done.
Cut them in half so that they will stand nicely. Scoop out the
inside, and mix the potato meal with some butter, pepper, and salt.
Make a little savoury meat by directions given for mince, and nearly
fill the potato skins with this. Put some of the potato on top, making
it look as rough and rocky as possible. Stand in the oven till quite
hot, and serve.

HARICOT BEANS AND BACON

* 1 pint Haricot Beans--2d.
*

* 1 teaspoonful Parsley
*

* 1/2 lb. Bacon
*

* Pepper and Salt--5d.
*

* Total Cost--7d.
*

* Time--Two Hours.
*

Soak the haricot beans and boil them by directions already given. Rub
them through a wire sieve. The bacon should be in thin rashers and very
fat. Cook it carefully in a small clean frying-pan, and as the fat runs
from it, pour it on the beans. Mash them up with this and a little
pepper and salt, and put them into a hot dish. Sprinkle over with
parsley and lay the bacon rashers on top. Serve hot.

ARTICHOKES, TO BOIL

* 2 lbs. Artichokes--4d.
*
* 1/2 pint White Sauce--1 1/2d.
*
* Total Cost--51/2 d.
*
* Time--One Hour
*

Wash and peel the artichokes and put them into some water; add a teaspoonful of vinegar and leave them for half an hour. Drain the water all away and put them into a saucepan, cover with cold water; add one gill of milk and some salt. Bring to the boil and cook slowly for about an hour. Take half a pint of the liquor in which the artichokes were boiled, and make a sauce; dish them and pour this over.

IMITATION SPINACH

Take the very young green shoots of the pumpkin plant. Wash them well and put them into a large saucepan, with a very little water seasoned with salt and a pinch of carbonate of soda; keep pressing them down into the water and boil till soft. Turn into a colander and squeeze very dry, put into a saucepan with one ounce of butter, pepper, salt, and a few drops of lemon juice. Stir about till thoroughly hot through, dish neatly, and serve.

BANANAS STEWED

* 1 doz. Green Bananas--3d.
*

* Lemon Juice
*

* 1/2 pint Brown Sauce
*

* Pepper and Salt--2d.
*

* Total Cost--5d.
*

* Time--Half an Hour.
*

Peel the bananas and put them in boiling water to which a few drops of lemon juice have been added; boil them for half an hour, or until soft. Make sauce by directions already given, flavour with lemon juice, pepper, and salt. Strain all the water from the bananas, dish, and pour over the sauce

POTATO CHIPS

To fry potatoes successfully, two things must be carefully attended to. First of all dry the potatoes thoroughly, and then have very hot fat. Peel the potatoes and dry them in a cloth. Cut into any shape--slices, strips, quarters, &c.--and dry again. Have a good quantity of very hot fat ready, put the chips into a frying basket, and plunge into the fat. Fry quickly, and directly they are brown enough they are done. Throw them on to some kitchen paper to drain off the fat. Pile high on a dish, sprinkle with salt, and serve very hot.

ITALIAN CABBAGE

* 1 Cabbage--2d.
*
* 1 oz. Butter--1d.
*
* 2 oz. Dry Cheese
*
* 1 spoonful Flour
*
* Pepper and Salt--1d.
*
* Total Cost--4d.
*
* Time--15 Minutes.
*

Boil the cabbage by directions given, strain away the water and press it very dry. Put the butter into a saucepan, and when it is dissolved, chop up the cabbage and put a layer at the bottom of the saucepan. Sprinkle over some grated cheese, pepper, and salt, then more cabbage and cheese, until all are used up. Simmer gently for fifteen minutes, slip it on to a hot dish, and serve.

SAVOURY POTATOES

* 5 or 6 Large Potatoes--1 1/2d.
*
* 2 oz. Cheese--1d.
*
* 1 spoonful of Milk
*
* 1 Egg
*
* Pepper and Salt--1d.
*
* Total Cost--31/2 d.
*
* Time--Two Hours.
*

Scrub the potatoes and bake them in the oven. Cut off the end, scoop out all the meal; grate up some dry pieces of cheese, beat it into the potatoes with the yolk of the egg, and some seasoning. Whip the white till stiff and stir lightly in; fill the potatoes with this mixture.
Lay in a baking sheet and bake for about twenty minutes. Garnish with parsley, and serve.

CAULIFLOWER FRITTERS

* Cold Cauliflower
*
* Frying Batter

* Hot Fat
*

* Total Cost--1 1/2 d.
*

* Time--5 Minutes.
*

Take any cold cauliflower that may be left, divide it into branches. Make the frying batter by directions given. Dip the pieces of cauliflower into it, and put into very hot fat. Fry a good colour and pile high on a dish. Garnish with fried parsley and serve very hot.

FRIED TOMATOES

* 1 doz. Tomatoes--4d.
*

* 1 gill Milk
*

* 1 oz. Butter
*

* Pepper and Salt--1 1/2d.
*

* Total Cost--51/2 d.
*

* Time--10 Minutes.
*

Slice up the tomatoes, mix a spoonful of flour with some pepper and salt; dip in the slices and fry quickly, pile on a dish. Pour the milk into the pan in which they were fried, stir until it boils, and pour over. Garnish with fried bread and serve hot.

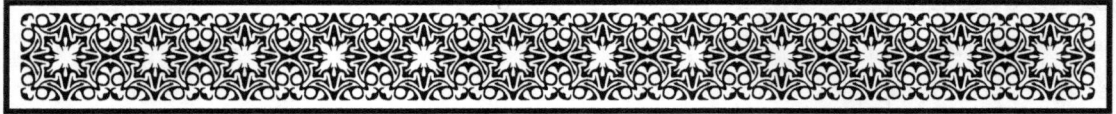

CHAPTER XXI.
FIFTY RECIPES FOR SALADS AND SAUCES

CURRY SAUCE

* 1 Onion
*
* 1 Apple
*
* 1/2 oz. Flour
*
* Lemon Juice
*
* Salt--1d
*
* 1/2 oz. Curry Powder
*
* 1 oz. Butter or Dripping
*
* 1 pint Gravy--1d
*
* Total Cost--2d.
*
* Time--Half an Hour.

Peel and chop up the apple and onion. Put the butter or dripping into a saucepan, and when it is melted put in the apple and onion, and fry for a few minutes; sprinkle over the curry powder and the flour. Pour over the gravy and stir until it boils. Simmer for half an hour, then strain, flavour with lemon juice and salt, boil up, and it is ready. If this sauce is for fish, use milk or fish stock instead of gravy.

MAITRE D'HOTEL SAUCE

* 1/2 pint Milk--1d.
*
* 1 oz. Butter--1d.
*
* Lemon Juice
*
* 1/2 oz. Flour
*
* 1 teaspoonful Parsley
*
* Pepper and Salt.--1d.
*
* Total Cost--3d.
*
* Time--5 Minutes.
*

Put the butter into a small saucepan, and when it is melted stir in the flour, and mix smoothly; pour in the milk and stir until it boils. Take the saucepan from the fire, add a few drops of lemon juice, a pinch of pepper and salt to taste, last of all the parsley. It is then ready to serve.

ONION SAUCE

* 3 Small Onions--1/2d.
*
* 1 oz. Butter--1d.
*
* Lemon Juice
*
* 1/2 pint Milk
*
* 1 oz. Bread Crumbs
*
* Pepper and Salt--1 1/2d.
*
* Total Cost--3d.
*
* Time--5 Minutes.
*

Peel the onions, put them into cold water, and let them boil for a minute. Strain away the water, cover again with cold water, boil up and cook till soft; take out the water, chop small. Put the butter and milk into a saucepan, and when it boils put in the bread crumbs and onions. Cook slowly for five minutes, season with pepper, salt, and a few drops of lemon juice, and it is ready to serve.

CREAM TOAST

* 4 Slices Toast--1d.
*

* Pepper and Salt

* 1/2 pint White Sauce--2d.
*

* Total Cost--3d.
*

* Time--**5** Minutes.
*

Make the toast and lay it in a dish. Make the sauce by directions given for white sauce. Season with pepper and salt, and pour over it; serve hot. If a richer dish is desired, a little butter may be put on the toast.

JAM SAUCE

* 1 tablespoonful Jam--1d.
*

* 1/2 pint Water
*

* 1 oz. Sugar
*

* 1 teaspoonful Cornflour
*

* 1/2 Lemon--1d.
*

* Total Cost--2d.

*

* Time--5 Minutes.

*

Put the water, jam, lemon juice, and sugar into a small
saucepan and boil it for five minutes. Mix the cornflour with a little
cold water and pour it in; stir till it boils up. Strain the jam out,
and it is ready to serve; a few drops of cochineal improve the colour.

TO CLARIFY DRIPPING

When the joint is served pour the dripping into a basin and stand away
till cold; then cut it out of the basin. The gravy that will be found
at the bottom is an excellent addition to hash or mince. Cut the
dripping into small pieces and pour over it sufficient boiling water to
dissolve it. Stir it well and leave till it is a solid cake of fat. Cut
it off the water, scrape the impurities from the bottom, and it will be
ready for use.

TO CLARIFY FAT

The fat from meat not required in dressing it, and the ends of chops,
&c., make excellent shortening for pies and cakes. Cut it into small
pieces and put it into an old saucepan with about one quart of water.
Boil until all the water is evaporated; the fat will then begin to
boil. Strain this melted fat into a basin, and continue to do so until
all the fat is extracted. This is a good substitute for butter and
lard.

MELTED BUTTER SAUCE

* 1/2 pint Water
*
* 1 oz. Butter
*
* 1/2 oz. Flour
*
* Salt
*
* Total Cost--1 1/2 d.
*
* Time--5 Minutes.
*

Put half the butter into a small saucepan, and when it is dissolved
stir in the flour and mix smoothly; pour in the cold water and
stir until it boils. Take the saucepan from the fire, stir in the rest
of the butter in small pieces, and some salt, it is then ready to
serve.

TO BOIL RICE

Wash the rice well in two or three waters; have a large saucepan on the
fire full of boiling water seasoned with salt. Throw in the rice and
boil very quickly for five or six minutes. Take up a grain, and if it
feels quite soft it is done; if not, boil another minute. Strain off
the water and pour over it some clean hot water to separate the grains.
If required immediately, put it back in the saucepan and toss over the

fire till dry. If not, spread it on a sieve or dish and dry on the stove, covered with a cloth, or in the oven with the door open.

TO FRY PARSLEY

The top or flower of parsley only should be used for frying. Pick it carefully and rub well in a damp cloth, and then in a dry cloth. Put into a frying basket and plunge into the fat when the fish, or whatever it is to be served with, has been fried; leave it in not more than one minute. Turn it on to some kitchen paper and stand for a minute on the stove to dry; it is then ready.

FRYING BATTER

* 1/4 lb. Flour--1/2d.
*
* 1/2 gill Tepid Water
*
* White of Egg
*
* 1 dessertspoonful Oil--1d.
*
* Total Cost--11/2 d.
*
* Time--5 Minutes.
*

Sift the flour into a basin, pour over it the oil, then the water, and beat into a smooth batter; stand away for an hour, if possible in a cool place. Whip the white of the egg to a stiff froth, and stir it in, and it is ready to use. This batter is useful for fritters and many dishes both sweet and savoury.

TOMATO SAUCE

* 6 Tomatoes--2d.
*
* 1 oz. Butter--1d.
*
* 1 1/2 oz. Flour
*
* 1/2 spoonful Sugar
*
* 1/2 spoonful Salt--1/2d.
*
* Total Cost--31/2 d.
*
* Time--5 Minutes.
*

If the tomatoes are ripe they need not be cooked; but if at all hard, boil them for five minutes. Then slice up and rub through a sieve. Put the butter into a small saucepan, and when it is dissolved stir in the flour and sugar; then pour in the tomato juice and stir until it boils; season with salt to taste. This is tomato sauce pure and simple; but it is often made with half stock and half tomato juice; it is suitable for chops, steaks, &c. If made thicker it is called a puree, and is served with braised and dressed meats.

WHITE SAUCE

* 1/2 pint Milk--1d.
*
* 1 oz. Butter--1d.
*
* 1/2 oz. Flour
*
* Salt and Pepper--1/2d.
*
* Total Cost--2 1/2 d.
*
* Time Minutes.
*

Put the butter into a small saucepan, and when it is dissolved put in the flour; mix well and pour on the cold milk and stir till it boils. Let it boil for two minutes and it is ready. It may be served either as a sweet or savoury sauce, putting either sugar or pepper and salt, as required.

BROWN GRAVY

Brown gravy can be made from any kind of stock. If the stock is good, put it into a saucepan and thicken every pint with 1 oz of flour. If the stock is not very good, boil some vegetables in it with any trimmings of meat and poultry available, and thicken with butter and flour; a few drops of lemon juice will bring up the flavour. It should be of a rich brown colour. It can be coloured with a little sugar burnt in a spoon, or with a few drops of caramel, a recipe for which will be found elsewhere.

BROWN SAUCE

* 1 pint Stock
*
* 1 oz. Butter
*
* 1/2 oz. Flour--1 1/2d.
*
* 1/2 Stalk of Celery
*
* 1 Carrot
*
* 1 Onion
*
* 1/2 Turnip
*
* 1 doz. Peppercorns--1d.
*
* Total Cost--21/2 d.
*
* Time--One Hour.
*

Put the butter into a saucepan, and when it is quite hot, slice up the vegetables and put them in with the peppercorns, and fry a good colour. Stir in the flour and brown that too, then pour in the stock and stir till it boils. Cover down and let it simmer slowly for an hour. Rub through a sieve, return to the saucepan; season with salt and lemon juice, boil up, and it is ready to serve.

CARAMEL

Put half a pound of sugar into a frying-pan and let it get very brown.
Pour over half a pint of water and stir till it boils; strain
into a bottle. It will keep good a long time, and is very useful for
colouring soup and gravies.

VEAL FORCEMEAT

* 2 oz. Suet (Beef)--1/2d.
*
* 3 oz. Bread Crumbs--1/2d.
*
* Pepper and Salt
*
* 1 Egg
*
* 1/2 teaspoonful Parsley
*
* 1/2 teaspoonful Sweet Herbs
*
* Half a Lemon--1 1/2d.
*
* Total Cost--21/2 d.
*

Shred the suet and mix it with the bread crumbs. Chop the parsley and
sweet herbs very finely and stir them in, then the grated rind of half
a lemon, and the pepper and salt; drop in the egg and bind into a
paste, and it is ready to use. This forcemeat is suitable for fowls,
turkeys, veal, and fish.

TO MAKE BROWN CRUMBS

Cut up some very stale bread and bake it in the oven till a nice colour. Put these pieces through a sausage machine and then rum them through a sieve; keep in a bottle for use. They are excellent for many savoury dishes, and it is good way of using up stale pieces of bread.

SALAD OF COLD VEGETABLES

Take any cold vegetables that there may be in the larder--such as potatoes, cauliflowers, peas, beans, haricots, &c. Slice up the potatoes, branch the cauliflower, and mix in the peas and beans; put all into a salad bowl. Take oil and vinegar in the proportion of one of oil to two of vinegar, blend them together and season with salt and pepper. Pour this over the vegetables, slice up one or two hard boiled eggs into very thin slices, and lay round as a garnish.

BANANA AND ORANGE SALAD

Peel and slice up some ripe bananas and oranges, removing the pips from the oranges, but saving the juice. Take a deep glass dish, lay at the bottom some bananas, then a layer of oranges. Sprinkle well with sugar, then some more bananas and oranges and sugar, until all the materials are used up. Cover and let it stand for an hour, then serve as a sweet.

COSMOPOLITAN SALAD

Take any fruits in season, such as oranges, mandarins, passion fruit, apricots, nectarines, pineapples, bananas, &c. Peel and slice them up, and put them into a glass dish in layers, with plenty of sugar between each layer. Stand in a cool place for an hour covered over, and it is ready to serve.

POTATO SALAD

Slice up some cold boiled potatoes. Sprinkle with salt, pepper, and chopped parsley. Mix the oil and vinegar together in the proportion of two of oil to one of vinegar; pour this over, let it stand for an hour, and serve.

VENETIAN RICE

* 1/2 lb. Rice--1d.
*
* 1/2 lb. Cheese--2d.
*
* 1 pint Stock
*
* 1 oz. Butter
*
* Pepper and Salt--1d.
*
* Total Cost--4d.

* Time--Three-quarters of an Hour.
*

Boil some rice, or take any cold rice that may be left, put it into a saucepan with the stock, and simmer till the stock is absorbed. Grate up some dry, hard pieces of cheese, stir them in with the butter, pepper and salt. Cover down by the side of the fire for about half an hour; pile on a dish, and serve.

TOMATOES AND EGGS

* 4 Eggs--4d.
*

* 1/2 pint Tomato Sauce--2d.
*

* Fried Bread
*

* 1 teaspoonful Parsley--1d.
*

* Total Cost--7d.
*

* Time--5 Minutes.
*

Take some thick tomato sauce and pour it on to a hot dish. Poach the eggs carefully and lay them on the sauce. Garnish with parsley and fried bread, and serve hot.

MACARONI CHEESE

* 2 oz. Macaroni--1 1/2d.
*
* 1/2 pint White Sauce--1 1/2d.
*
* 3 oz. Dry Cheese
*
* Pepper and Salt--1d.
*
* Total Cost--4d.
*
* Time--10 Minutes.
*

Put the macaroni into boiling salt and water, and boil for half an hour or until soft; strain off the water and cut into pieces about 1 1/2 inch long. Make the sauce by directions given elsewhere. Mix in half the cheese and some pepper and salt. Take a dish in which it can be served, and lay at the bottom some macaroni; then some sauce and a little of the dry cheese. Continue in this way till all the materials are used up, leaving plenty of dry cheese for the top. Put in the oven for five or ten minutes till a nice colour. Serve hot.

MAYONNAISE

* 2 Eggs--2d.
*
* 1 gill Oil--2d.
*

* 1/2 gill Vinegar
*
* Salt--1/2d.
*
* Total Cost--41/2 d.
*
* Time--Three-quarters of an Hour.
*

Put the yolks of the eggs into a basin, sprinkle over the salt, begin to stir them with a wooden spoon, dropping in the oil very slowly. The sauce must be kept thick, and the oil added very slowly. When it is quite thick and smooth, pour in the vinegar slowly, and it is ready for use. This is considered the finest of all salad dressings. If made some time before it is required for table, it must be kept cool. It ought to stand in ice, and the vinegar should be added just before serving. It may be used for any kind of salad instead of the ordinary dressing.

HINTS ON SALAD

Salads form such a pleasant item in the menu, particularly during the hot season, that they should be regarded as a daily dish. There are no scraps of fish, poultry, meat, or cold boiled vegetables, but what can be turned to account in this way. If these are utilised, a great variety can be obtained at a very trifling cost; in fact these dainty tit-bits can often be made of food that otherwise would be thrown away. Cold cauliflowers, beans, peas, and potatoes are particularly nice in salads.

FISH SALAD

* Cold Boiled Fish--4d.
*
* 1 Lettuce--1/2d.
*
* 1 Egg--1d.
*
* Salad Dressing, or Remoulade Sauce--4d.
*
* Total Cost--91/2 d.
*

Make a salad dressing the same as that given for lettuce salad; flake
up the fish free from skin and bone. Wash and dry the lettuce and shred
it up, mix the fish with the dressing. Put a layer of lettuce at the
bottom of the bowl, then one of fish and dressing. Do this
alternatively, leaving plenty of lettuce for the top; garnish with hard
boiled eggs cut into slices.

LETTUCE SALAD

* 2 Lettuces--1d.
*
* 1 tablespoonful Condensed Milk
*
* 2 teaspoonful Mustard--1d.
*
* 2 Eggs--2d.
*

* 1/2 gill Vinegar--1/2d.
*

* 1/4 gill Oil
*

* Pepper and Salt--1/2d.
*

* Total Cost--5d.
*

Boil the eggs hard; take the yolk of one and put it into a basin and work it quite smooth with a spoon. Then add the mustard made with vinegar instead of water, the condensed milk, pepper, and salt, and then the oil slowly; last of all the vinegar. Mix it all very thoroughly. Cut off the outside leaves of the lettuce, and pull it all to pieces, wash in cold water and dry thoroughly in a cloth. Break into small pieces and put into a salad bowl, pour over the dressing. Garnish with the other egg and the white that was not used in the dressing. These should be cut into slices and placed round. A few of the best pieces of lettuce should be laid over the dressing.

BEETROOT AND MACARONI SALAD

* 3 oz. Macaroni--2d.
*

* 2 tablespoonsful Oil--1d.
*

* 1 bunch Beetroot
*

* Pepper and Salt
*

* 2 tablespoonful Vinegar--2d.
*

* Total Cost--5d.
*

Boil both the macaroni and the beetroot by directions given elsewhere. When quite cold, peel and slice up the beetroot and cut the macaroni into pieces about two inches long; arrange them in alternate layers on a dish. Blend the oil and vinegar with the salt and pepper and pour it over; let it stand for an hour, basting continually with the oil and vinegar. By that time it should be of a bright red colour. It is then ready to serve.

PRAWN SALAD

* 1 pint Prawns--9d.
*

* 6 Tomatoes--2d.
*

* Mayonnaise or Salad Dressing--4d.
*

* Total Cost--1s. 3d.
*

Pick the prawns, leaving the skin on a few fine ones for a garnish. Peel and slice up the tomatoes and arrange them on a dish; put over them the prawns, and pour over all some mayonnaise or salad dressing. Place the other prawns round as a garnish with a few lettuce leaves broken up.

SALAD OF CORNED BEEF

* Slices of Corned Beef
*
* 1 Lettuce--1/2.
*
* 2 Eggs--2d.
*
* Mayonnaise or Salad Dressing--4d.
*
* Total Cost--61/2 d.
*

Take some slices of cold corned beef, dip them in a salad dressing, and lay them in a dish with alternate layers of lettuce leaves. Garnish with hard boiled eggs cut in slices.

EGG SALAD

* 6 Eggs--6d.
*
* 1 Lettuce--1d.
*
* 1 bunch Watercress--1d.
*
* Mayonnaise or Salad Dressing--4d.
*
* 1 Beetroot--1/2d.
*
* Total Cost--1s. 0 1/2 d.

Put the eggs into boiling water and boil fifteen minutes. Plunge into cold water till quite cold, peel and cut into quarters. Wash and cleanse the watercress and lettuce and cut into pieces. Put a layer of this at the bottom of the bowl, then one of eggs dipped in the dressing, then another of lettuce and egg until all are used up, leaving plenty of lettuce for the top. Garnish with sprigs of watercress and slices of beetroot alternately.

CELERY SALAD

* 1 Head of Celery--1d.
*
* 1 Lettuce--1/2d.
*
* Salad Dressing--4d.
*
* Total Cost--51/2 d.
*

Pull the celery to pieces, wash it, and cut into small pieces; shred up some lettuce and lay it at the bottom the dish. Stir the celery into the dressing and lay it on the top of the lettuce. Cover with more lettuce, and serve.

SARDINE SALAD

* 1/2 tin Sardines--4d.
*
* 2 Eggs--2d.
*
* 1 Lettuce--1/2d.
*
* Salad Dressings--4d.
*
* Total Cost--101/2 d.
*

Split the sardines open and remove the bone. Break some of the lettuce into a bowl, lay on this the sardines. Chop up one of the eggs and sprinkle over them, pour on the dressing. Cover with the rest of the lettuce, and garnish with the other egg cut in slices, and a little watercress or beetroot.

OYSTER SALAD

* 1 bottle Oysters--1s.
*
* 1 Lettuce--1d.
*
* Half a Lemon
*
* Mayonnaise or Salad Dressing--4d.
*
* Total Cost--1s. 5d.

Strain away the liquor from a bottle of oysters; put it into a saucepan, and when it boils put in the oysters and cook for five minutes; let them get cold in the liquor. Wash and break up the lettuce and put some of the bottom of a bowl. Strain the liquor from the oysters and mix a little with the dressing, stir in the oysters and spread over the lettuce. Cover with more lettuce and garnish with slices of lemon and red radishes.

BLUE COD SALAD

Any remains of smoked blue cod that may have been left from a meal make an excellent salad either with just a simple dressing of oil and vinegar and a lettuce, or with a mayonnaise or salad dressing. Follow the directions for fish salad, but do not put any salt, as the fish is usually salt enough.

ITALIAN SALAD

* 1 Salt Herring
*

* Cold slices of Meat
*

* 1 teaspoonful Mustard
*

* 1 Beetroot--1 1/2d.
*

* 4 tablespoonsful Oil--1d.
*

* 3 tablespoonsful Tarragon Vinegar
*

* 1/2 oz. Capers
*

* 3 Boiled Potatoes--2d.
*

* Total Cost--4 1/2d.
*

Wash the herring in cold water and soak it in milk for an hour; cut it open and take out the bone and slice up both the fish and the meat. Arrange in a bowl, chop the capers and put over. Put the mustard into a basin, add gradually the oil and vinegar; pour this, when well mixed, over the fish and meat, and cover with slices of cold potatoes. Garnish with any cold vegetables in the larder or with some green pickles from a bottle of pickles, a little chopped parsley, and some small radishes.

MACARONI AND CHEESE SALAD

* 1/4 lb. Macaroni--2 1/2d.
*

* 1/4 lb. Cheese--1 1/2d.
*

* 1 teaspoonful French Mustard
*

* 3 tablespoonsful Oil--1d.
*

* 3 tablespoonsful Vinegar--1/2d.
*

* 1/2 Head of Celery--1/2d.
*

* 1/2 Lettuce--1/2d.

* Total Cost--6 1/2 d.
*

Boil the macaroni, or use any cold that may be in the larder. Cut it into pieces about three inches long, cut the cheese into very thin slices, and cut the celery into very small pieces. Lay these alternately in a bowl with some shredded lettuce. Make a dressing of the mustard, oil, and vinegar, and pour it over. Garnish with a little beetroot, and serve.

CHEESE SAVOURY

Take some dry, hard cheese and some dry crusts of bread. Pour a little boiling milk over the bread, cover it down till quite soft, then beat it with a fork; grate up the cheese and beat it in with the yolk of an egg and some pepper and salt. Beat the white of the egg to a stiff froth and stir it lightly in, pour into a buttered pie-dish and bake in a quick oven for twenty minutes. Serve hot.

TURNIP SALAD

* 4 Young Turnips
*

* 2 Spring Onions--1 1/2d.
*

* 2 Boiled Potatoes--1/2d.
*

* Half a Lettuce--1/2d.
*

* Salad Dressing--4d.

* Total Cost--6 1/2 d.
*

Peel and slice up the turnips and boil them for twenty minutes,
or until soft. Let them get quite cold. Shred up very small the onions,
and slice up the potatoes. Break up half a lettuce. Arrange these
neatly in a bowl and pour over a simple salad dressing or remoulade
sauce.

EAST INDIAN SALAD SAUCE

* 2 Eggs--2d.
*

* 1 teaspoonful Curry Powder--1/2d.
*

* 1/2 gill Oil
*

* 1/4 gill Vinegar--1 1/2d.
*

* Total Cost--4d.
*

Boil the eggs hard; put the yolks into a bowl and work them till they
are quite smooth. Work in gradually the curry powder, oil, and vinegar.
Blend well, and it is ready. It may be used sometimes instead of
mayonnaise or ordinary salad dressing.

BREAD SALAD

* 5 slices Stale Bread
*

* 1/2 gill Oil
*

* 3 Pickled Onions
*

* 1 piece Pickled Cauliflower--2d.
*

* 2 Eggs--2d.
*

* 1 Beetroot
*

* 2 slices Cold Mutton
*

* 1 tablespoonful Vinegar--1d.
*

* Mustard and Cress--1/2d.
*

* Total Cost--51/2 d.
*

Trim off the crust and cut the bread into dice, put into a bowl and pour over the oil. Let it stand till all the oil is absorbed; then mince up the onion, cauliflower, eggs, and meat, and strew them over. Season with pepper and salt. Well wash the mustard and cress and arrange on the top. Cut the beetroot into neat shapes and arrange as a garnish.

BREAKFAST SALAD

* 2 Tomatoes--1/2d.
*
* 1 Cucumber--2d.
*
* 1 tablespoonful Oil--1/2d.
*
* 1 Spring Onion
*
* Half a Lettuce
*
* 2 tablespoonsful Vinegar--1/2d.
*
* Total Cost--31/2 d.
*

Scald the tomatoes and take off the skin, and put them into cold water or on to the ice until quite cold. Cut them up the same as an orange; peel and cut up the cucumber into very thin slices and mince up the onion. Sprinkle these with pepper and salt, pour over the oil and vinegar. Shred up the lettuce and lay on the top, it is then ready to serve.

CAULIFLOWER SALAD

* 1 Cauliflower--3d.
*
* Half a Lettuce--1/2d.
*
* 2 Eggs--2d.
*
* 1/2 gill Oil and Vinegar--1d.
*
* Total Cost--61/2 d.
*

Boil the cauliflower by directions given elsewhere and branch it carefully. Boil the eggs hard, separate the whites from the yolks; chop the whites small and cut the yolks in slices. Shred up the lettuce in a bowl and put the branches of cauliflower all round it, and the slices of yolk of egg outside as a border. Pour on the salad dressing and put the white of egg in little heaps on the lettuce. It is then ready to serve.

CARROT SALAD

* 2 or 3 Cold Boiled Carrots--1/2d.
*
* 1/2 lb. Cold Boiled Mutton
*
* 1 stalk Celery
*
* 6 Capers--1 1/2d.

* Half a teaspoonful Parsley--1/2d.
*
* Salad Dressing--3d.
*
* Total Cost--51/2 d.
*

Cut up some cold boiled mutton into small pieces and lay them in a salad bowl. Mince up the celery and capers and strew over it, then pour over the dressing. Slice up the cold carrots and lay them on top; garnish with the chopped parsley, and serve.

CALF'S FOOT SALAD

Calves' feet that have been boiled down for jelly make a good salad. They must, of course, be boiled very thoroughly for at least eight hours. Strain off the stock, remove the bones, and put the meat on one side till quite cold. Then cut up into neat pieces and put into a salad bowl. Pour over a salad dressing or just oil and vinegar; shred over it a nice white lettuce, and garnish with sliced beetroot.

REMOULADE SALAD DRESSING

This is a good dressing when mayonnaise is not liked. It is made in the same way as mayonnaise, using hard boiled eggs (yolks) instead of raw ones. Put the yolks into a basin and work very smoothly with the bowl of a wooden spoon; add the oil gradually, using about one gill to every two yolks. A little French mustard and vinegar may be added before using.

SOUP MEAT SALAD

The meat which has been boiled down for soup makes a nice salad. When the stock has been poured off, press the meat into a basin with about a gill of jelly stock, and some salt and pepper. When cold and firm, cut it into neat pieces and lay in a salad bowl. Pour over it some remoulade sauce and shred on top some nice white lettuce leaves; it may be garnished with beetroot or hard boiled eggs.

LAMB SALAD

* Cold Roast Lamb
*
* 2 Lettuces--1d.
*
* 1 Tomato--1/2d.
*
* 12 Capers--1/2d.
*
* 2 Eggs--2d.
*
* Remoulade Dressing--3d.
*
* Total Cost--7d.
*

Cut the lamb into small pieces and lay it in a bowl. Cut the tomato into thin slices and lay it over, then the capers chopped small. Pour over the dressing, break up the lettuces and put over, and garnish with the hard boiled eggs cut in slices.

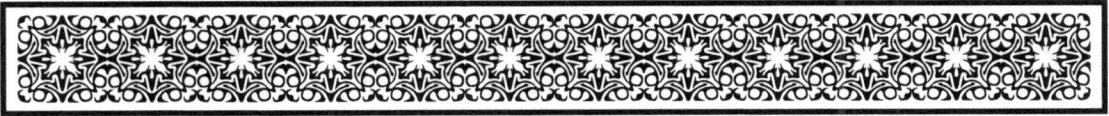

CHAPTER XXII.
FIFTY RECIPES FOR SWEETS

APPLE AND TAPIOCA

* 6 Apples--3d.
*
* 1 1/2 oz. Tapioca--1/2d.
*
* 1/2 Lemon--1/2d.
*
* 2 oz. Sugar
*
* 1 1/4 pints Water
*
* A few drops of Cochineal--1/2d.
*
* Total Cost--41/2 d.
*
* Time--Half an Hour
*

Peel and quarter the apples and remove the core, put them into a saucepan with the lemon juice, sugar, and a spoonful of water, and stew till soft but not broken. Place them in a glass dish. Wash the tapioca in cold water, put it in a saucepan, pour over it 1 1/4 pints of water, and stir till it boils. Cook it till quite clear, sweeten and flavour with a few drops of lemon juice, and colour with cochineal. Pour over the apples and put away till cold; it is then ready to serve.

SHORT PASTRY--No. 1

* 1 lb. Flour
*
* 6 or 8 oz. Dripping
*
* 1 gill Water
*
* Total Cost--2d.
*

Sift the flour into a basin, rub in the dripping very lightly until it is quite fine, mix into a very stiff dough with the water, turn on to a floured board, and knead into a smooth paste. Roll out to the required thickness, and it is ready at once. This will be found an exceedingly nice paste for everyday pies, and it is very wholesome. The dripping should be clarified, directions for which are given elsewhere.

SHORT PASTRY--No. 2

* 1 lb. Flour--2d.
*
* 8 oz. Butter
*
* 1 gill Water

*

* Juice of Half a Lemon--6d.

*

* Total Cost--8d.

*

Sift the flour into a basin, rub the butter lightly in, until it is
fine as bread crumbs; make a well in the centre, and strain the lemon
juice. Mix into a stiff paste with the water, knead for a few minutes
until it is quite smooth, it is then ready for use. A crust may be made
with lard just in the same way; this is much lighter of digestion than
a butter crust, and should always be given to anyone suffering from a
weak digestion.

FLAKY CRUST

* 1 lb. Flour--2d.

*

* 4 oz. Butter--3d.

*

* 4 oz. Lard

*

* 1/2 pint Water

*

* Juice of Half a Lemon--2d.

*

* Total Cost--7d.

*

Sift the flour into a basin, cut about one ounce of the lard into it
with a knife, then mix into a paste with the water; it should be about
the same consistency as the butter. Roll it out evenly, and lay on it
small pieces of the butter and lard, sprinkle with flour and roll into

three; roll out again and proceed as before. It is ready for use at once if required, but it is much improved by standing in a cool place for an hour. This kind of pastry requires a very quick oven; and if used for meat pies, a piece of buttered paper should be laid over the top as soon as it has rise, to prevent it getting too brown.

SUET PASTRY--No. 1

* 1 lb. Flour--2d.
*
* 10 oz. Beef Suet
*
* 1/2 pint Water--3d.
*
* Total Cost--5d.
*

Sift the flour into a basin, and make it into a firm paste with the water. Free the suet from skin, and put it twice through a sausage machine. Roll the paste out, and put half over it in very tiny pieces; sprinkle with flour and fold into three. Double the ends over till they meet, roll out again, and put on the rest of the suet and proceed as before. It is then ready for use, but is much improved by standing for an hour in a cold place. This is a very wholesome pastry, and particularly nice for meat pies. If it is properly made, it ought to rise like the best puff pastry; it is an easy crust to make in hot weather, when the puff crusts made with butter are troublesome.

SUET PASTRY--No. 2

* 1 lb. Flour--2d.
*

* 8 oz. Suet
*

* 1/2 pint Water
*

* Pinch of Salt--3d.
*

* Total Cost--5d.
*

Sift the flour into a basin; prepare the suet by cutting it into very thin slices and then shredding it up very fine indeed; mix it in with the flour. Stir in the water until it is a firm consistency, but do not use too much water, or the paste will be tough. Suet crust should be kept as dry as possible. Turn it on to a floured board and knead for a few minutes. It is then ready for use; this crust is suitable for all kinds of boiled puddings, such as meat, apple, jam, & c. These puddings require to be boiled for a very long time. They must always be plunged into boiling water, and kept boiling and covered with water all the time they are cooking.

SUET PUDDING

* 1 lb. Flour--2d.
*
* 8 or 10 oz. Suet
*
* 1/4 teaspoonful Salt
*
* 1/2 pint Water
*
* 2 Cold Potatoes--3d.
*
* Total Cost--5d.
*
* Time--Two Hours and a Half.
*

Sift the flour and salt into a basin, mash the potatoes or rub them
through a sieve, and stir them in. Shred the suet finely and mix in
thoroughly with a knife; make into rather a stiff paste with the water,
dip a pudding cloth into boiling water. Put the pudding into the
centre, and tie up tightly. Plunge into boiling water and boil steadily
for two hours; turn out of the cloth carefully into a hot dish, and
serve. This pudding is delicious with roast meat, or it may be served
as a sweet; jam sauce is nice poured round it. A recipe for this will
be found elsewhere.

HASTY PUDDING SOUFFLE

* 1 pint Milk--2d.
*

* 2 Eggs--2d.
*

* 1 oz. Flour
*

* 1 oz. Sugar
*

* Flavourings--1d.
*

* Total Cost--5d.
*

* Time--40 Minutes
*

Put the milk on to boil, mix the flour smoothly with a little cold milk; when the milk in the saucepan nearly boils stir this in and stir until it boils. Then take off the fire and beat in the sugar, flavouring, and the yolks of the eggs. Whisk the whites to a stiff froth and stir them lightly in, pour into a buttered pie-dish, and bake in a brisk oven for forty minutes; serve hot.

CHEESE CAKES

* 1 pint Sour Milk--2d.
*

* 2 Eggs--2d.
*

* 1/2 lb. Flaky Pastry--3d.
*

* 2 oz. Sugar
*

* Flavouring--1d.
*

* Total Cost--8d.
*

* Time--15 Minutes.
*

Pour the milk through a sieve and use only the thick curd which does not run through into the basin; beat in the sugar, yolks of the eggs, and flavouring to taste. Roll our some flaky pastry and line some patty pans with it; fill them with rice or crusts of bread, and bake for about ten minutes. Then take out the rice or crusts and fill with the cheese cake mixture. Finish baking, and stand on a sieve till cool. Sprinkle well with sugar, and serve cold.

BANANA SOUFFLE

* 6 Bananas--2d.
*

* 2 oz. Sugar--1/2d.
*

* 1/2 pint Milk--1d.
*

* 2 Eggs--2d.
*

* Total Cost--51/2 d.
*

* Time--5 Minutes.

Choose ripe bananas, peel and slice them up, and lay them in a glass dish, sprinkle with sugar. Make a custard with the milk and yolks of the eggs by directions for boiled custard, flavour with a pinch of ginger, and pour it over the bananas. Let it stand till quite cold, then whip the whites to a very stiff froth and heap them on top; sprinkle with sugar, and serve.

BOILED CUSTARD

* 1 pint Milk--2d.
*
* 3 Eggs--3d.
*
* 1 1/2 oz. Sugar
*
* Flavouring--1d.
*
* Total Cost--6d.
*
* Time--5 Minutes
*

Put the yolks of the eggs into a basin and whisk them. Put the milk into a saucepan, and when it is boiling pour it over the eggs, stirring all the time. Strain back into the saucepan and whist well till it comes to boiling point; draw away from the fire, but continue whisking for a few minutes. Then pour into a basin, sweeten and flavour to taste, and it is ready for use.

CORNFLOUR CUSTARD

* 1/2 pint Milk--1d.
*
* 1 Egg--1d.
*
* 1 dessertspoonful Cornflour
*
* Sugar and Flavouring--1d.
*
* Total Cost--3d.
*
* Time--5 Minutes.
*

Put the milk into a saucepan to boil, mix the cornflour with a spoonful of cold milk, and when the milk in the saucepan is nearly boiling, stir it in and continue stirring till it boils. Let it boil two or three minutes, then draw the saucepan away from the fire, beat in the yolk of the egg and flavouring. Put back on the fire and bring to boiling point; it is then ready for use. This is a good sauce for plum or other puddings and fruit tarts.

BACHELOR'S BUTTONS

* 5 oz. Flour--1/2d.
*
* 2 oz. Sugar--1/2d.
*
* 1/2 teaspoonful Carbonate of Soda

* 1 oz. Butter
*

* 1 teaspoonful Cream of Tartar
*

* 6 drops Essence of Almonds--2d.
*

* Total Cost--3d.
*

* Time--10 Minutes.
*

Rub the butter into the flour, stir in the sugar, carbonate of soda, and cream of tartar; mix into a stiff dough with the egg and flavouring. Roll into small balls about the size of a marble; toss in coarse sugar, put on to a greased baking sheet, and bake from five to eight minutes.

PRINCE OF WALES CAKES

* 1/4 lb. Flour--1/2d.
*

* 1/4 lb. Cornflour--1d.
*

* 1 gill Milk--1/2d.
*

* 1/2 teaspoonful Baking Powder--1/2d.
*

* 2 oz. Butter--2d.
*

* 1 Egg--1d.
*

* Flavouring--1/2d.

* 2 oz. Sugar--1/2d.
*

* Total Cost--61/2 d.
*

* Time--20 Minutes.
*

Mix the flour, cornflour, and baking powder together, beat the butter
and sugar to a cream, beat in the egg, flavouring, and milk, then the
flour, &c., and continue to beat for five minutes. Butter some small
bun tins, half fill them with the mixture, put into a moderate oven and
bake for about twenty minutes; stand on a sieve till cold.

NORMANDY PUDDING

* 2 Stale Buns--2d.
*

* 1 Egg--1d.
*

* 1/2 pint Milk--1d.
*

* Sugar--1/2d.
*

* Total Cost--41/2 d.
*

* Time--One Hour and a Half.
*

Boil the milk and pour it over the beaten egg, sweeten to
taste. Put the buns into a pie-dish, pour over the custard, cover and
leave for an hour. Then put into a moderate oven and bake for about
half an hour. Serve hot.

RUSK PUDDING

* 1 slice of Dry Bread
*
* 2 Eggs--2d.
*
* 1 oz. Sugar--1/2d.
*
* Half a Lemon--1/2d.
*
* 1 1/2 pints of Milk--4d.
*
* 1 tablespoonful Jam--1d.
*
* 1/2 tablespoonful Cornflour--1/2d.
*
* Total Cost--81/2 d.
*
* Time--One Hour.
*

Take a piece of very stale bread and cut it into small squares, bake it in the oven till a good colour. Break the eggs into a pie-dish, beat in the sugar and grated rind of the lemon, pour in one pint of milk, and mix well. Drop in the rusks and put into a cool oven and bake till firm; then spread on the top a layer of jam. Put half a pint of milk into a saucepan, and when it nearly boils, stir in the cornflour which has been mixed with a little lemon peel and sugar, and pour it on top of the pudding. Put it back in the oven for a few minutes, then stand away till cold.

BEDFORD PUDDING

* Dry Crusts of Bread
*
* 1/2 pint of Milk--1d.
*
* 1 tablespoonful Jam--1d.
*
* 2 Eggs--2d.
*
* 1 1/2 oz. Sugar--1/2d.
*
* Total Cost--41/2 d.
*
* Time--Three-quarters of an Hour.
*

Soak the bread in cold water till quite soft, put it into a cloth and squeeze all the water out of it; turn into a basin and beat it smooth with a spoon. Then beat in the yolks of the eggs, sugar, milk, and a little grated lemon peel. Pour into a pie dish and bake till quite firm, then take from the oven and spread the jam on the top. Whip the whites to a stiff froth and spread over the jam; put back in the oven for a few minutes till brown, then sprinkle with sugar and serve either hot or cold.

DE MESTRE PUDDING

* 1/2 lb. Flour--1d.
*
* 1/4 lb. Raisins--2d.
*
* 1/4 lb. Sugar--1d.
*
* 1 oz. Dripping
*
* 1 teaspoonful Carbonate of Soda
*
* 1 gill Boiling Water--1/2d.
*
* Total Cost--41/2 d.
*
* Time--Three Hours.
*

Put the flour into a basin; stone the raisins and cut them in half, mix in the sugar and carbonate of soda. Dissolve the dripping in the water, pour in and make into a dough; leave it to stand all night. Dip a cloth in boiling water and tie the pudding up tightly. Plunge into plenty of boiling water, and keep it boiling steadily for three hours; turn into a hot dish. A little custard sauce served with this pudding is a great improvement.

YANKEE PUDDING

* 1 Egg, and its Weight in Flour--1 1/2d.
*
* Sugar--1/2d.
*
* Bread Crumbs--1/2d.
*
* 1 tablespoonful Marmalade--1d.
*
* 1/2 teaspoonful Carbonate of Soda
*
* 1/2 gill Milk--1/2d.
*
* Total Cost--4d.
*
* Time--One Hour.
*

Mix the flour, sugar, and bread crumbs together; stir in the marmalade. Make the milk just warm, dissolve in it the soda. Beat up the egg and mix together, pour this over the dry ingredients, beat for a few minutes; turn into a buttered basin. Tie over it a cloth, plunge into boiling water, and boil one hour. Serve either hot or cold. A spoonful of marmalade placed on the top of this pudding just before serving is an improvement.

SPONGE ROLL

* 3 tablespoonsful Flour--1/2d.
*
* 3 tablespoonsful Sugar--1d.
*
* 3 Eggs--3d.
*
* 2 teaspoonsful Baking Powder--1d.
*
* 3 teaspoonsful Jam--1 1/2d.
*
* Total Cost--7d.
*
* Time--10 Minutes.
*

Beat the eggs and sugar together for five minutes, mix the flour and baking powder together and stir them lightly in. Pour into a well-buttered tin and bake in a quick oven for eight or ten minutes. Turn on to a damp cloth and roll up directly; warm the jam in a saucepan while the roll is cooking, and if it is very stiff mix in a spoonful of water. Take the roll out of the cloth and lay flat on a piece of sugared paper, spread the jam on quickly and roll up again; place on a sieve till cold.

SEED CAKE

* 1 lb. Flour--2d.
*
* 6 oz. Dripping
*
* 6 oz. Sugar--1 1/2d.
*
* 1 1/2 teaspoonsful Caraway Seeds--1/2d.
*
* 1 Egg--1d.
*
* 2 teaspoonsful Baking Powder
*
* 1 gill Milk or Water--1 1/2d.
*
* Total Cost--61/2 d.
*
* Time--One Hour and a Half.
*

Sift the flour into a basin and rub in the dripping; carefully stir in the sugar, baking powder, and caraway seeds.

Beat up the egg and milk or water, and mix the dry ingredients into a dough; beat for two or three minutes. Turn into a cake tin which has been well rubbed with dripping, stand on a baking sheet and place in a moderate oven. Bake for one hour and a half or longer, test it by running a skewer right through the centre; if it comes out clean the cake is done. Turn it out of the tine carefully and stand on a sieve till cold.

SCONES--No. 1

* 3/4 lb. Flour--1 1/2d.
*
* 1/2 pint Milk--1d.
*
* 1 oz. Butter--1d.
*
* 2 teaspoonsful Baking Powder--1 1/2d.
*
* Total Cost--5d.
*
* Time--10 Minutes.
*

Rub the butter into the flour, stir in the baking powder, and make into a very light dough with the milk; turn on to a floured board, knead for a few minutes, roll out about half an inch thick. Cut into shapes, put on to a floured tin, and bake in a quick oven for about ten minutes. Serve either hot or cold.

SCONES--No. 2

* 1 lb. Flour--2d.
*
* 1/2 pint Sour Milk
*
* 3 teaspoonsful Baking Powder
*
* 1 teaspoonful Salt--1 1/2d.

*

* Total Cost--31/2 d.
*

* Time--5 Minutes.
*

Mix the flour, baking powder, and salt together, mix into a very light dough with the milk, adding a little more milk if necessary; turn on to a floured board and knead till smooth, roll out half an inch thick. Cut into small rounds and bake for about five minutes.

SCONES--No. 3

* 1 lb. Flour--2d.
*

* 2 oz. Dripping
*

* 1 oz. Sugar
*

* 1/2 pint Sour Milk
*

* 1 teaspoonful Cream of Tartar
*

* 1/2 teaspoonful Carbonate of Soda--1 1/2d.
*

* Total Cost--31/2 d.
*

* Time--20 Minutes.
*

Rub the dripping into the flour; stir in the sugar, cream of tartar, and soda. Mix into a very light dough with the milk, turn on to a floured board; divide into two parts. Flatten these out into two cakes, divide each one into four pieces, brush over with milk. Put on to a floured tin and bake in a hot oven from fifteen to twenty minutes.

POTATO FRITTERS

* Cold Potatoes
*
* 1 Egg
*
* 2 oz. Sugar
*
* Nutmeg or Lemon Peel
*
* Hot Fat
*
* Total Cost--11/2 d.
*
* Time--5 Minutes.
*

Mash up the potatoes very smoothly, beat in the sugar and a flavouring of nutmeg or grated lemon peel. Beat up the egg and pour over the potatoes and mix into a paste; form into small round cakes. Fry in very hot fat till brown; pile high on a dish, sprinkle with sugar and serve. One egg is sufficient for about 1 lb., potatoes.

APPLE FRITTERS

* 3 Apples--2d.
*
* Frying Batter--1d.
*
* Hot Fat
*
* Sugar
*
* Lemon--1d.
*
* Total Cost--4d.
*
* Time--5 Minutes.
*

Peel and slice up the apples into rounds, take out the core with a small round cutter. Make frying batter by directions given elsewhere, and flavour with lemon juice. Dip in the pieces of apple, plunge into plenty of hot fat, and fry till a good colour. Drain on kitchen paper, pile high on a dish, and sprinkle well with sugar; serve very hot.

SWEET OMELET

* 2 Eggs--2d.
*
* 1/2 oz. Butter--1/2d.
*
* 1 teaspoonful Jam--1/2d.
*
* Sugar--1/2d.
*
* Total Cost--31/2 d.
*
* Time--5 Minutes.
*

Put the yolks of the eggs into a basin and beat in half the sugar, put the whites on to a plate with a little sugar, and whip till stiff; mix with the yolks. Put the butter into a small frying-pan, and when it is dissolved pour in the mixture; leave over the fire for about three minutes. Then hold the pan in front of the fire for a minute or two to brown the top. Put the jam on to a hot plate, slip the omelet on the top; serve at once.

TAPIOCA MERINGUE

* 1 pint Milk--2d.
*
* 1 1/2 oz. Tapioca--1/2d.
*
* 1 oz. Sugar--1/2d.

*
* Whites of 2 Eggs--1d.
*
* Flavouring--1/2d.
*
* 1 oz. Beef Suet--1/2d.
*
* Total Cost--5d.
*
* Time--Two Hours.
*

Wash the tapioca well in cold water, strain off the water, and put it into a pie dish. Chop the suet very finely and mix it in with the sugar; flavour with grated lemon peel or nutmeg, pour over the milk and mix well, stand in a very cool oven for two hours. Whip the whites of the eggs to a very stiff froth, flavour the same as the pudding, spread these on top, sprinkle with sugar, and stand in the oven till set; serve cold. This meringue is very much improved if a few macaroons are broken up and laid on the top before the eggs are put on, or if a spoonful of raspberry jam is spread over.

HASTY PUDDING

* 1 pint Milk--2d.
*
* 1 oz. Butter--1d.
*
* 3 oz. Flour
*
* 2 oz. Sugar--1d.
*

* Total Cost--4d.
*

* Time--5 Minutes.
*

Put the milk on the fire to boil, and when boiling stir in the flour quickly; it should be rather lumpy. Pour it into a dish, melt the butter and sugar, and pour it in the middle of the pudding. A little flavouring of grated lemon peel may be put into the milk, or jam served with the pudding.

QUICK PUDDING

* 1 Egg
*

* 1 tablespoonful Flour--1d.
*

* 1 tablespoonful Jam
*

* 1 teaspoonful Sugar
*

* 1 teaspoonful Baking Powder--2d.
*

* Total Cost--3d.
*

* Time--5 Minutes.
*

Mix the flour and baking powder together, beat the egg till very light, whisk in the sugar, and stir in the flour. Pour into a buttered tin, and bake five minutes; turn on to a sugared paper spread with jam. Roll up and serve. Custard sauce is nice with this.

STANLEY PUDDING

* 1 pint Milk
*
* 2 oz. Flour--2d.
*
* 1 oz. Sugar--1d.
*
* 2 Eggs--2d.
*
* 2 spoonful Jam--1d.
*
* Total Cost--6d.
*
* Time--One Hour.
*

Put the milk into a saucepan, mix the flour with a little cold milk; and when the milk in the saucepan is nearly boiling, stir it in, and let it boil up. Pour into a basin and beat in the yolks of the eggs and the sugar; turn into a pie dish and bake till firm. Spread a spoonful of jam on the top; whip the whites of the eggs to a stiff froth and spread them over, sprinkle with sugar, and put back in the oven to set. Serve cold.

IMITATION OMELET

* 1 Egg--1d.
*
* 1/2 gill Milk--1/2d.

*

* 1 teaspoonful Sugar

*

* 1 teaspoonful Jam

*

* 1 teaspoonful Flour--1d.

*

* Total Cost--21/2 d.

*

* Time--5 Minutes.

*

Beat the yolk and white of egg separately; beat the flour and milk together, and mix in the sugar and yolk of egg. Stir in the white, butter a saucer, put the jam at the bottom. Pour in the mixture, bake in the oven for five minutes, sprinkle with sugar, and serve.

OXFORDSHIRE PUDDING

* 1 pint Milk--2d.

*

* 1 1/2 oz. Rice--1/2d.

*

* 1 oz. Sugar

*

* Rind of Half a Lemon--1/2d.

*

* Total Cost--3d.

*

* Time--Two Hours.

*

Wash the rice well, strain off the water and put it into a pie-dish.

Mix in the sugar and the rind of the lemon; pour over the milk, and let it sand for half an hour. Put it into a very slow oven, and bake till firm. This is a very delicious pudding if properly made; it should be firm, but not dry.

MILK BISCUITS

* 1/2 lb. Flour--1d.
*
* 1 gill Milk--1/2d.
*
* 1 oz. Butter
*
* 1/4 saltspoonful Salt--1d.
*
* Total Cost--21/2 d.
*
* Time--10 Minutes.
*

Rub the butter into the flour, sprinkle in the salt, and make into a dough with the milk; knead till smooth, roll out very thin. Cut into small rounds, prick well with a fork, put on to a floured tin and bake for about ten minutes. They should not get brown.

SODA CAKE

* 1 lb. Flour--2d.
*
* 1/2 lb. Currants--2d.
*
* 1/2 lb. Sugar--1d.
*
* 6 oz. Dripping
*
* 1 1/2 teaspoonsful Carbonate of Soda
*
* 1/2 pint Milk--2d.
*
* Total Cost--7d.
*
* Time--Two Hours.
*

Rub the dripping and the flour together; clean and stir in the currants
and sugar. Stir in the soda and mix into a dough with the milk, beat
for a few minutes. Pour into a tin which has been well rubbed with
dripping, bake in a moderate oven for two hours.

DIGESTIVE BISCUITS

* 1/2 lb. Brown Meal
*
* 1/4 lb. Flour--1 1/2d.
*

* 1 1/2 gills Water
*

* 1 oz. Butter or Lard
*

* 1 oz. Sugar--1d.
*

* Total Cost--21/2 d.
*

* Time--5 Minutes.
*

Mix the meal and flour together, rub in the butter or lard and the sugar; mix into a dry paste with water, knead till smooth. Roll out very thin, cut into rounds, and bake in rather a slow oven.

LEMON PUDDING

* 1/2 lb. Flour--1d.
*

* 3 oz. Suet--1d.
*

* 1 Egg--1d.
*

* 2 Lemons--1d.
*

* 2 oz. Sugar
*

* 1/2 gill Water--1/2d.
*

* Total Cost--41/2 d.

* Time--Two Hours.
*

Sift the flour, chop the suet finely, and mix together. Stir in the sugar and the grated rind of the lemons, beat up the egg, add the juice of one lemon, and mix the pudding into a dough with this, and a little water if required. Dip a cloth in boiling water, tie the pudding in it; plunge into boiling water and boil two hours. Take out of the cloth and turn on to a hot dish, and pour round it the following sauce: Squeeze the juice of the other lemon into a small saucepan, stir in some sugar and a gill of water, and boil up; it is then ready.

BLACK CAP PUDDING

* 1 pint Milk--2d.
*

* 2 Eggs
*

* 1 oz. Currants--2d.
*

* 1/2 lb. Flour--1d.
*

* Total Cost--5d.
*

* Time--One Hour.
*

Put the eggs into a basin, beat in the flour, and then the milk, pour into a battered basin. Clean the currents and drop them in; steam for one hour, turn out of the basin, sprinkle with sugar, and serve.

ROCK CAKES

* 1/2 lb. Flour
*
* 2 oz. Dripping--1d.
*
* 1/4 lb. Sugar--1d.
*
* 2 oz. Currants--1d.
*
* 1 Egg--1d.
*
* 1 oz. Peel--1d.
*
* 1 teaspoonful Baking Powder--1/2d.
*
* Total Cost--51/2 d.
*
* Time--15 Minutes.
*

Rub the dripping and flour together, stir in the sugar, currants (well cleaned), the baking powder, and the peel. Beat up the egg and pour it in, and make into a very stiff dough; take up in rough pieces and lay on a greased tin, bake in rather a quick oven for fifteen minutes.

KINGSWOOD PUDDING

* 1/4 lb. Flour--1/2d.
*
* 1/4 lb. Bread Crumbs--1d.
*
* 1/4 lb. Raisins--2d.
*
* 6 oz. Suet--1 1/2d.
*
* 1/4 lb. Sultanas--2d.
*
* 1/4 lb. Sugar--1d.
*
* 2 Apples--1d.
*
* Total Cost--9d.
*
* Time--Six Hours.
*

Mix the flour and bread crumbs together. Any dry pieces of bread will
do if put through the sausage machine; shred the suet finely and mix it
in with the sugar. Stone the raisins and pull them in half, and clean
the sultanas; mix these in. Peel and core the apples; put in the pips,
chop the apples finely, and add them. Let it stand for an hour, and
then mix it into a paste; the juice from the applies and the sugar will
be found sufficient. Press into a basin, tie down tightly, and boil at
least six hours. This will be found an excellent pudding if
well boiled.

DELHI PUDDING

* 1 pint Milk--2d.
*
* 1 oz. Almonds--1d.
*
* 2 oz. Sugar
*
* 1 1/2 oz. Arrowroot--2d.
*
* Total Cost--5d.
*
* Time--5 Minutes.
*

Blanch and chop the almonds very small, mix them with the sugar and arrowroot. Put the milk on to boil, and when it boils pour it on to the arrowroot and stir; if it does not get thick enough, pour back into the saucepan and boil for a minute. Turn into a wet mould and stand away till firm; then turn out and serve with jam or custard sauce, or it may be served plainly.

ROTHSAY PUDDING

* 1/4 lb. Flour--1/2d.
*
* 1/4 lb. Bread Crumbs--1d.
*
* 1/4 lb. Suet--1d.

* 1 oz. Sugar
*

* 1 tablespoonful Vinegar--1/2d.
*

* 1 gill Milk--1d.
*

* 1 tablespoonful Raspberry Jam--2d.
*

* 1 Egg
*

* 1/2 teaspoonful Carbonate of Soda--1d.
*

* Total Cost--7d.
*

* Time--Two Hours.
*

Mix the flour, crumbs, finely chopped suet, and sugar in a basin, then stir in the jam. Beat up the egg and milk, and stir it in. Mix up the carbonate of soda and the vinegar together; beat it in, and when well mixed pour it into a buttered basin. Tie up carefully, and boil for two hours; turn out on to a hot dish, and serve either with sifted sugar or custard sauce.

RHUBARB MOULD

* 1 bundle Rhubarb--3d.
*

* 6 oz. Sugar--1 1/2d.
*

* 1/4 lb. Sago

* 1/2 pint Water--1 1/2d.
*

* Total Cost--6d.
*

* Time--20 Minutes
*

Wipe and cut up the rhubarb and put it on to boil with one gill water, and boil for about ten minutes. Wash the sago and soak it in one gill warm water, then add to the rhubarb. Stir in also the sugar, and boil for about ten minutes or longer, stirring constantly. Pour into a basin or mould which has been dipped in cold water, and stand away till cold and firm, then turn out and serve. A little boiled custard is a great improvement to this dish.

APPLES AND RICE

* 3 Large Apples--2d.
*

* 2 oz. Rice--1d.
*

* 2 oz. Sugar--1/2d.
*

* 1 tablespoonful Jam--1d.
*

* 1 Egg--1d.
*

* 1/2 pint Milk--1d.
*

* Total Cost--61/2 d.
*

* Time--Half an Hour.

Peel the apples and scoop out the core and fill in with jam; put into a pie-dish and bake till the apples are soft. While they are baking, boil the rice and milk together till the rice is soft and the milk absorbed. Beat in the egg and sugar, pour over the apples; brush over with milk, and bake till a nice colour. Serve either hot or cold.

RICE BLACMANGE

* 1 pint Milk--2d.
*

* 1 1/2 oz. Ground Rice--1/2d.
*

* 1 oz. Sugar
*

* Flavouring--1d.
*

* Total Cost--31/2 d.
*

* Time--5 Minutes.
*

Put the milk on to boil with a strip of lemon peel in it; when nearly boiling mix the rice in a spoonful of cold water and pour it in. Stir till it boils, and let it boil two or three minutes; pour into a mould which has been dipped in cold water, and stand away till firm. Turn out when cold, and serve with jam, stewed fruit, or custard sauce.

DEVONSHIRE JUNKET

* 1 quart Milk--4d.
*
* 1 tablespoonful Rennet
*
* 1 oz. Sugar--1d.
*
* Nutmeg--1/2d.
*
* Total Cost--51/2 d.
*
* Time--Two Hours.
*

Make the milk tepid, stir in the sugar and a spoonful of rennet or a rennet tablet; pour into a dish and stand on the stove till solid. Grate a little nutmeg on top and serve cold. Rennet can be bought at the chemist's ready for use; but rennet tables, which answer very nicely, can be used instead. These can be bought in many places, and keep good a long time.

BANBURY CAKES

* 1/2 lb. Pastry--5d.
*
* 1 oz. Currants
*
* 1 oz. Raisins

* Half a Lemon

* Half an Orange--2d.
*

* 1 oz. Cake or Bread Crumbs--1/2d.
*

* 1 oz. Sugar--1/2d.
*

* Total Cost--8d.
*

* Time--20 Minutes.
*

Stone the raisins and chop them lightly, put them into a basin with the currants cleaned, the sugar, and the cake or bread crumbs. Mix together, grate over the rind of half a lemon, and half an orange. Strain in the juice, and let it stand for an hour. Roll out the pastry and cut into rounds about three inches long. Lay a little of the mixture in the centre, close over the pastry, turn the cake over, flatten it out in the middle. Brush over with sugar, and bake in rather a quick oven. Serve warm.

LEMON BISCUITS

* 1/2 lb. Flour
*

* 3 oz. Dripping--1d.
*

* 1 teaspoonful Baking Powder
*

* 3 oz. Sugar--1d.

* 1 Lemon--1d.
*

* 1 Egg--1d.
*

* Total Cost--4d.
*

* Time--10 Minutes.
*

Rub the dripping into the flour, stir in the sugar and baking powder, and grate over the rind of the lemon. Beat up the egg and strain in the lemon juice; add these to the dry ingredients, mix into a stiff dough, and knead for a few minutes. Roll out, cut into small biscuits, and bake in a quick oven for about ten minutes.

YORKSHIRE TEA CAKES

* 3/4 lb. Flour--1 1/2d.
*

* 1 Egg--1d.
*

* 1 1/2 gills Milk--1d.
*

* 1 tablespoonful Yeast
*

* 1/2 tablespoonful Sugar--1/2d.
*

* 1 oz. Butter--1d.
*

* Total Cost--5d.
*

* Time--One Hour and a Quarter

Rub the butter and flour together, make a well in the centre, sprinkle in the sugar, and drop in the egg. Mix the yeast and sugar in a basin, make the milk just tepid, and pour it over the yeast. Strain into the flour and egg and work into a light dough, divide into two parts. Rub a little butter over two small tins, and put one cake in each tin. Cover with thin paper, and stand the tins near the stove for an hour, or until they have risen to at least three times their original size; then bake in a quick oven for fifteen minutes. Serve either plain, or toasted and buttered.

TEA CAKE

* 1 lb. Flour--2d.
*
* 1/2 pint Milk--1d.
*
* 2 oz. Butter--1 1/2d.
*
* 1 Egg--1d.
*
* 2 teaspoonsful Baking Powder
*
* 1 teaspoonful Sugar--1 1/2d.
*
* Total Cost--7d.
*
* Time--20 Minutes.
*

Rub the butter into the flour, stir in the sugar and baking powder. Beat up the egg and milk, and mix the dry ingredients into a dough with them; divide into two pieces and form each into a flat cake. Cut lightly across into four with a knife, put on to a buttered tin, and bake twenty minutes. Cut open, butter, and serve.

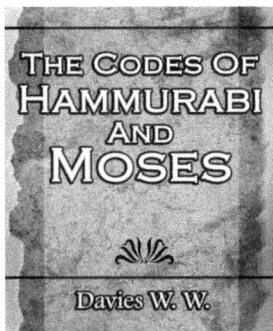

The Codes Of Hammurabi And Moses
W. W. Davies

QTY

The discovery of the Hammurabi Code is one of the greatest achievements of archaeology, and is of paramount interest, not only to the student of the Bible, but also to all those interested in ancient history...

Religion   **ISBN:** *1-59462-338-4*   **Pages:132**
MSRP $12.95

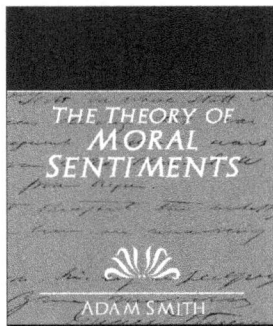

The Theory of Moral Sentiments
Adam Smith

QTY

This work from 1749. contains original theories of conscience amd moral judgment and it is the foundation for systemof morals.

Philosophy   **ISBN:** *1-59462-777-0*   **Pages:536**
MSRP $19.95

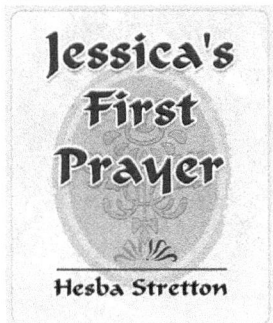

Jessica's First Prayer
Hesba Stretton

QTY

In a screened and secluded corner of one of the many railway-bridges which span the streets of London there could be seen a few years ago, from five o'clock every morning until half past eight, a tidily set-out coffee-stall, consisting of a trestle and board, upon which stood two large tin cans, with a small fire of charcoal burning under each so as to keep the coffee boiling during the early hours of the morning when the work-people were thronging into the city on their way to their daily toil...

Pages:84

Childrens   **ISBN:** *1-59462-373-2*   **MSRP $9.95**

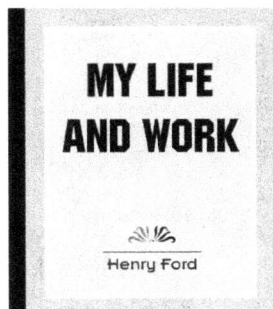

My Life and Work
Henry Ford

QTY

Henry Ford revolutionized the world with his implementation of mass production for the Model T automobile. Gain valuable business insight into his life and work with his own auto-biography... "We have only started on our development of our country we have not as yet, with all our talk of wonderful progress, done more than scratch the surface. The progress has been wonderful enough but..."

Pages:300

Biographies/   **ISBN:** *1-59462-198-5*   **MSRP $21.95**

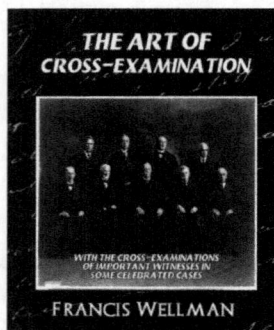

The Art of Cross-Examination
Francis Wellman

QTY

I presume it is the experience of every author, after his first book is published upon an important subject, to be almost overwhelmed with a wealth of ideas and illustrations which could readily have been included in his book, and which to his own mind, at least, seem to make a second edition inevitable. Such certainly was the case with me; and when the first edition had reached its sixth impression in five months, I rejoiced to learn that it seemed to my publishers that the book had met with a sufficiently favorable reception to justify a second and considerably enlarged edition. ..

Reference   ISBN: *1-59462-647-2*

Pages:412

MSRP $19.95

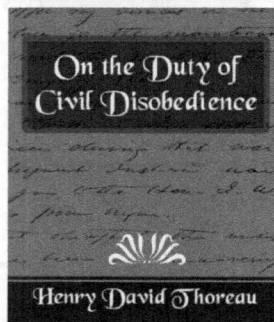

On the Duty of Civil Disobedience
Henry David Thoreau

QTY

Thoreau wrote his famous essay, On the Duty of Civil Disobedience, as a protest against an unjust but popular war and the immoral but popular institution of slave-owning. He did more than write—he declined to pay his taxes, and was hauled off to gaol in consequence. Who can say how much this refusal of his hastened the end of the war and of slavery ?

Law   ISBN: *1-59462-747-9*

Pages:48

MSRP $7.45

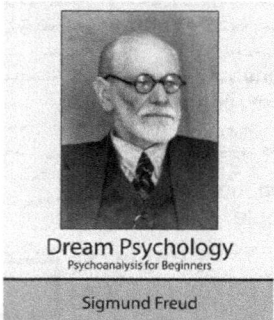

Dream Psychology Psychoanalysis for Beginners
Sigmund Freud

QTY

Sigmund Freud, born Sigismund Schlomo Freud (May 6, 1856 - September 23, 1939), was a Jewish-Austrian neurologist and psychiatrist who co-founded the psychoanalytic school of psychology. Freud is best known for his theories of the unconscious mind, especially involving the mechanism of repression; his redefinition of sexual desire as mobile and directed towards a wide variety of objects; and his therapeutic techniques, especially his understanding of transference in the therapeutic relationship and the presumed value of dreams as sources of insight into unconscious desires.

Psychology   ISBN: *1-59462-905-6*

Pages:196

MSRP $15.45

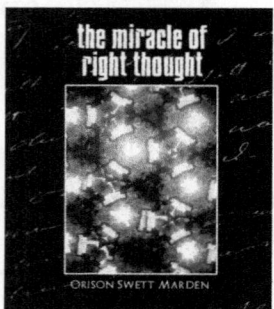

The Miracle of Right Thought
Orison Swett Marden

QTY

Believe with all of your heart that you will do what you were made to do. When the mind has once formed the habit of holding cheerful, happy, prosperous pictures, it will not be easy to form the opposite habit. It does not matter how improbable or how far away this realization may see, or how dark the prospects may be, if we visualize them as best we can, as vividly as possible, hold tenaciously to them and vigorously struggle to attain them, they will gradually become actualized, realized in the life. But a desire, a longing without endeavor, a yearning abandoned or held indifferently will vanish without realization.

Self Help   ISBN: *1-59462-644-8*

Pages:360

MSRP $25.45

QTY

The Rosicrucian Cosmo-Conception Mystic Christianity *by Max Heindel*   ISBN: *1-59462-188-8*   **$38.95**
The Rosicrucian Cosmo-conception is not dogmatic, neither does it appeal to any other authority than the reason of the student. It is: not controversial, but is: sent forth in the, hope that it may help to clear...   New Age/Religion Pages 646

Abandonment To Divine Providence *by Jean-Pierre de Caussade*   ISBN: *1-59462-228-0*   **$25.95**
"The Rev. Jean Pierre de Caussade was one of the most remarkable spiritual writers of the Society of Jesus in France in the 18th Century. His death took place at Toulouse in 1751. His works have gone through many editions and have been republished...   Inspirational/Religion Pages 400

Mental Chemistry *by Charles Haanel*   ISBN: *1-59462-192-6*   **$23.95**
Mental Chemistry allows the change of material conditions by combining and appropriately utilizing the power of the mind. Much like applied chemistry creates something new and unique out of careful combinations of chemicals the mastery of mental chemistry...   New Age Pages 354

The Letters of Robert Browning and Elizabeth Barret Barrett 1845-1846 vol II   ISBN: *1-59462-193-4*   **$35.95**
by Robert Browning and Elizabeth Barrett   Biographies Pages 596

Gleanings In Genesis (volume I) *by Arthur W. Pink*   ISBN: *1-59462-130-6*   **$27.45**
Appropriately has Genesis been termed "the seed plot of the Bible" for in it we have, in germ form, almost all of the great doctrines which are afterwards fully developed in the books of Scripture which follow...   Religion/Inspirational Pages 420

The Master Key *by L. W. de Laurence*   ISBN: *1-59462-001-6*   **$30.95**
In no branch of human knowledge has there been a more lively increase of the spirit of research during the past few years than in the study of Psychology, Concentration and Mental Discipline. The requests for authentic lessons in Thought Control, Mental Discipline and...   New Age/Business Pages 422

The Lesser Key Of Solomon Goetia *by L. W. de Laurence*   ISBN: *1-59462-092-X*   **$9.95**
This translation of the first book of the "Lernegton" which is now for the first time made accessible to students of Talismanic Magic was done, after careful collation and edition, from numerous Ancient Manuscripts in Hebrew, Latin, and French...   New Age/Occult Pages 92

Rubaiyat Of Omar Khayyam *by Edward Fitzgerald*   ISBN:*1-59462-332-5*   **$13.95**
Edward Fitzgerald, whom the world has already learned, in spite of his own efforts to remain within the shadow of anonymity, to look upon as one of the rarest poets of the century, was born at Bredfield, in Suffolk, on the 31st of March, 1809. He was the third son of John Purcell...   Music Pages 172

Ancient Law *by Henry Maine*   ISBN: *1-59462-128-4*   **$29.95**
The chief object of the following pages is to indicate some of the earliest ideas of mankind, as they are reflected in Ancient Law, and to point out the relation of those ideas to modern thought.   Religiom/History Pages 452

Far-Away Stories *by William J. Locke*   ISBN: *1-59462-129-2*   **$19.45**
"Good wine needs no bush, but a collection of mixed vintages does. And this book is just such a collection. Some of the stories I do not want to remain buried for ever in the museum files of dead magazine-numbers an author's not unpardonable vanity..."   Fiction Pages 272

Life of David Crockett *by David Crockett*   ISBN: *1-59462-250-7*   **$27.45**
"Colonel David Crockett was one of the most remarkable men of the times in which he lived. Born in humble life, but gifted with a strong will, an indomitable courage, and unremitting perseverance...   Biographies/New Age Pages 424

Lip-Reading *by Edward Nitchie*   ISBN: *1-59462-206-X*   **$25.95**
Edward B. Nitchie, founder of the New York School for the Hard of Hearing, now the Nitchie School of Lip-Reading, Inc, wrote "LIP-READING Principles and Practice". The development and perfecting of this meritorious work on lip-reading was an undertaking...   How-to Pages 400

A Handbook of Suggestive Therapeutics, Applied Hypnotism, Psychic Science   ISBN: *1-59462-214-0*   **$24.95**
by Henry Munro   Health/New Age/Health/Self-help Pages 376

A Doll's House: and Two Other Plays *by Henrik Ibsen*   ISBN: *1-59462-112-8*   **$19.95**
Henrik Ibsen created this classic when in revolutionary 1848 Rome. Introducing some striking concepts in playwriting for the realist genre, this play has been studied the world over.   Fiction/Classics/Plays 308

The Light of Asia *by sir Edwin Arnold*   ISBN: *1-59462-204-3*   **$13.95**
In this poetic masterpiece, Edwin Arnold describes the life and teachings of Buddha. The man who was to become known as Buddha to the world was born as Prince Gautama of India but he rejected the worldly riches and abandoned the reigns of power when...   Religion/History/Biographies Pages 170

The Complete Works of Guy de Maupassant *by Guy de Maupassant*   ISBN: *1-59462-157-8*   **$16.95**
"For days and days, nights and nights, I had dreamed of that first kiss which was to consecrate our engagement, and I knew not on what spot I should put my lips..."   Fiction/Classics Pages 240

The Art of Cross-Examination *by Francis L. Wellman*   ISBN: *1-59462-309-0*   **$26.95**
Written by a renowned trial lawyer, Wellman imparts his experience and uses case studies to explain how to use psychology to extract desired information through questioning.   How-to/Science/Reference Pages 408

Answered or Unanswered? *by Louisa Vaughan*   ISBN: *1-59462-248-5*   **$10.95**
Miracles of Faith in China   Religion Pages 112

The Edinburgh Lectures on Mental Science (1909) *by Thomas*   ISBN: *1-59462-008-3*   **$11.95**
This book contains the substance of a course of lectures recently given by the writer in the Queen Street Hail, Edinburgh. Its purpose is to indicate the Natural Principles governing the relation between Mental Action and Material Conditions...   New Age/Psychology Pages 148

Ayesha *by H. Rider Haggard*   ISBN: *1-59462-301-5*   **$24.95**
Verily and indeed it is the unexpected that happens! Probably if there was one person upon the earth from whom the Editor of this, and of a certain previous history, did not expect to hear again...   Classics Pages 380

Ayala's Angel *by Anthony Trollope*   ISBN: *1-59462-352-X*   **$29.95**
The two girls were both pretty, but Lucy who was twenty-one who supposed to be simple and comparatively unattractive, whereas Ayala was credited, as her Bombwhat romantic name might show, with poetic charm and a taste for romance. Ayala when her father died was nineteen...   Fiction Pages 484

The American Commonwealth *by James Bryce*   ISBN: *1-59462-286-8*   **$34.45**
An interpretation of American democratic political theory. It examines political mechanics and society from the perspective of Scotsman James Bryce   Politics Pages 572

Stories of the Pilgrims *by Margaret P. Pumphrey*   ISBN: *1-59462-116-0*   **$17.95**
This book explores pilgrims religious oppression in England as well as their escape to Holland and eventual crossing to America on the Mayflower, and their early days in New England...   History Pages 268

QTY

The Fasting Cure *by Sinclair Upton*   ISBN: *1-59462-222-1* **$13.95**
In the Cosmopolitan Magazine for May, 1910, and in the Contemporary Review (London) for April, 1910, I published an article dealing with my experiences in fasting. I have written a great many magazine articles, but never one which attracted so much attention... New Age/Self Help/Health Pages 164

Hebrew Astrology *by Sepharial*   ISBN: *1-59462-308-2* **$13.45**
In these days of advanced thinking it is a matter of common observation that we have left many of the old landmarks behind and that we are now pressing forward to greater heights and to a wider horizon than that which represented the mind-content of our progenitors... Astrology Pages 144

Thought Vibration or The Law of Attraction in the Thought World   ISBN: *1-59462-127-6* **$12.95**
by William Walker Atkinson   Psychology/Religion Pages 144

Optimism *by Helen Keller*   ISBN: *1-59462-108-X* **$15.95**
Helen Keller was blind, deaf, and mute since 19 months old, yet famously learned how to overcome these handicaps, communicate with the world, and spread her lectures promoting optimism. An inspiring read for everyone... Biographies/Inspirational Pages 84

Sara Crewe *by Frances Burnett*   ISBN: *1-59462-360-0* **$9.45**
In the first place, Miss Minchin lived in London. Her home was a large, dull, tall one, in a large, dull square, where all the houses were alike, and all the sparrows were alike, and where all the door-knockers made the same heavy sound... Childrens/Classic Pages 88

The Autobiography of Benjamin Franklin *by Benjamin Franklin*   ISBN: *1-59462-135-7* **$24.95**
The Autobiography of Benjamin Franklin has probably been more extensively read than any other American historical work, and no other book of its kind has had such ups and downs of fortune. Franklin lived for many years in England, where he was agent... Biographies/History Pages 332

Name	
Email	
Telephone	
Address	
City, State ZIP	

☐ **Credit Card**   ☐ **Check / Money Order**

Credit Card Number	
Expiration Date	
Signature	

Please Mail to: Book Jungle
PO Box 2226
Champaign, IL 61825
or Fax to: 630-214-0564

ORDERING INFORMATION

web: *www.bookjungle.com*
email: *sales@bookjungle.com*
fax: *630-214-0564*
mail: *Book Jungle PO Box 2226 Champaign, IL 61825*
or PayPal *to sales@bookjungle.com*

Please contact us for bulk discounts

DIRECT-ORDER TERMS

**20% Discount if You Order
Two or More Books**
Free Domestic Shipping!
Accepted: Master Card, Visa,
Discover, American Express

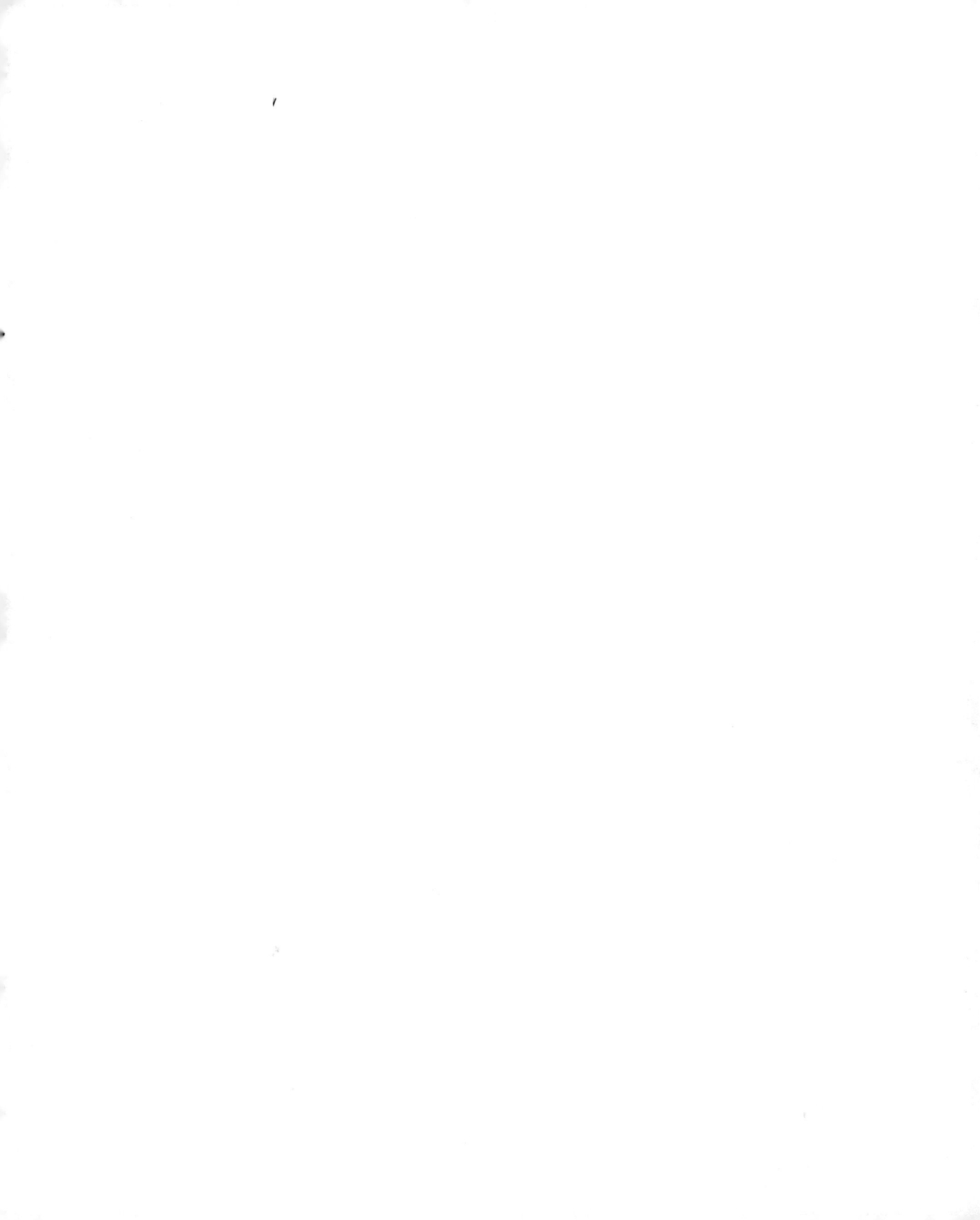

www.ingramcontent.com/pod-product-compliance
Lightning Source LLC
Chambersburg PA
CBHW080409270326

41929CB00018B/2951